Neonatal-Perinatal Infections: An Update

Editors

P. BRIAN SMITH
DANIEL K. BENJAMIN Jr

CLINICS IN PERINATOLOGY

www.perinatology.theclinics.com

Consulting Editor
LUCKY JAIN

March 2015 • Volume 42 • Number 1

ELSEVIER

1600 John F. Kennedy Boulevard • Suite 1800 • Philadelphia, Pennsylvania, 19103-2899

http://www.theclinics.com

CLINICS IN PERINATOLOGY Volume 42, Number 1
March 2015 ISSN 0095-5108, ISBN-13: 978-0-323-37637-2

Editor: Kerry Holland
Developmental Editor: Casey Jackson

Clinics in Perinatology (ISSN 0095-5108) is published quarterly by Elsevier Inc., 360 Park Avenue South, New York, NY 10010-1710. Months of issue are March, June, September, and December. Business and Editorial Offices: 1600 John F. Kennedy Blvd., Ste. 1800, Philadelphia, PA 19103-2899. Customer Service Office: 3251 Riverport Lane, Maryland Heights, MO 63043. Periodicals postage paid at New York, NY and additional mailing offices. Subscription prices are $285.00 per year (US individuals), $445.00 per year (US institutions), $340.00 per year (Canadian individuals), $545.00 per year (Canadian institutions), $420.00 per year (international individuals), $545.00 per year (international institutions), $135.00 per year (US students), and $195.00 per year (Canadian and international students). International air speed delivery is included in all Clinics subscription prices. All prices are subject to change without notice. **POSTMASTER:** Send address changes to *Clinics in Perinatology*, Elsevier Health Sciences Division, Subscription Customer Service, 3251 Riverport Lane, Maryland Heights, MO 63043. **Customer Service: Telephone: 1-800-654-2452** (U.S. and Canada); **1-314-447-8871** (outside U.S. and Canada). **Fax: 1-314-447-8029.** E-mail: **journalscustomerservice-usa@elsevier.com** (for print support); **journalsonlinesupport-usa@elsevier.com** (for online support).

Reprints. For copies of 100 or more, of articles in this publication, please contact the Commercial Reprints Department, Elsevier Inc., 360 Park Avenue South, New York, NY 10010-1710. Tel. 212-633-3874; Fax: 212-633-3820; E-mail: reprints@elsevier.com.

Clinics in Perinatology is also pubilshed in Spanish by McGraw-Hill Interamericana Editores S.A., P.O. Box 5-237, 06500 Mexico D.F., Mexico.

Clinics in Perinatology is covered in *MEDLINE/PubMed (Index Medicus) Current Contents, Excepta Medica, BIOSIS and ISI/BIOMED.*

Printed in the United States of America.

Contributors

CONSULTING EDITOR

LUCKY JAIN, MD, MBA
Richard W. Blumberg Professor and Executive Vice Chairman, Department of Pediatrics, Emory University School of Medicine; Executive Medical Director, Children's Healthcare of Atlanta Faculty Practices, Atlanta, Georgia

EDITORS

P. BRIAN SMITH, MD, MPH, MHS
Associate Professor of Pediatrics, Duke University Medical Center, Durham, North Carolina

DANIEL K. BENJAMIN Jr, MD, MPH, PhD
Kiser Arena Distinguished Professor of Pediatrics, Duke University Medical Center, Durham, North Carolina

AUTHORS

MEHREEN ARSHAD, MD
Division of Infectious Diseases, Department of Pediatrics, Duke University School of Medicine, Durham, North Carolina

JULIE AUTMIZGUINE, MD, MHS, FRCPC
Infectious Diseases Division, Department of Pediatrics, Centre hospitalier universitaire Sainte Justine, University of Montreal; Department of Pharmacology, University of Montreal; Research Center, Centre hospitalier universitaire Sainte-Justine, Montreal, Quebec, Canada

DANIEL K. BENJAMIN Jr, MD, MPH, PhD
Kiser Arena Distinguished Professor of Pediatrics, Duke University Medical Center, Durham, North Carolina

KRISTY M. BIALAS, PhD
Human Vaccine Institute, Duke University Medical Center, Duke University School of Medicine, Durham, North Carolina

ANA C. BLANCHARD, MDCM
Department of Pediatrics, Centre hospitalier universitaire Sainte Justine, University of Montreal, Montreal, Quebec, Canada

KIM A. BOGGESS, MD
Professor, Department of Obstetrics & Gynecology, University of North Carolina School of Medicine, Chapel Hill, North Carolina

JOSEPH B. CANTEY, MD
Fellow, Divisions of Neonatal/Perinatal Medicine and Infectious Diseases, Department of Pediatrics, University of Texas Southwestern Medical Center, Dallas, Texas

SARAH A. COGGINS, BA
School of Medicine, Vanderbilt University, Nashville, Tennessee

MICHAEL COHEN-WOLKOWIEZ, MD, PhD
Associate Professor, Department of Pediatrics, Duke Clinical Research Institute, Durham, North Carolina

C. MICHAEL COTTEN, MD, MHS
Associate Professor of Pediatrics; Medical Director, Neonatology Clinical Research, Duke University Medical Center, Durham, North Carolina

JENNIFER DUCHON, MDCM, MPH
Clinical Fellow, Division of Pediatric Infectious Disease, New York-Presbyterian Morgan Stanley Children's Hospital, New York, New York

JESSICA E. ERICSON, MD
Pediatric Infectious Diseases Fellow, Department of Pediatrics, Duke Clinical Research Institute, Duke University, North Carolina

SCOTT H. JAMES, MD
Assistant Professor, Division of Infectious Diseases, Department of Pediatrics, University of Alabama at Birmingham, Birmingham, Alabama

MATTHEW S. KELLY, MD, MPH
Fellow in Infectious Diseases, Department of Pediatrics, Duke University; Duke Clinical Research Institute, Durham, North Carolina

DAVID W. KIMBERLIN, MD
Professor, Division of Infectious Diseases, Department of Pediatrics, University of Alabama at Birmingham, Birmingham, Alabama

LAWRENCE C. KU, MD
Fellow, Department of Pediatrics, Duke Clinical Research Institute, Durham, North Carolina

MATTHEW M. LAUGHON, MD, MPH
Associate Professor, Department of Pediatrics, UNC Hospitals, The University of North Carolina at Chapel Hill, Chapel Hill, North Carolina

AARON M. MILSTONE, MD, MHS
Associate Professor of Pediatrics, Division of Infectious Diseases, Department of Pediatrics, Johns Hopkins University School of Medicine, Baltimore, Maryland

HEATHER M. MONK, PharmD
Department of Pharmacy, Children's Hospital of Philadelphia, Philadelphia, Pennsylvania

NATALIE NEU, MD, MPH
Associate Professor of Pediatrics, Division of Pediatric Infectious Disease, Columbia University Medical Center, New York, New York

SALLIE R. PERMAR, MD, PhD
Department of Pediatrics, Human Vaccine Institute, Duke University Medical Center, Duke University School of Medicine, Durham, North Carolina

LESLIE C. PINEDA, MD
Neonatal-Perinatal Medicine Fellow, Department of Pediatrics, Duke University Medical Center, Duke University, Durham, North Carolina

CAROLINE QUACH, MD, MSc, FRCPC
Division of Infectious Diseases, Department of Medical Microbiology; Department of Pediatrics, The Montreal Children's Hospital, McGill University Health Centre; Department of Epidemiology, Biostatistics and Occupational Health, McGill University, Montreal, Quebec, Canada

PATRICK C. SEED, MD, PhD
Division of Infectious Diseases, Department of Pediatrics, Duke University School of Medicine, Durham, North Carolina

P. BRIAN SMITH, MD, MPH, MHS
Associate Professor of Pediatrics, Duke University Medical Center, Durham, North Carolina

GEETA K. SWAMY, MD
Division of Maternal-Fetal Medicine, Department of Obstetrics and Gynecology, Duke University Medical Center, Duke University, Durham, North Carolina

KELLY C. WADE, MD, PhD, MSCE
Associate Professor of Clinical Pediatrics, Division of Neonatology, Department of Pediatrics, Perelman School of Medicine, Children's Hospital of Philadelphia Newborn Care at Pennsylvania Hospital, Philadelphia, Pennsylvania

KEVIN M. WATT, MD
Assistant Professor, Department of Pediatrics, Duke Clinical Research Institute, Duke University Medical Center, Duke University, Durham, North Carolina

JÖRN-HENDRIK WEITKAMP, MD
Assistant Professor of Pediatrics, Division of Neonatology, Department of Pediatrics, Monroe Carell Jr. Children's Hospital at Vanderbilt, Vanderbilt University, Nashville, Tennessee

JAMES L. WYNN, MD
Assistant Professor, Department of Pediatrics, Monroe Carell Jr. Children's Hospital at Vanderbilt, Vanderbilt University, Nashville, Tennessee

PHILIP ZACHARIAH, MD
Clinical Fellow, Division of Pediatric Infectious Disease, New York-Presbyterian Morgan Stanley Children's Hospital, New York, New York

Contents

Foreword: Neonatal-Perinatal Infections: Are We Losing the Battle?   xv

Lucky Jain

Preface: Neonatal-Perinatal Infections: An Update   xix

P. Brian Smith and Daniel K. Benjamin Jr

Bloodstream Infections: Epidemiology and Resistance   1

Joseph B. Cantey and Aaron M. Milstone

> Bloodstream infections in the neonatal intensive care unit (NICU) are asso-
> ciated with many adverse outcomes in infants, including increased length
> of stay and cost, poor neurodevelopmental outcomes, and death. Atten-
> tion to the insertion and maintenance of central lines, along with careful
> review of when the catheters can be safely discontinued, can minimize
> central-line–associated bloodstream infections rates. Good antibiotic
> stewardship can further decrease the incidence of bloodstream infections,
> minimize the emergence of drug-resistant organisms or *Candida* as path-
> ogens in the NICU, and safeguard the use of currently available antibiotics
> for future infants.

Urinary Tract Infections in the Infant   17

Mehreen Arshad and Patrick C. Seed

> Urinary tract infection (UTI) in an infant may be the first indication of an un-
> derlying renal disorder. Early recognition and initiation of adequate therapy
> for UTI is important to reduce the risk of long-term renal scarring. Ampicillin
> and gentamicin are traditionally the empiric treatment of choice; however,
> local antibiotic resistance patterns should be considered. Maternal anti-
> biotics during pregnancy also increase the risk of resistant pathogens
> during neonatal UTI. Long-term management after the first UTI in infants
> remains controversial because of lack of specific studies in this age group
> and the risk-benefit issues for antibiotic prophylaxis between reduced
> recurrent disease and emergent antibiotic resistance.

Bacterial Meningitis in Infants   29

Lawrence C. Ku, Kim A. Boggess, and Michael Cohen-Wolkowiez

> Neonatal bacterial meningitis is uncommon but devastating. Morbidity
> among survivors remains high. The types and distribution of pathogens
> are related to gestational age, postnatal age, and geographic region. Con-
> firming the diagnosis is difficult. Clinical signs are often subtle, lumbar
> punctures are frequently deferred, and cerebrospinal fluid (CSF) cultures
> can be compromised by prior antibiotic exposure. Infants with bacterial
> meningitis can have negative blood cultures and normal CSF parameters.
> Promising tests such as the polymerase chain reaction require further
> study. Prompt treatment with antibiotics is essential. Clinical trials

investigating a vaccine for preventing neonatal Group B Streptococcus infections are ongoing.

Neonatal Herpes Simplex Virus Infection: Epidemiology and Treatment   47

Scott H. James and David W. Kimberlin

Herpes simplex virus types 1 (HSV-1) and 2 (HSV-2) are highly prevalent viruses capable of establishing lifelong infection. Genital herpes in women of childbearing age represents a major risk for mother-to-child transmission (MTCT) of HSV infection, with primary and first-episode genital HSV infections posing the highest risk. The advent of antiviral therapy with parenteral acyclovir has led to significant improvement in neonatal HSV disease mortality. Further studies are needed to improve the clinician's ability to identify infants at increased risk for HSV infection and prevent MTCT, and to develop novel antiviral agents with increased efficacy in infants with HSV infection.

Perinatal Cytomegalovirus and Varicella Zoster Virus Infections: Epidemiology, Prevention, and Treatment   61

Kristy M. Bialas, Geeta K. Swamy, and Sallie R. Permar

Mother-to-child transmission of cytomegalovirus (CMV) and varicella zoster virus (VZV) can lead to severe birth defects and neurologic impairment of infants. Congenital CMV complicates up to 1% of all pregnancies globally. Although antiviral treatment of infants congenitally infected with CMV can ameliorate the CMV-associated hearing loss and developmental delay, interventions to prevent congenital CMV infection and the associated neurologic impairments are still being evaluated. Congenital VZV infection is rare. Active and passive immunization strategies to prevent perinatal CMV infection with similar efficacy to those established to prevent perinatal VZV infections are critically needed in pediatric health.

TORCH Infections   77

Natalie Neu, Jennifer Duchon, and Philip Zachariah

TORCH infections classically comprise toxoplasmosis, *Treponema pallidum*, rubella, cytomegalovirus, herpesvirus, hepatitis viruses, human immunodeficiency virus, and other infections, such as varicella, parvovirus B19, and enteroviruses. The epidemiology of these infections varies; in low-income and middle-income countries, TORCH infections are major contributors to prenatal, perinatal, and postnatal morbidity and mortality. Evidence of infection may be seen at birth, in infancy, or years later. For many of these pathogens, treatment or prevention strategies are available. Early recognition, including prenatal screening, is key. This article covers toxoplasmosis, parvovirus B19, syphilis, rubella, hepatitis B virus, hepatitis C virus, and human immunodeficiency virus.

The Epidemiology and Diagnosis of Invasive Candidiasis Among Premature Infants   105

Matthew S. Kelly, Daniel K. Benjamin Jr, and P. Brian Smith

Invasive candidiasis is a leading infectious cause of morbidity and mortality in premature infants. Improved recognition of modifiable risk factors and antifungal prophylaxis has contributed to the recent decline in the incidence of this infection among infants. Invasive candidiasis typically occurs in the first 6 weeks of life and presents with nonspecific signs of sepsis. Definitive diagnosis relies on the growth of *Candida* in blood culture or cultures from other normally sterile sites, but this may identify fewer than half of cases. Improved diagnostics are needed to guide the initiation of antifungal therapy in premature infants.

Staphylococcal Infections in Infants: Updates and Current Challenges   119

Ana C. Blanchard, Caroline Quach, and Julie Autmizguine

Staphylococci are common pathogens in the neonatal period. Increased survival of premature infants leads to prolonged hospital stay with associated risk factors for developing invasive staphylococcal disease. Challenges of diagnosing coagulase-negative staphylococcal infections result in conflicting definitions and inconsistent clinical practice. Resistance to methicillin influences the choice of empirical therapy.

Infectious Causes of Necrotizing Enterocolitis   133

Sarah A. Coggins, James L. Wynn, and Jörn-Hendrik Weitkamp

Necrotizing enterocolitis (NEC) is the most common gastrointestinal emergency among premature infants. Although a large body of research has focused on understanding its pathogenesis, the exact mechanism has not been elucidated. Of particular interest is the potential causative role of infectious culprits in the development of NEC. A variety of reports describe bacterial, viral, and fungal infections occurring in association with NEC; however, no single organism has emerged as being definitively involved in NEC pathogenesis. In this review, the authors summarize the literature on infectious causes of NEC.

Chorioamnionitis: Implications for the Neonate   155

Jessica E. Ericson and Matthew M. Laughon

Chorioamnionitis (CA) is characterized by inflammation of the fetal membranes. The incidence increases with decreasing gestational age at birth. When suspected on clinical criteria, pathologic assessment of the placenta should be performed. Although the mechanisms are not entirely clear, CA predisposes to premature birth, neonatal sepsis, and intraventricular hemorrhage. Its role in respiratory distress syndrome, bronchopulmonary dysplasia, and neurodevelopmental impairment is mixed. Prevention and treatment are ill-defined; antibiotics for preterm premature rupture of membranes reduce the incidence and increase the length of time to delivery. Antibiotics are recommended for infants exposed to CA while laboratory studies are being performed.

New Antibiotic Dosing in Infants   167

Leslie C. Pineda and Kevin M. Watt

To prevent the devastating consequences of infection, most infants admitted to the neonatal intensive care unit are exposed to antibiotics. However, dosing regimens are often extrapolated from data in adults and older children, increasing the risk for drug toxicity and lack of clinical efficacy because they fail to account for developmental changes in infant physiology. However, newer technologies are emerging with minimal-risk study designs, including ultra-low-volume assays, pharmacokinetic modeling and simulation, and opportunistic drug protocols. With minimal-risk study designs, pharmacokinetic data and dosing regimens for infants are now available for ampicillin, clindamycin, meropenem, metronidazole, and piperacillin/tazobactam.

New Antifungal and Antiviral Dosing   177

Kelly C. Wade and Heather M. Monk

Neonatal fungal and viral infections are associated with mortality and neurologic impairment among survivors. Advances in pharmacokinetics (PK) and pharmacodynamics (PD) of antimicrobial medications have led to improved dosing guidance for neonates. This article discusses the basic PK/PD properties and dosing of the most common antifungal and antiviral medications used in neonates.

Antibiotic Stewardship: Reassessment of Guidelines for Management of Neonatal Sepsis   195

C. Michael Cotten

In 2010, the Centers for Disease Control and Prevention (CDC) provided updated guidelines for prevention of perinatal group B streptococcus disease. In 2012, the American Academy of Pediatrics' Committee on the Fetus and Newborn (COFN) provided a clinical report which suggested approaches to infants with risk factors for EOS which would increase empirical antibiotic use beyond the CDC guidelines. This Clinics article reviews the CDC guidelines and 2012 COFN report, summarizes the 2014 commentary provided by COFN members which provided a revised clinical algorithm, and discusses mechanisms which could reduce the number of well-appearing term infants exposed to empirical antibiotics.

Index   207

PROGRAM OBJECTIVE

The goal of *Clinics in Perinatology* is to keep practicing perinatologists, neonatologists, obstetricians, practicing physicians and residents up to date with current clinical practice in perinatology by providing timely articles reviewing the state of the art in patient care.

TARGET AUDIENCE

Perinatologists, neonatologists, obstetricians, practicing physicians, residents and healthcare professionals who provide patient care utilizing findings from *Clinics in Perinatology*.

LEARNING OBJECTIVES

Upon completion of this activity, participants will be able to:

1. Review new antibiotics, antifungal and antiviral dosing guidelines for infants.
2. Discuss neonatal-perinatal Infections including infections of the blood, bacterial meningitis, and urinary tract infections.
3. Review updates and current challenges of staphylococcal infections in infants

ACCREDITATION

The Elsevier Office of Continuing Medical Education (EOCME) is accredited by the Accreditation Council for Continuing Medical Education (ACCME) to provide continuing medical education for physicians.

The EOCME designates this enduring material for a maximum of 15 *AMA PRA Category 1 Credit*(s)™. Physicians should claim only the credit commensurate with the extent of their participation in the activity.

All other health care professionals requesting continuing education credit for this enduring material will be issued a certificate of participation.

DISCLOSURE OF CONFLICTS OF INTEREST

The EOCME assesses conflict of interest with its instructors, faculty, planners, and other individuals who are in a position to control the content of CME activities. All relevant conflicts of interest that are identified are thoroughly vetted by EOCME for fair balance, scientific objectivity, and patient care recommendations. EOCME is committed to providing its learners with CME activities that promote improvements or quality in healthcare and not a specific proprietary business or a commercial interest.

The planning committee, staff, authors and editors listed below have identified no financial relationships or relationships to products or devices they or their spouse/life partner have with commercial interest related to the content of this CME activity:

Mehreen Arshad, MD; Julie Autmizguine, MD MHS, FRCPC; Kristy M. Bialas, PhD; Ana C. Blanchard, MDCM; Kim A. Boggess, MD; Joseph B. Cantey, MD; Sarah A. Coggins; C. Michael Cotten, MD, MHS; Jennifer Duchon, MDCM, MPH; Jessica E. Ericson, MD; Kerry Holland; Brynne Hunter; Lucky Jain, MD, MBA; Scott H. James, MD; Matthew S. Kelly, MD, MPH; David W. Kimberlin, MD; Lawrence C. Ku, MD; Matthew M. Laughon, MD, MPH; Sandy Lavery; Aaron M. Milstone, MD MHS; Heather M. Monk, PharmD; Palani Murugesan; Natalie Neu, MD, MPH; Sallie R. Permar, MD, PhD; Leslie C. Pineda, MD; Caroline Quach, MD, MSc, FRCPC; Patrick C. Seed, MD, PhD; Megan Suermann; Geeta K. Swamy, MD; Kelly C. Wade, MD, PhD, MSCE; Kevin M. Watt, MD; Jörn-Hendrik Weitkamp, MD; James L. Wynn, MD; Philip Zachariah, MD.

The planning committee, staff, authors and editors listed below have identified financial relationships or relationships to products or devices they or their spouse/life partner have with commercial interest related to the content of this CME activity:

Daniel K. Benjamin Jr, MD, MPH, PhD is a consultant/advisor for Astellas Pharma US, Inc., Cempra, Inc., Cubist Pharmaceuticals, Inc., Johnson & Johnson, The Medicines Company, Merck & Co., Inc., and Pfizer, Inc.

Michael Cohen-Wolkowiez, MD, PhD is a consultant/advisor for Cempra, Inc., GlaxoSmithKline plc, The Medicines Company, Special Products Limited, and Tetraphase Pharmaceuticals.

P. Brian Smith, MD, MPH, MHS is a consultant/advisor for Astellas Pharma US, Inc., GlaxoSmithKline plc, Mission Pharma, and Pfizer, Inc.

UNAPPROVED/OFF-LABEL USE DISCLOSURE

The EOCME requires CME faculty to disclose to the participants:

1. When products or procedures being discussed are off-label, unlabelled, experimental, and/or investigational (not US Food and Drug Administration (FDA) approved); and
2. Any limitations on the information presented, such as data that are preliminary or that represent ongoing research, interim analyses, and/or unsupported opinions. Faculty may discuss information about pharmaceutical agents that is outside of FDA-approved labelling. This information is intended solely for CME

and is not intended to promote off-label use of these medications. If you have any questions, contact the medical affairs department of the manufacturer for the most recent prescribing information.

TO ENROLL

To enroll in the *Clinics in Perinatology* Continuing Medical Education program, call customer service at 1-800-654-2452 or sign up online at http://www.theclinics.com/home/cme. The CME program is available to subscribers for an additional annual fee of $235 USD.

METHOD OF PARTICIPATION

In order to claim credit, participants must complete the following:

1. Complete enrolment as indicated above.
2. Read the activity.
3. Complete the CME Test and Evaluation. Participants must achieve a score of 70% on the test. All CME Tests and Evaluations must be completed online.

CME INQUIRIES/SPECIAL NEEDS

For all CME inquiries or special needs, please contact elsevierCME@elsevier.com.

CLINICS IN PERINATOLOGY

FORTHCOMING ISSUES

June 2015
**Genetics Diagnosis, Inborn Errors of
Metabolism and Newborn Screening:
An Update**
Michael J. Gambello and V. Reid Sutton,
Editors

September 2015
**Bronchopulmonary Dysplasia and Chronic
Lung Disease**
Suhas G. Kallapur and Gloria S. Pryhuber,
Editors

December 2015
**Neonatal Hematology and Transfusion
Medicine**
Robert D. Christensen, Sandra E. Juul,
and Antonio Del Vecchio, *Editors*

RECENT ISSUES

December 2014
Current Controversies in Perinatology
Robert H. Lane and Robert M. Kliegman,
Editors

September 2014
Renal and Urologic Issues
Michelle N. Rheault and
Larry A. Greenbaum, *Editors*

June 2014
Current Concepts in Neonatal Nutrition
Brenda Poindexter and Heidi Karpen,
Editors

Foreword

Neonatal-Perinatal Infections: Are We Losing the Battle?

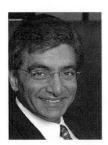

Lucky Jain, MD, MBA
Consulting Editor

The December 3, 2014 edition of *The New York Times*[1] carried an alarming story: "Superbugs Kill India's Babies and Pose an Overseas Threat." The article describes a deadly epidemic "that is quietly sweeping India and could have global implications." Among its victims are "tens of thousands of newborns who are dying because once-miraculous cures no longer work." Bacterial infections in these newborns are resistant to most (if not all) of the antibiotics available for use in these areas. The result: 58,000 newborn deaths in 2013 from drug-resistant infections in India, far in excess of the nearly 24,000 or so annual newborn deaths in the United States from all causes combined.[2]

Similar trends, albeit not as striking, are being reported from many other countries as well. Multiple factors have contributed to this escalation of deaths from multi-drug-resistant pathogens. *First* (and foremost) is the overuse of broad spectrum antibiotics. Clinicians working in affected areas feel compelled to use the most powerful antimicrobials available to them when working with sick patients at high risk of death or disability. However, prudent use of antimicrobials and true antimicrobial stewardship can help achieve the multiple goals of treating the infection, protecting the native microbiome, preventing emergence of resistant pathogens, and minimizing other risks associated with antibiotic overuse (**Box 1**).[3,4] Antibiotic overprescribing is a huge problem in primary care given the large number of viral infections that do not require treatment but pose diagnostic challenges for busy practitioners.[3] Multifaceted interventions are needed to reduce the overuse, including prohibition of the over-the-counter sale of antibiotics, use of antibiotic stewardship programs, use of rapid point-of-care tests, and audits/reporting of antibiotic usage patterns.[3]

There is more bad news: the lack of new antimicrobials that can treat tough infections is pretty daunting. The pipeline for antibiotics has a paucity of promising new

Clin Perinatol 42 (2015) xv–xvii
http://dx.doi.org/10.1016/j.clp.2014.12.002
0095-5108/15/$ – see front matter © 2015 Published by Elsevier Inc.

Box 1
Risks associated with overuse of antibiotics

Increased antimicrobial resistance

Increased severity of infections

Increase in length of disease and hospital stay

Increase in risk of complications

Increased mortality

Increase in health care costs

Increased risk of adverse effects of antibiotics

Increased risk of rehospitalizations

Increased medicalization of self-limiting infectious and noninfectious conditions

Adapted from Llor C, Bjerrum L. Antimicobial resistance: risk associated with antibiotic overuse and initiatives to reduce the problem. Ther Adv Drug Saf 2014;5:231; with permission.

---

candidates with the exception of small molecule antibiotics currently in development. Strategies being considered include revival of old antibiotics. For neonatologists, combinations such as ampicillin and gentamycin have withstood the test of time for initial sepsis treatment. Yet, clinicians often choose other combinations, sometimes to the detriment of the patient.[5]

There is also the need to better understand the antibiotic resistome and the factors that influence evolution of resistance genes along with the spread of mobile resistance elements.[6] These and many other important issues related to perinatal infections have been extensively covered by the many authors recruited by Drs Smith and Benjamin. With renewed concern about bloodstream infections, necrotizing enterocolitis, and fungal and viral infections, this issue of the *Clinics in Perinatology* is very timely. In addition to the editors and contributing authors, I am grateful to the publishing staff at Elsevier, particularly Kerry Holland and Casey Jackson, for their support. I am also grateful to you, the readers, for your support of the *Clinics in Perinatology* and ongoing feedback about topics relevant to you.

Lucky Jain, MD, MBA
Department of Pediatrics
Emory University School of Medicine and
Children's Healthcare of Atlanta
2015 Uppergate Drive
Atlanta, GA 30322, USA

E-mail address:
ljain@emory.edu

REFERENCES

1. Harris G. Superbugs kill India's babies and pose an overseas threat. The New York Times 2014.
2. Gregory EC, MacDorman MF, Martin JA. Trends in fetal and perinatal mortality in the United States, 2006-2012. NCHS Data Brief 2014;169:1–7.
3. Llor C, Bjerrum L. Antimicobial resistance: risk associated with antibiotic overuse and initiatives to reduce the problem. Ther Adv Drug Saf 2014;5:229–41.

4. Brooks BD, Brooks AE. Therapeutic strategies to combat antibiotic resistance. Adv Drug Deliv Rev 2014;78C:14–27.
5. Clark RH, Bloom BT, Spitzer AR, et al. Empiric use of ampicillin and cefotaxime, compared with ampicillin and gentamycin, for neonates at risk for sepsis is associated with an increased risk of neonatal death. Pediatrics 2006;117:67–74.
6. Perry JA, Westman EL, Wright GD. The antibiotic resistome: what's new? Curr Opin Microbiol 2014;21:45–50.

Preface

Neonatal-Perinatal Infections: An Update

 CrossMark

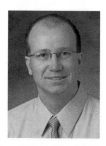 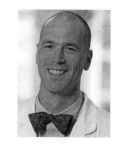

P. Brian Smith, MD, MPH, MHS   Daniel K. Benjamin Jr, MD, MPH, PhD
Editors

Infants are uniquely susceptible to infections. The immature neonatal immune system contributes to the wide variety of organisms affecting this population, and infections in this period can have life-long consequences even when recognized early and treated appropriately. Physicians evaluating potentially infected infants should carefully consider the timing of the presentation in addition to thoroughly reviewing the maternal and perinatal history.

In this issue of *Clinics in Perinatology*, we provide a contemporary look at the epidemiology, clinical manifestations, treatment, and outcomes for neonatal-perinatal infections. Contributors include neonatologists, infectious disease specialists, and critical care specialists with a wide variety of research interests in this arena.

Readers will be exposed to the latest information on dosing of antibiotics, antivirals, and antifungals. This information is critical in the infant population given the rapid changes in physiology, metabolic pathways, and renal elimination that occur over the first months of life. There is an extensive examination of infectious processes that commonly present in infants, including meningitis, bloodstream infections, and urinary tract infections. Additional topics include infectious processes affecting the newborn (chorioamnionitis and TORCH infections) and premature infants (necrotizing enterocolitis). Specific pathogens are highlighted in articles on HSV, CMV/VZV, staphylococcal species, and *Candida*. Finally, the rationale for the most recent changes to guidelines for initiating therapy for early-onset neonatal sepsis is reviewed.

Clin Perinatol 42 (2015) xix–xx
http://dx.doi.org/10.1016/j.clp.2014.12.001
0095-5108/15/$ – see front matter © 2015 Published by Elsevier Inc.

perinatology.theclinics.com

We are excited about this issue and each author's contributions to this important topic. We would like to thank the authors for their work. We would also like to thank Dr Lucky Jain for inviting us to participate and the Elsevier staff for their oversight of this project.

P. Brian Smith, MD, MPH, MHS
Duke University Medical Center
Box 17969, DCRI
Durham, NC 27715, USA

Daniel K. Benjamin Jr, MD, MPH, PhD
Duke University Medical Center
Box 17969, DCRI
Durham, NC 27715, USA

E-mail addresses:
brian.smith@duke.edu (P.B. Smith)
danny.benjamin@duke.edu (D.K. Benjamin)

Bloodstream Infections
Epidemiology and Resistance

 CrossMark

Joseph B. Cantey, MD[a,b,*], Aaron M. Milstone, MD, MHS[c]

KEYWORDS

- Antibiotic stewardship • Central-line–associated bloodstream infection
- Infection control • Multidrug resistance • Neonate • NICU

KEY POINTS

- Among hospitalized infants, bloodstream infections are associated with increased mortality, as well as increased length of stay, health care costs, and adverse neurodevelopmental outcome in survivors.
- Risk factors for bloodstream infections include prematurity, indwelling catheters or other medical devices, exposure to prolonged empiric antibiotic therapy, acid-blocking medications, or steroids, and overcrowding or understaffing.
- Gram-positive organisms, particularly coagulase-negative *Staphylococcus*, account for most bloodstream infections, but gram-negative and *Candida* infections are associated with higher morbidity and mortality.
- Drug-resistant bacteria account for an increasing proportion of infections and outbreaks in the neonatal intensive care unit. Good antibiotic stewardship and infection prevention practices are of paramount importance to slow the increase in resistant organisms.

INTRODUCTION

Bloodstream infections (BSI) are a common cause of morbidity and mortality in neonatal intensive care units (NICUs) worldwide. **Table 1** highlights the adverse outcomes associated with BSI in infants, including increased length of stay, poor neurodevelopmental outcome, and higher mortality.[1–5] BSI can be divided into early-onset or late-onset sepsis (LOS), with LOS occurring greater than 3 days after delivery. The purpose of this review is to focus on the epidemiology of BSI in the NICU, with a focus on prevention.

Disclosures: The authors have no financial disclosures or conflicts of interest to report.
^a Division of Neonatal/Perinatal Medicine, Department of Pediatrics, University of Texas Southwestern Medical Center, 5323 Harry Hines Boulevard, Dallas, TX 75390, USA; ^b Division of Infectious Diseases, Department of Pediatrics, University of Texas Southwestern Medical Center, 5323 Harry Hines Boulevard, Dallas, TX 75390, USA; ^c Division of Infectious Diseases, Johns Hopkins University School of Medicine, 200 North Wolfe Street, Room 3141, Baltimore, MD 21287, USA
* Corresponding author. 5323 Harry Hines Boulevard, Dallas, TX 75390.
E-mail address: joseph.cantey@utsouthwestern.edu

Clin Perinatol 42 (2015) 1–16
http://dx.doi.org/10.1016/j.clp.2014.10.002
0095-5108/15/$ – see front matter
perinatology.theclinics.com

Table 1
Selected adverse outcomes associated with bloodstream infection in very low-birth-weight infants in the neonatal intensive care unit

Adverse Outcome	Study	Adjusted Effect
Mortality	Stoll et al.[1] (1996)	2.4-fold increase (17% vs 7%)
	Stoll et al.[2] (2002)	2.6-fold increase (18% vs 7%)
	Makhoul[53] (2002)	2.0-fold increase (17% vs 9%)
Poor neurodevelopmental outcome	De Haan[90] (2013)	OR 4.8 (1.5–15.9), for gram-negative BSI[a]
	Mitha[4] (2013)	OR 2.2 (1.5–3.1)[b]
	Schlapbach[91] (2011)	OR 3.2 (1.2–8.5)[b]
	Stoll[5] (2004)	OR 1.4 (1.3–2.2)[a]
Length of stay	Stoll et al.[1] (1996)	19–22 d mean increase
	Stoll et al.[2] (2002)	18.6 d mean increase
	Makhoul[53] (2002)	27 d mean increase
	Atif[92] (2008)	9.2 d mean increase
Increased cost	Payne et al.[3] (2004)	$54,539 mean increase
	Donovan[93] (2013)	$16,800 mean increase

All studies adjusted for gestational age.
Abbreviation: OR, odds ratio.
[a] Bayley-II motor or cognitive score less than 85, blindness, deafness, or cerebral palsy.
[b] Cerebral palsy.

EPIDEMIOLOGY AND DEFINITIONS

In addition to early-onset and late-onset, BSI in the NICU frequently are further categorized to facilitate benchmarking rates between and within hospitals. Hospital-acquired BSIs (HABSI) are defined by the Centers for Disease Control and Prevention's National Healthcare Safety Network (NHSN) as BSI not present on admission, in which blood culture yields a proven pathogen at least once or a possible pathogen (ie, coagulase-negative *Staphylococcus* [CoNS]) on 2 or more occasions.[6] BSI may be associated with infection at another site, such as necrotizing enterocolitis (NEC) or a urinary tract infection. BSIs may also be associated with an indwelling catheter. These "central-line–associated" BSI (CLABSIs) are a subset of HABSI and are defined by the NHSN as HABSIs in which the initial positive culture occurs at least 2 days after the placement of a central line that is in situ or was removed less than 2 days before the positive culture, and the positive blood culture is not attributable to infection at another site.[6] Traditionally, CLABSIs are reported as occurrences per 1000 central-line–days. By monitoring CLABSI incidence rates, institutions can improve their prevention efforts and their quality of care. In 2010, the Patient Protection and Affordable Care Act created a policy of non-reimbursement for hospital charges that result from CLABSI care.[7] Data suggest that CLABSI rates are underreported. Relying on physician coding to identify CLABSI is unreliable because of different interpretations of criteria for BSI.[8,9] Furthermore, adjudicating whether a possible CLABSI is a contaminant or may be "attributable to infection at another site" can be subjective, and discordance has been demonstrated between trained professionals reviewing the same case.[10–12] For these reasons, it has been suggested that HABSIs may be a more generalizable method for reporting BSI in the NICU setting.[13] Others have recommended the use of an adjusted CLABSI rate that takes gestational age or severity of illness into account; currently, CLABSI reporting to the NHSN is stratified only by birth weight.[14–16]

RISK FACTORS
Prematurity

Prematurity is a strong predictor of BSI in the NICU. Stoll and colleagues[2] reported an LOS rate of 46% for infants less than 25 weeks' gestation; 28% for infants 25 to 28 weeks' gestation, and 10% for infants 29 to 32 weeks' gestation. These rates are virtually unchanged from a similar network study 6 years earlier.[1] Extremely premature infants are predisposed to BSI because of their immature immune function and decreased skin and mucosal integrity. They also frequently require the support of indwelling devices (**Table 2**), empiric antibiotic therapy, or acid-blocking medications, all of which have been associated with higher incidence of BSI. Finally, premature infants are at higher risk of complications resulting from prematurity, most notably NEC and bronchopulmonary dysplasia, which are associated with BSI even after adjustment for gestational age.[1,2] As survival of premature infants improves, the total number of BSIs will increase even if the rate per 1000 line-days remains constant.[17]

Central Lines and Risk of Bloodstream Infections

Central venous catheters are frequently used for blood sampling, delivery of parenteral fluid or hyperalimentation, and medication delivery in the critically ill infant. Despite their advantages, central lines increase the risk of BSI by providing multiple entryways through the skin barrier, both along the external surface of the cannula and through the

Table 2
Supportive devices or medical care associated with increased risk for bloodstream infection in the neonatal intensive care unit

Type of Support	Study	Adjusted Risk (95% CI)[a]
Mechanical ventilation	Stoll[2] (2002)	6.8 (5.9–7.8)
	Makhoul[53] (2002)	1.7 (1.4–2.1)
	Smith[28] (2010)	4.2 (1.4–12.4)
Central line (any duration)	Stoll[2] (2002)	6.1 (5.0–7.4)
	Perlman[94] (2007)	9.3 (5.9–14.8)
Central line (>7 d)	Stoll[2] (2002)	6.2 (5.0–7.6)
	Mahieu[18] (2001)	3.5 (1.3–9.2)
Central line (>21 d)	Stoll[2] (2002)	6.1 (4.6–8.0)
	Graham[40] (2006)	80.6 (6.9–944.6)
Umbilical catheter (>7 d)	Stoll[2] (2002)	1.9 (1.7–2.1)
PICC (>7 d)	Stoll[2] (2002)	2.9 (2.5–3.3)
Peripheral arterial line (>7 d)	Stoll[2] (2002)	3.7 (3.0–4.6)
Hyperalimentation (>7 d)	Holmes[95] (2008)	14.2 (8.8–22.9)
	Stoll[2] (2002)	12.9 (9.7–17.2)
	Mahieu[18] (2001)	7.1 (2.8–18.1)
	Perlman[94] (2007)	4.7 (2.2–9.9)
Vancomycin	Smith[28] (2010)	6.1 (1.9–20.1)
Dexamethasone	Stoll[96] (1999)	1.8 (1.0–3.3)
	Mahieu[18] (2001)	4.8 (1.7–13.2)
H2-blocker or proton pump inhibitor use	Bianconi[39] (2007)	6.7 (3.8–12.9)
	Stoll[96] (1999)	3.1 (1.3–7.6)
	Smith[28] (2010)	7.9 (2.8–21.1)
	Graham[40] (2006)	3.1 (1.0–10.2)

[a] Adjusted for gestational age.

lumen. Absence of colonizing bacteria at the line site and hub has excellent negative predictive value for CLABSI.[18] Mahieu and colleagues[19] reported that central lines in their NICU were manipulated an average of 30 times a day (range, 1–300); every manipulation of the central line is a risk for infection.[18] Extra care must be taken to minimize risk to the patient at insertion, maintenance, and removal of all central lines (**Box 1**). By "bundling" the care of central lines, a steady decrease has been seen in CLABSI rates in the NICU over the last decade (**Fig. 1**).

Umbilical venous and arterial catheters are placed in greater than 50% of infants less than 1500 g and virtually all infants less than 1000 g at birth. The risk of umbilical catheter infection increases with longer dwell times, with as much as a 20% higher risk per day.[20,21] As a result, some centers have focused on limiting umbilical catheter duration to no more than 7 days, with placement of a peripherally inserted central catheter (PICC) if central access is still needed. This approach may result in a lower CLABSI rate.[22]

Box 1
Elements of evidence-based central line bundles to minimize risk of central-line associated bloodstream infections in the neonatal intensive care unit

Education

- Emphasis on hand hygiene, with prospective audit and feedback
- Prohibition of artificial nails, nail polish, or complex rings
- Training sessions on proper catheter placement and management techniques
- Update staff monthly on CLABSI rate

Insertion

- Specific individuals trained for insertion and maintenance of catheters
- Establish central line kit or cart with all items necessary
- Maximal barrier precautions, sterile procedure
- Skin antisepsis regimen before insertion

Maintenance

- Minimize access ports
- Sterilize access ports before entry ($\geq$15 seconds)
- Minimize entry to line
- Limit dressing changes to when dressing is soiled/compromised or when catheter needs to be adjusted
- Sterile technique for placement, adjustment, and dressing changes

Removal

- Daily discussion on rounds regarding need for catheter
- Surgical lines removed within 48 hours of discontinuation of use

Surveillance

- Monitoring CLABSI rate
- Committee to review data, monitor medical literature, and update protocols
- Monitoring hand hygiene compliance

Adapted from Refs.[83–86]

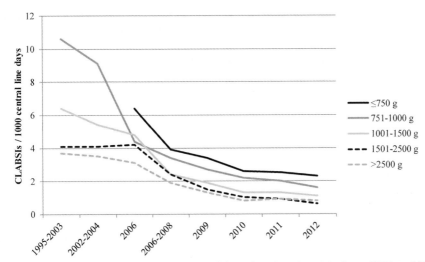

Fig. 1. Incidence of CLABSI per 1000 central line–days in US NICUs from 1995 to 2012, stratified by birth weight. (*Data from* Dudeck MA, Weiner LM, Allen-Bridson K. National Healthcare Safety Network (NHSN) report, data summary for 2012, Device-associated module. Am J Infect Control 2013;41:1148–66.)

PICC lines are used most frequently for infants requiring central access beyond the first week of life. The CLABSI rate per 1000 line-days is lower for PICCs than for umbilical catheters.[23] Whether dwell times are associated with higher risk of infection is controversial,[24] but most studies support an association between longer PICC dwell time and higher risk of CLABSI.[25–29] Site of insertion (eg, lower extremity vs upper extremity) is not associated with risk of infection.[30]

Medications Associated with Increased Risk of Bloodstream Infections

For premature infants with sterile blood cultures, prolonged ($\geq$5 days) empiric antibiotic therapy has been associated with LOS, NEC, and death.[31,32] Infants receiving third-generation cephalosporins are at higher risk for colonization and infection with *Candida*.[33,34] Both of these adverse outcomes may be the result of selective pressure on the infant microbiome, leading to decreased diversity of gut bacteria and selection for *Enterobacteriaceae* and *Candida* spp.[35,36] Minimizing antibiotic use, particularly with broad-spectrum agents, is critical to reduce BSI in the NICU.[37]

There are several medications other than antibiotics that have been associated with increased rates of BSI in the NICU. H2 blockers and proton pump inhibitors have been associated with higher risks of LOS, particularly from gram-negative organisms or NEC.[38–40] Recently, Gupta and colleagues[41] demonstrated that H2 blockers narrow the diversity of the neonatal microbiome and select for Proteobacteria. This pattern is also seen with antibiotic use.

Neonatal Intensive Care Units Environment

Understaffing of nurses in the NICU has been associated with higher rates of nosocomial infection, including BSI. Using data from the Vermont-Oxford Network, Rogowski and colleagues[42] showed that a 1 standard-deviation-higher understaffing level (approximately 0.1 nurse per infant) was associated with a 40% increase in nosocomial infections. Other studies have shown similar reductions in BSI when NICUs are staffed appropriately according to national guidelines.[43,44] Appropriate space for infant beds (minimum of 150 ft^2 for intensive care) or single-infant rooms is recommended.[45] These associations likely are due to multiple causes. Understaffing and crowding both reflect increased patient census. More work for health care providers may mean less attention to routine infection control practices, including hand washing. Some risk may be attributable to physical space as well; less floor space between isolettes means less distance an organism has to travel on contaminated equipment to reach another host. Although the patient census is not under the control of NICU administration, maintaining adequate space and staffing ratios are.

CAUSATIVE AGENTS

Gram-positive organisms, particularly CoNS, are the most common organisms causing BSI in the NICU, accounting for approximately two-thirds of all BSI in the NICU (**Fig. 2**).[1,2] Of these, approximately 70% are CoNS, followed by *Staphylococcus aureus*, *Enterococcus* spp, and group B *Streptococcus*. Gram-negative organisms include the *Enterobacteriaceae* and less commonly *Pseudomonas*, *Serratia*, and others. *Candida* spp account for 5% to 10% of BSI on average, but the incidence varies widely between NICUs.

Coagulase-negative Staphylococcus

CoNS includes a variety of species, including *Staphylococcus epidermidis, Staphylococcus capitis, Staphylococcus hominis,* and *Staphylococcus haemolyticus.* They account for almost 50% of BSI in the NICU and an even higher proportion of CLABSIs because of their presence on the skin and the ability to form biofilms on indwelling plastic.[46] Most CoNS isolates are resistant to semisynthetic penicillins such as oxacillin or nafcillin because of the presence of the *mecA* gene, which alters the penicillin-binding proteins that are their targets. The *mecA* gene is also present in

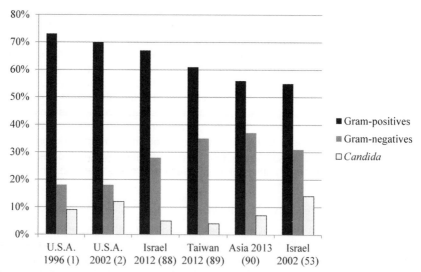

Fig. 2. Distribution of organisms causing late-onset BSI in the neonatal intensive care unit. Country and year of study shown on x-axis, with reference number in parentheses. (*Data from* Refs.[1,2,53,87–89])

methicillin-resistant *S aureus* (MRSA), and CoNS is thought to have been the origin of the *mecA* gene in *S aureus*.[47] Given the predominance of CoNS as a cause of late-onset BSI, many NICUs include vancomycin as part of their empiric antibiotic therapy for late-onset infection. However, CoNS is also a common contaminant, and even proven CoNS infections are associated with increased morbidity but not mortality. Therefore, some NICUs follow a vancomycin-reduction protocol that includes oxacillin or nafcillin empirically rather than vancomycin, which is only used for a proven CoNS infection ($\geq$2 positive blood cultures for CoNS) or when MRSA is suspected.[48]

Staphylococcus aureus

Similar to CoNS, *S aureus* is found on the skin and mucosal surfaces. *S aureus* is a less frequent cause of BSI in the NICU, accounting for only 4% to 8% of infections. Unlike CoNS, *S aureus* infections are associated with significant morbidity and mortality, including a case-fatality rate for BSI that approaches 25%.[49] In a large multicenter review of *S aureus* infections in the NICU, Shane and colleagues[49] found that there were no significant differences between infants with MRSA infections and those with methicillin-susceptible *S aureus* infections, suggesting that local bacterial epidemiology rather than patient-specific risk factors dictates which organism infants are at risk for. See the full review by Julie Autmizguine in this issue for more information.

Enterococcus

Enterococcus faecalis and *Enterococcus faecium* account for approximately 3% of BSI in the NICU. All *Enterococci* are intrinsically resistant to oxacillin and nafcillin. Vancomycin is an effective treatment of *Enterococci* resistant to ampicillin unless the isolates harbor *Van-A* or *Van-B* genes. These genes confer vancomycin resistance by altering the amino acid residues of the bacterial cell wall and prevent vancomycin from binding and inhibiting cell wall growth.[50] Such isolates are called vancomycin-resistant *Enterococcus* (VRE). Similar to MRSA, VRE have been associated with NICU outbreaks.

Gram-Negatives

Gram-negative organisms account for approximately one-third of BSIs in the NICU. *Escherichia coli* is second only to group B streptococcal infections as a cause of EOS and meningitis in the NICU, but other gram-negative organisms including *Klebsiella, Enterobacter, Pseudomonas, Serratia, Acinetobacter, Citrobacter*, and more are also frequent pathogens. These organisms are present in the infant microbiome and can be selected for by prolonged antibiotic use. Smith and colleagues[28] obtained prospective stool surveillance cultures on very low-birth-weight infants and found that subsequent BSI due to gram-negatives were attributable to organisms previously identified in the infant's gastrointestinal tract. These findings are consistent with a previous study, in which gram-negative organisms isolated from blood cultures were genotypically identical to those present in paired or previously obtained rectal cultures in 95% of cases.[51] Gram-negative organisms are also present in the environment and can be easily transmitted on the hands of health care workers, contaminated medical equipment, or visitors. The role of postnatal parent-to-child transmission is unknown but is an important consideration given increasing prevalence in the community. Regardless of how these organisms are introduced, close attention to hand hygiene and careful environmental cleaning are paramount to prevent horizontal transmission of organisms from infant to infant.

Candida

Candida BSIs are less common than either gram-positive or gram-negative BSI, accounting for approximately 10% of BSI in the NICU.[52,53] However, *Candida* is associated with high morbidity and mortality, with a case-fatality rate exceeding 30% and poor neurodevelopmental outcomes in survivors.[54,55] Prematurity and exposure to antibiotics, particularly third-generation cephalosporins, are risk factors for colonization with and infection from *Candida* isolates. Prophylactic fluconazole has been shown to reduce colonization and infection with *Candida* in extremely low-birth-weight infants,[56] but a recent randomized controlled trial did not demonstrate a reduction in the combined outcomes of death or invasive candidiasis.[57] Fluconazole prophylaxis is not a substitute for good antibiotic stewardship practices. See the full review by Danny Benjamin in this issue for more information.

RESISTANCE

The proportion of drug-resistant organisms causing infection in the NICU, including BSIs, is increasing. A Medline search for MRSA, VRE, extended-spectrum β-lactamase (ESBL), and carbapenemase-producing organisms shows a sharp increase in the number of NICU-specific publications regarding these resistant organisms (**Fig. 3**), often in the setting of an outbreak. Review of the worldwide database of health care–associated outbreaks found ESBL producing gram-negative organisms and MRSA listed as the causative pathogens of more than 15% of NICU outbreaks, some of which have led to unit closure during the outbreak period.[58–60] Moreover, the incidence of resistant infections is increasing, as demonstrated by the 300% increase in late-onset MRSA infections in US NICUs between 1995 and 2004.[61] Even in the non-outbreak setting, these organisms are constantly introduced, from health care workers, contaminated medical equipment, and parents or other visitors,

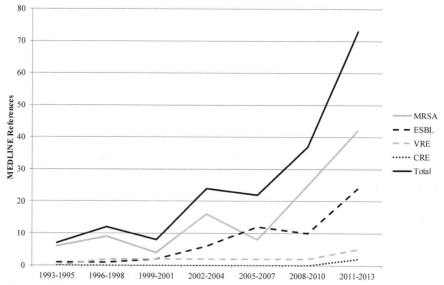

Fig. 3. Publications describing antibiotic-resistant organisms in the NICU, 1993–2013. CRE, carbapenemase-resistant *Enterobacteriaceae*.

and close attention to hand hygiene is paramount to prevent horizontal transmission of these agents to and between infants.[62,63] Approximately one-third of infants colonized with a resistant organism will develop an infection with the same organism.[28,64,65] Commonly used empiric therapy in most NICUs does not routinely cover these resistant organisms, leading to a potential "bug-drug" mismatch, a delay in effective therapy, and poor outcomes.[66,67] However, administering broad-spectrum empiric therapy to all infants as a matter of routine will further drive resistance. Careful monitoring of the prevalence of resistant organisms in the NICU can inform appropriate empiric antibiotic selection.

Good antibiotic stewardship practices can help to minimize the prevalence of resistant organisms in the NICU.[68] There is a clear association between the use of broad-spectrum antibacterial agents, particularly third-generation cephalosporins, and the rapid development of resistant organisms within an NICU.[69] Antibiotic use drives resistance by selecting for organisms with antibiotic-resistant genes. These genes are transmitted by several mechanisms:

- Genes may be present on the bacterial chromosome
  - All members of the species may carry a gene (ie, *AmpC*)
    - Gene can be active at all times, OR
    - Gene can be de-repressed by exposure to antibiotics
  - Certain strains can acquire a gene by mobile elements such as cassettes (ie, *mecA*)
  - De novo mutations can lead to antibiotic resistance[70]
- Genes may be shared between bacteria
  - Via plasmid
  - Via transformation, whereby DNA fragments from dead bacteria are absorbed
    - Both processes are accelerated following antibiotic exposure.[71,72]

Antibiotic-resistant organisms can emerge in an infant's skin or gastrointestinal microbiota. Antibiotic therapy can eliminate susceptible commensal organisms and enable resistant organisms to rapidly become the dominant strain.[73] Furthermore, elimination of commensals may predispose the infant to colonization with resistant organisms in the NICU environment, which can occupy mucosal space that has been cleared of commensals.[74,75] Empiric antibiotic therapy for BSI in a given NICU should be the narrowest possible spectrum of activity, while still accounting for that specific unit's epidemiology and resistance patterns. If the MRSA prevalence is low, then oxacillin or nafcillin in combination with an aminoglycoside is an appropriate choice for suspected late-onset BSI.[48] If the prevalence of MRSA requires empiric MRSA coverage, then vancomycin in combination with an aminoglycoside should be empiric therapy, and the vancomycin should be narrowed or discontinued once MRSA infection is excluded. Given the association with increased *Candida* and resistant gram-negative organisms, third-generation cephalosporin use should be reserved for suspected gram-negative meningitis.[33] Unit-specific epidemiology can inform when broader therapy, such as cephalosporins or carbapenems, is needed for high-risk infants.

The proliferation of resistant organisms is jeopardizing the use of available antibiotics and is concerning given the limited number of new agents to combat these organisms in the pipelines of the pharmaceutical industry, particularly in infants in whom available antibiotics are often not US Food and Drug Administration–approved or have little available pharmacokinetic data.[76] Drug resistance in gram-negative organisms is accelerating, highlighted by the recent emergence of carbapenemase-producing *Enterobacteriaceae*. Infections with gram-negative organisms account for the highest attributable morbidity and mortality and will only become more challenging to manage as treatment options become increasingly limited. The focus must be on preventing the horizontal transfer of these organisms and practicing good antibiotic stewardship to limit selective pressure.[77,78]

INFECTION CONTROL AND PREVENTION

As detailed above, infection control and antibiotic stewardship are essential to prevent infections and the emergence of antibiotic-resistant organisms in the NICU. In addition to antibiotic-driven selection pressure within the NICU, there is a consistent low rate of gram-negative multidrug-resistant organisms that are introduced to the NICU from other parts of the hospital or the community.[62] Close attention to good infection prevention practice can prevent horizontal transmission of these organisms.[63] Good infection prevention practices include the following:

- Hand hygiene practices
  - Soap or hand gel before and after patient contact
  - No artificial nails, complex rings, or nail polish
  - Prospective audit of hand hygiene practice with feedback
- Environmental control
  - Proper bed space cleaning, with audit and feedback
  - Environmental cleaning
  - Minimizing crowding
    - American Academy of Pediatrics recommends a minimum of 150 ft^2 for critically ill infants
- Antibiotic stewardship
  - Limiting empiric therapy to the narrowest-spectrum agents that cover likely pathogens circulating in unit
  - Avoiding prolonged or unnecessary antibiotic therapy for suspected or proven infections
  - Prospective surveillance of antibiotic use, with feedback and interventions[79]
- Multidisciplinary approach
  - Involvement of neonatologists, infection preventionists, nurses, and unit managers, respiratory therapy, environmental services, and microbiology
    - Proven benefit in outbreak setting and in routine prevention[80,81]
  - Hospital administration and health department can expedite processes in the outbreak setting.[82]

SUMMARY

BSIs in the NICU are associated with a variety of adverse outcomes in infants, including increased length of stay and cost, poor neurodevelopmental outcomes, and death. BSI are more common in preterm infants, many of whom require the support of indwelling devices such as catheters. Meticulous attention to the insertion and maintenance of central lines, along with careful review of when the catheters can be safely discontinued, has been shown to minimize CLABSI rates. Minimizing prolonged or unnecessary antibiotic exposure can further decrease the incidence of BSI, minimize the emergence of drug-resistant organisms or Candida as pathogens in the NICU, and safeguard the use of currently available antibiotics for future infants. An understanding of infection control and prevention as well as local epidemiology can help minimize emerging resistance or outbreaks and optimize empiric antimicrobial selection.

Best practices

What is the current practice?

Neonatal bloodstream infection

Best practice/guideline/care path objectives

- Promptly diagnose with performance of adequate volume (≥1 mL)
- Begin antibiotics without delay to reduce mortality
- Bundled care for insertion and maintenance of central lines
- Discontinue central lines as soon as no longer needed

What changes in current practice are likely to improve outcomes?

- Minimize scenarios associated with increased CLABSI rates, including:
  - Avoid unnecessary or prolonged antibiotic therapy
  - Minimize use of acid-blocking medications
  - Avoid overstaffing or overcrowding

Major recommendations

- Obtain appropriate-volume (≥1 mL) blood cultures for infants with suspected BSI (grade 1A)
- Begin empiric antibiotics in all cases of suspected BSI (grade 1A)
  - Consider empiric ampicillin and gentamicin for early-onset sepsis if meningitis is not suspected
  - Consider empiric oxacillin and gentamicin for LOS if meningitis is not suspected and infant not colonized with MRSA
- Adjust therapy as additional clinical information becomes available (grade 1A)
- Remove central lines as soon as no longer needed or CLABSI is diagnosed (grade 1A)
  - Exception: Coagulase-negative staphylococcal CLABSI that responds promptly to therapy may not require line discontinuation (grade 2)

Summary statement

- Appropriate blood cultures (≥1 mL) and prompt empiric antibiotic therapy is essential when BSI is suspected. Practices that minimize CLABSI rates are critical to minimize the morbidity and mortality from BSI in preterm infants.

REFERENCES

1. Stoll BJ, Gordon T, Korones SB, et al. Late-onset sepsis in very low birth weight neonates: a report from the National Institute of Child Health and Human Development Neonatal Research Network. J Pediatr 1996;129(1):63–71.
2. Stoll BJ, Hansen N, Fanaroff AA, et al. Late-onset sepsis in very low birth weight neonates: the experience of the NICHD Neonatal Research Network. Pediatrics 2002;110(2 Pt 1):285–91.
3. Payne NR, Carpenter JH, Badger GJ, et al. Marginal increase in cost and excess length of stay associated with nosocomial bloodstream infections in surviving very low birth weight infants. Pediatrics 2004;114(2):348–55.
4. Mitha A, Foix-L'Helias L, Arnaud C, et al. Neonatal infection and 5-year neurodevelopmental outcome of very preterm infants. Pediatrics 2013;132(2):e372–80.
5. Stoll BJ, Hansen NI, Adams-Chapman I, et al. Neurodevelopmental and growth impairment among extremely low-birth-weight infants with neonatal infection. JAMA 2004;292(19):2357–65.

6. Centers for Disease Control and Prevention. CDC/NHSN surveillance definitions for specific types of infections. Available at: http://www.cdc.gov/nhsn/pdfs/Accessed July pscmanual/17pscnosinfdef_curent.pdf. Accessed July 31, 2014.

7. Centers for Medicare and Medicaid Services. Medicaid program payment adjustments for provider-preventable conditions including health care acquired conditions. Final rule. Fed Regist 2011;76(108):32816–38.

8. Rich KL, Reese SM, Bol KA, et al. Assessment of the quality of publicly reported central line-associated bloodstream infection data in Colorado, 2010. Am J Infect Control 2013;41(10):874–9.

9. Patrick SW, Davis MM, Sedman AB, et al. Accuracy of hospital administrative data in reporting central line-associated bloodstream infections in newborns. Pediatrics 2013;131(Suppl 1):S75–80.

10. Thompson ND, Yeh LL, Magill SS, et al. Investigating systematic misclassification of central line-associated bloodstream infection (CLABSI) to secondary bloodstream infection during health care-associated infection reporting. Am J Med Qual 2013;28(1):56–9.

11. Seybold U, Reichardt C, Halvosa JS, et al. Clonal diversity in episodes with multiple coagulase-negative Staphylococcus bloodstream isolates suggesting frequent contamination. Infection 2009;37(3):256–60.

12. Niedner MF, National Association of Children's Hospitals and Related Institutions. The harder you look, the more you find: catheter-associated bloodstream infection surveillance variability. Am J Infect Control 2010;38(8):585–95.

13. Folgori L, Bielicki J, Sharland M. A systematic review of strategies for reporting of neonatal hospital-acquired bloodstream infections. Arch Dis Child Fetal Neonatal Ed 2013;98(6):F518–23.

14. Phillips P, Cortina-Borja M, Gilbert R, et al. Risk stratification by level of care for comparing bloodstream infection rates in neonatal intensive care units. J Hosp Infect 2009;72(2):181–3.

15. Leighton P, Cortina-Borja M, Millar M, et al. Risk-adjusted comparisons of bloodstream infection rates in neonatal intensive-care units. Clin Microbiol Infect 2012; 18(12):1206–11.

16. Barbadoro P, Marigliano A, D'Errico MM, et al. Gestational age as a single predictor of health care-associated bloodstream infections in neonatal intensive care unit patients. Am J Infect Control 2011;39(2):159–62.

17. Zafar N, Wallace CM, Kieffer P, et al. Improving survival of vulnerable infants increases neonatal intensive care unit nosocomial infection rate. Arch Pediatr Adolesc Med 2001;155(10):1098–104.

18. Mahieu LM, De Muynck AO, Ieven MM, et al. Risk factors for central vascular catheter-associated bloodstream infections among patients in a neonatal intensive care unit. J Hosp Infect 2001;48(2):108–16.

19. Mahieu LM, De Dooy JJ, Lenaerts AE, et al. Catheter manipulations and the risk of catheter-associated bloodstream infection in neonatal intensive care unit patients. J Hosp Infect 2001;48(1):20–6.

20. Yumani DF, van den Dungen FA, van Weissenbruch MM. Incidence and risk factors for catheter-associated bloodstream infections in neonatal intensive care. Acta Paediatr 2013;102(7):e293–8.

21. Zingg W, Posfay-Barbe KM, Pfister RE, et al. Individualized catheter surveillance among neonates: a prospective, 8-year, single-center experience. Infect Control Hosp Epidemiol 2011;32(1):42–9.

22. Butler-O'Hara M, D'Angio CT, Hoey H, et al. An evidence-based catheter bundle alters central venous catheter strategy in newborn infants. J Pediatr 2012;160(6):972–7.e2.

23. de Brito CS, de Brito DV, Abdallah VO, et al. Occurrence of bloodstream infection with different types of central vascular catheter in critically neonates. J Infect 2010;60(2):128–32.
24. Smith PB, Benjamin DK Jr, Cotten CM, et al. Is an increased dwell time of a peripherally inserted catheter associated with an increased risk of bloodstream infection in infants? Infect Control Hosp Epidemiol 2008;29(8):749–53.
25. Ohki Y, Maruyama K, Harigaya A, et al. Complications of peripherally inserted central venous catheter in Japanese neonatal intensive care units. Pediatr Int 2013;55(2):185–9.
26. Milstone AM, Reich NG, Advani S, et al. Catheter dwell time and CLABSIs in neonates with PICCs: a multicenter cohort study. Pediatrics 2013;132(6):e1609–15.
27. Sengupta A, Lehmann C, Diener-West M, et al. Catheter duration and risk of CLABSI in neonates with PICCs. Pediatrics 2010;125(4):648–53.
28. Smith A, Saiman L, Zhou J, et al. Concordance of gastrointestinal tract colonization and subsequent bloodstream infections with gram-negative bacilli in very low birth weight infants in the neonatal intensive care unit. Pediatr Infect Dis J 2010; 29(9):831–5.
29. Hsu JF, Tsai MH, Huang HR, et al. Risk factors of catheter-related bloodstream infection with percutaneously inserted central venous catheters in very low birth weight infants: a center's experience in Taiwan. Pediatr Neonatol 2010;51(6):336–42.
30. Wrightson DD. Peripherally inserted central catheter complications in neonates with upper versus lower extremity insertion sites. Adv Neonatal Care 2013; 13(3):198–204.
31. Cotten CM, Taylor S, Stoll B, et al. Prolonged duration of initial empirical antibiotic treatment is associated with increased rates of necrotizing enterocolitis and death for extremely low birth weight infants. Pediatrics 2009;123(1):58–66.
32. Kuppala VS, Meinzen-Derr J, Morrow AL, et al. Prolonged initial empirical antibiotic treatment is associated with adverse outcomes in premature infants. J Pediatr 2011;159(5):720–5.
33. Cotten CM, McDonald S, Stoll B, et al. The association of third-generation cephalosporin use and invasive candidiasis in extremely low birth-weight infants. Pediatrics 2006;118(2):717–22.
34. Saiman L, Ludington E, Dawson JD, et al. Risk factors for Candida species colonization of neonatal intensive care unit patients. Pediatr Infect Dis J 2001; 20(12):1119–24.
35. Mai V, Torrazza RM, Ukhanova M, et al. Distortions in development of intestinal microbiota associated with late onset sepsis in preterm infants. PLoS One 2013;8(1):e52876.
36. Torrazza RM, Ukhanova M, Wang X, et al. Intestinal microbial ecology and environmental factors affecting necrotizing enterocolitis. PLoS One 2013;8(12): e83304.
37. Cantey JB, Patel SJ. Antimicrobial stewardship in the NICU. Infect Dis Clin North Am 2014;28(2):247–61.
38. Guillet R, Stoll BJ, Cotten CM, et al. Association of H2-blocker therapy and higher incidence of necrotizing enterocolitis in very low birth weight infants. Pediatrics 2006;117(2):e137–42.
39. Bianconi S, Gudavalli M, Sutija VG, et al. Ranitidine and late-onset sepsis in the neonatal intensive care unit. J Perinat Med 2007;35(2):147–50.
40. Graham PL 3rd, Begg MD, Larson E, et al. Risk factors for late onset gram-negative sepsis in low birth weight infants hospitalized in the neonatal intensive care unit. Pediatr Infect Dis J 2006;25(2):113–7.

41. Gupta RW, Tran L, Norori J, et al. Histamine-2 receptor blockers alter the fecal microbiota in premature infants. J Pediatr Gastroenterol Nutr 2013;56(4):397–400.
42. Rogowski JA, Staiger D, Patrick T, et al. Nurse staffing and NICU infection rates. JAMA Pediatr 2013;167(5):444–50.
43. Cimiotti JP, Haas J, Saiman L, et al. Impact of staffing on bloodstream infections in the neonatal intensive care unit. Arch Pediatr Adolesc Med 2006;160(8):832–6.
44. Leistner R, Thurnagel S, Schwab F, et al. The impact of staffing on central venous catheter-associated bloodstream infections in preterm neonates - results of nation-wide cohort study in Germany. Antimicrob Resist Infect Control 2013;2(1):11.
45. Lockwood CJ, Lemons JA, editors. Guidelines for perinatal care. 6th edition. Elk Grove Village (IL): American Academy of Pediatrics; 2007.
46. Otto M. Virulence factors of the coagulase-negative staphylococci. Front Biosci 2004;9:841–63.
47. Garza-Gonzalez E, Morfin-Otero R, Llaca-Diaz JM, et al. Staphylococcal cassette chromosome mec (SCC mec) in methicillin-resistant coagulase-negative staphylococci. A review and the experience in a tertiary-care setting. Epidemiol Infect 2010;138(5):645–54.
48. Chiu CH, Michelow IC, Cronin J, et al. Effectiveness of a guideline to reduce vancomycin use in the neonatal intensive care unit. Pediatr Infect Dis J 2011;30(4):273–8.
49. Shane AL, Hansen NI, Stoll BJ, et al. Methicillin-resistant and susceptible Staphylococcus aureus bacteremia and meningitis in preterm infants. Pediatrics 2012;129(4):e914–22.
50. Mascini EM, Bonten MJ. Vancomycin-resistant enterococci: consequences for therapy and infection control. Clin Microbiol Infect 2005;11(Suppl 4):43–56.
51. Graham PL 3rd, Della-Latta P, Wu F, et al. The gastrointestinal tract serves as the reservoir for Gram-negative pathogens in very low birth weight infants. Pediatr Infect Dis J 2007;26(12):1153–6.
52. Benjamin DK Jr, Stoll BJ, Gantz MG, et al. Neonatal candidiasis: epidemiology, risk factors, and clinical judgment. Pediatrics 2010;126(4):e865–73.
53. Makhoul IR, Sujov P, Smolkin T, et al. Epidemiological, clinical, and microbiological characteristics of late-onset sepsis among very low birth weight infants in Israel: a national survey. Pediatrics 2002;109(1):34–9.
54. Benjamin DK Jr, Stoll BJ, Fanaroff AA, et al. Neonatal candidiasis among extremely low birth weight infants: risk factors, mortality rates, and neurodevelopmental outcomes at 18 to 22 months. Pediatrics 2006;117(1):84–92.
55. Adams-Chapman I, Bann CM, Das A, et al. Neurodevelopmental outcome of extremely low birth weight infants with Candida infection. J Pediatr 2013;163(4):961–7.e3.
56. Manzoni P, Stolfi I, Pugni L, et al. A multicenter, randomized trial of prophylactic fluconazole in preterm neonates. N Engl J Med 2007;356(24):2483–95.
57. Benjamin DK Jr, Hudak ML, Duara S, et al. Effect of fluconazole prophylaxis on candidiasis and mortality in premature infants: a randomized clinical trial. JAMA 2014;311(17):1742–9.
58. Maragakis LL, Winkler A, Tucker MG, et al. Outbreak of multidrug-resistant Serratia marcescens infection in a neonatal intensive care unit. Infect Control Hosp Epidemiol 2008;29(5):418–23.
59. Stone PW, Gupta A, Loughrey M, et al. Attributable costs and length of stay of an extended-spectrum beta-lactamase-producing Klebsiella pneumoniae outbreak in a neonatal intensive care unit. Infect Control Hosp Epidemiol 2003;24(8):601–6.

60. Gastmeier P, Loui A, Stamm-Balderjahn S, et al. Outbreaks in neonatal intensive care units - they are not like others. Am J Infect Control 2007;35(3):172–6.

61. Lessa FC, Edwards JR, Fridkin SK, et al. Trends in incidence of late-onset methicillin-resistant Staphylococcus aureus infection in neonatal intensive care units: data from the National Nosocomial Infections Surveillance System, 1995–2004. Pediatr Infect Dis J 2009;28(7):577–81.

62. Toltzis P, Dul MJ, Hoyen C, et al. Molecular epidemiology of antibiotic-resistant gram-negative bacilli in a neonatal intensive care unit during a nonoutbreak period. Pediatrics 2001;108(5):1143–8.

63. Mammina C, Di Carlo P, Cipolla D, et al. Surveillance of multidrug-resistant gram-negative bacilli in a neonatal intensive care unit: prominent role of cross transmission. Am J Infect Control 2007;35(4):222–30.

64. Carey AJ, Della-Latta P, Huard R, et al. Changes in the molecular epidemiological characteristics of methicillin-resistant Staphylococcus aureus in a neonatal intensive care unit. Infect Control Hosp Epidemiol 2010;31(6):613–9.

65. Singh N, Patel KM, Leger MM, et al. Risk of resistant infections with Enterobacteriaceae in hospitalized neonates. Pediatr Infect Dis J 2002;21(11):1029–33.

66. Sick AC, Tschudin-Sutter S, Turnbull AE, et al. Empiric combination therapy for gram-negative bacteremia. Pediatrics 2014;133:e1148–55.

67. Tsai MH, Chu SM, Hsu JF, et al. Risk factors and outcomes for multidrug-resistant gram-negative bacteremia in the NICU. Pediatrics 2014;133(2):e322–9.

68. Moro ML, Gagliotti C. Antimicrobial resistance and stewardship in long-term care settings. Future Microbiol 2013;8(8):1011–25.

69. de Man P, Verhoeven BA, Verbrugh HA, et al. An antibiotic policy to prevent emergence of resistant bacilli. Lancet 2000;355(9208):973–8.

70. Hughes D, Andersson DI. Selection of resistance at lethal and non-lethal antibiotic concentrations. Curr Opin Microbiol 2012;15(5):555–60.

71. Charpentier X, Kay E, Schneider D, et al. Antibiotics and UV radiation induce competence for natural transformation in Legionella pneumophila. J Bacteriol 2011;193(5):1114–21.

72. Dorer MS, Fero J, Salama NR. DNA damage triggers genetic exchange in Helicobacter pylori. PLoS Pathog 2010;6(7):e1001026.

73. Tourneur E, Chassin C. Neonatal immune adaptation of the gut and its role during infections. Clin Dev Immunol 2013;2013:270301.

74. Almuneef MA, Baltimore RS, Farrel PA, et al. Molecular typing demonstrating transmission of gram-negative rods in a neonatal intensive care unit in the absence of a recognized epidemic. Clin Infect Dis 2001;32(2):220–7.

75. Goldmann DA, Leclair J, Macone A. Bacterial colonization of neonates admitted to an intensive care environment. J Pediatr 1978;93(2):288–93.

76. Bush K. Alarming beta-lactamase-mediated resistance in multidrug-resistant Enterobacteriaceae. Curr Opin Microbiol 2010;13(5):558–64.

77. Centers for Disease Control and Prevention. Guidance for control of infections with carbapenem-resistant or carbapenemase-producing Enterobacteriaceae in acute care facilities. MMWR Morb Mortal Wkly Rep 2009;58(10):256–60.

78. Roy S, Viswanathan R, Singh A, et al. Gut colonization by multidrug-resistant and carbapenem-resistant Acinetobacter baumannii in neonates. Eur J Clin Microbiol Infect Dis 2010;29(12):1495–500.

79. Dellit TH, Owens RC, McGowan JE Jr, et al. Infectious Diseases Society of America and the Society for Healthcare Epidemiology of America guidelines for developing an institutional program to enhance antimicrobial stewardship. Clin Infect Dis 2007;44(2):159–77.

80. Ransjo U, Lytsy B, Melhus A, et al. Hospital outbreak control requires joint efforts from hospital management, microbiology and infection control. J Hosp Infect 2010;76(1):26–31.

81. Enoch DA, Summers C, Brown NM, et al. Investigation and management of an outbreak of multidrug-carbapenem-resistant Acinetobacter baumannii in Cambridge, UK. J Hosp Infect 2008;70(2):109–18.

82. Cantey JB, Sreeramoju P, Jaleel M, et al. Prompt control of an outbreak caused by extended-spectrum beta-lactamase-producing Klebsiella pneumoniae in a neonatal intensive care unit. J Pediatr 2013;163(3):672–9.e1-3.

83. Bizzarro MJ, Sabo B, Noonan M, et al. A quality improvement initiative to reduce central line-associated bloodstream infections in the neonatal intensive care unit. Infect Control Hosp Epidemiol 2010;31(3):241–8.

84. Leboucher B, Leblanc M, Berlie I, et al. Effectiveness of an informative report on the prevention of nosocomial bloodstream infections in a neonatal intensive care unit. Arch Pediatr 2006;13(5):436–41.

85. Schulman J, Stricof R, Stevens TP, et al. Statewide NICU central-line-associated bloodstream infection rates decline after bundles and checklists. Pediatrics 2011; 127(3):436–44.

86. Fisher D, Cochran KM, Provost LP, et al. Reducing central line-associated bloodstream infections in North Carolina NICUs. Pediatrics 2013;132(6):e1664–71.

87. Grisaru-Soen G, Friedman T, Dollberg S, et al. Late-onset bloodstream infections in preterm infants: a 2-year survey. Pediatr Int 2012;54(6):748–53.

88. Lim WH, Lien R, Huang YC, et al. Prevalence and pathogen distribution of neonatal sepsis among very-low-birth-weight infants. Pediatr Neonatol 2012; 53(4):228–34.

89. Al-Taiar A, Hammoud MS, Cuiqing L, et al. Neonatal infections in China, Malaysia, Hong Kong and Thailand. Arch Dis Child Fetal Neonatal Ed 2013;98(3):F249–55.

90. de Haan TR, Beckers L, de Jonge RC, et al. Neonatal gram negative and Candida sepsis survival and neurodevelopmental outcome at the corrected age of 24 months. PLoS One 2013;8(3):e59214.

91. Schlapbach LJ, Aebischer M, Adams M, et al. Impact of sepsis on neurodevelopmental outcome in a Swiss National Cohort of extremely premature infants. Pediatrics 2011;128(2):e348–57.

92. Atif ML, Sadaoui F, Bezzaoucha A, et al. Prolongation of hospital stay and additional costs due to nosocomial bloodstream infection in an Algerian neonatal care unit. Infect Control Hosp Epidemiol 2008;29(11):1066–70.

93. Donovan EF, Sparling K, Lake MR, et al. The investment case for preventing NICU-associated infections. Am J Perinatol 2013;30(3):179–84.

94. Perlman SE, Saiman L, Larson EL. Risk factors for late-onset health care-associated bloodstream infections in patients in neonatal intensive care units. Am J Infect Control 2007;35(3):177–82.

95. Holmes A, Dore CJ, Saraswatula A, et al. Risk factors and recommendations for rate stratification for surveillance of neonatal healthcare-associated bloodstream infection. J Hosp Infect 2008;68(1):66–72.

96. Stoll BJ, Temprosa M, Tyson JE, et al. Dexamethasone therapy increases infection in very low birth weight infants. Pediatrics 1999;104(5):e63.

Urinary Tract Infections in the Infant

Mehreen Arshad, MD, Patrick C. Seed, MD, PhD*

KEYWORDS

- Infants • Urinary tract infection • *Escherichia coli* • Renal imaging
- Antibiotic resistance • Vesicoureteral reflux

KEY POINTS

- Uncircumcised boys have the highest risk of urinary tract infection.
- *Escherichia coli* is the most common pathogen.
- Premature infants are at increased risk for *Candida* urinary tract infections.
- Infants with urinary tract infection are at risk for concomitant bacteremia and meningitis.
- Prophylaxis may increase the risk of antibiotic resistance for recurrent urinary tract infection.

INTRODUCTION

Urinary tract infections (UTIs) in infants are common. UTIs may be the sentinel event for underlying renal abnormality, although normal anatomy is most common. Prompt diagnosis and initiation of treatment is important in preventing long-term renal scarring. However, increasing antibiotic resistance may delay initiation of appropriate therapy. Antibiotic prophylaxis remains controversial.

EPIDEMIOLOGY AND RISK FACTORS FOR URINARY TRACT INFECTIONS IN INFANTS
Occurrence of Urinary Tract Infections in the First 3 Days of Life Is Exceedingly Rare

The true incidence of UTI in the first days of life is difficult to assess, as most large studies have included such cases in the broader age categories (7%–9%).[1–4] Small studies indicate the incidence in the febrile infant is between 10.7% and 15.4%.[5,6] Occurrence of UTIs in the first 3 days of life is reportedly rare (0%–1%) in the United States[7,8] and up to 1.8% in developing countries.[9,10] Even in premature infants, virtually no cases are detected in the first 24 hours of life.[8]

Disclosures: None.
Division of Infectious Diseases, Department of Pediatrics, Duke University School of Medicine, DUMC 3499, Durham, NC 27710, USA
* Corresponding author.
E-mail address: patrick.seed@duke.edu

Clin Perinatol 42 (2015) 17–28
http://dx.doi.org/10.1016/j.clp.2014.10.003
0095-5108/15/$ – see front matter © 2015 Elsevier Inc. All rights reserved.

Escherichia coli Is the Most Common Cause of Neonatal Urinary Tract Infection

The most common bacterial etiology for neonatal UTIs, similar to other age groups, is *Escherichia coli*.[3,11–14] However, some studies found that the overall burden of disease by *E. coli* was lower in this age group (about 50% of all positive cultures) compared with older age groups in which *E. coli* is responsible for up to 80% of UTIs.[10,15] In particular, male infants with vesicoureteral reflux (VUR) were more likely to present with UTIs caused by other pathogens.[3,5,12,15] These pathogens include other gram-negative organisms: *Klebsiella pneumoniae, Klebsiella oxytoca, Proteus mirabilis, Proteus vulgaris, Enterobacter aerogenes, Pseudomonas aeruginosa*, and *Morganella morganii*.[5,12] Neonatal UTI with gram-positive organisms is rare, but cases of *Enterococcus faecalis, Staphylococcus aureus*, Group B *streptococcus*, and *Streptococcus pneumonia* have been reported.[6,16–18] Coagulase-negative staphylococci may be causative agents in premature infants, with isolation of the organism in 14% of catheterized urine culture samples from infants with suspected infection and 18% concordance with positive blood cultures.[19] However, this finding remains controversial; one study, which included mostly premature infants, showed a less than 1% incidence of coagulase-negative staphylococci UTI.[20] *Candida* UTIs occur more commonly in extremely premature infants. One study reported that 42% of UTIs in a neonatal intensive care unit were caused by *Candidia* spp, with *Enterobacter cloacae* being the second most common.[21] **Table 1** lists the most common pathogens associated with neonatal UTI.

Uncircumcised Male Infants Have the Highest Risk of Urinary Tract Infection

A clear male predominance has been associated with neonatal UTI, with boys making up approximately 70% to 90% of all cases.[5,11,12] This finding is also true in premature infants.[22,23] To evaluate the effect of circumcision on male risk for infantile UTI, Zorc and colleagues[3] conducted a prospective multicenter trial, which included approximately 1000 febrile infants less than 60 days of age whose evaluation for sepsis included a urine culture and urinalysis. Infants who had growth of a single organism

Table 1		
Common pathogens isolated in neonatal UTI		
Organism	**Incidence (%)**	**References**
Gram-negative rods		
E. coli	40–72	5,12,42
Klebsiella spp	7–40	5,35
Enterobacter cloacae	3–8	5,42
Proteus vulgaris	3	5
Serratia marcescens	1–7	5,35
Pseudomonas aeruginosa	1	5
Gram-positive cocci		
Enterococcus spp	10–16	5,42
Staphylococcus aureus	1–5	5,42
Group B *streptococcus*	1–3	5,70
Staphylococcus, coagulase negative	1	5
Viridans streptococcus	1	5
Yeast		
Candida spp	25–42	21,71

in the urine culture were included in the subsequent evaluation. Uncircumcised boys had the highest incidence of UTIs (21%), whereas circumcised boys (2%) and girls (5%) has similar incidences. These results were similar to those in a meta-analysis,[1] in which 20% of the uncircumcised boys less than 90 days of age with fever had a UTI compared with 2% of circumcised boys and 8% of girls. Phimosis, limited retraction of the foreskin, is significantly associated with an increase in UTIs in male infants.[24] A recent study in older children that examined the periurethral flora in boys between the ages of 6 weeks and 96 months before and after circumcision found that the presence of the prepuce results in a significantly higher burden of uropathogens.[25]

Underlying Renal Abnormalities Increase the Risk of Neonatal Urinary Tract Infection

VUR is associated with approximately 20% of neonatal cases of UTI,[5,26] although the incidence of VUR is not significantly different between genders, birth weight, gestational age, or mode of delivery.[26,27] A study of infants less than 2 months of age in a neonatal intensive care unit with a median gestation age of 28 weeks reported a less than 5% rate of anatomic abnormalities in patients with UTI. VUR was, however, associated with a younger age at UTI presentation and was 4-fold higher in infants with *Klebsiella* UTI compared with *E coli* UTI.[5,26] A study of 45 male infants with a first UTI renal ultrasound scan (RUS) and voiding cystourethrogram (VCUG) found a renal abnormality in half of the infants, the most common being VUR and other abnormalities, including duplicated collecting system, posterior urethral valves, ureteropelvic junction stricture, and renal atrophy and scarring.[28] The dimercaptosuccinic acid (DMSA) scan was abnormal almost exclusively in those with grade 3 or higher VUR. These results are similar to those in a recent study, in which 47% of febrile infants less than 30 days of age with a UTI had renal abnormalities, most of them hydronephrosis (27%) and pelviectasis (20%).[5] However, even in the absence of any abnormalities on the RUS or VCUG, infants with UTI can have an abnormal DMSA scan, indicating renal cortical damage, although that may be an effect rather than a cause of a UTI.[29] Representative images for RUS and VCUG in infants are shown in **Figs. 1** and **2**.

Maternal History of Urinary Tract Infection Is Associated with a Higher Risk of Urinary Tract Infection in the Infant

A history of maternal UTI during pregnancy has been associated with up to a 5.9-fold higher risk of UTI in infants.[30,31] Milas and colleagues[31] also observed a higher incidence of UTIs in febrile infants born after premature rupture of membranes. This

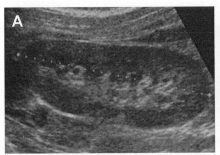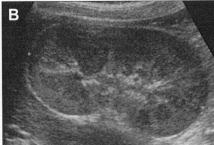

Fig. 1. Ultrasound appearance of neonatal hydronephrosis. (*A*) Right kidney in an infant showing normal structures. (*B*) Left kidney in the same infant with edematous swollen slightly hyperechoic right kidney. (*Courtesy of* Dr T.S.A. Geertsma, Ziekenhuis Gelderse Vallei, Ede, The Netherlands.)

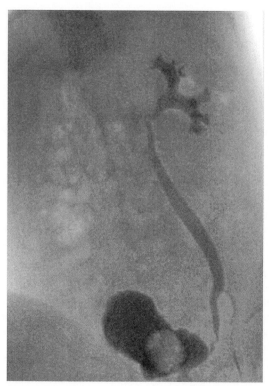

Fig. 2. Grade III vesicoureteric reflux during micturition: reflux into the ureter and the calices with mild dilatation. (*Courtesy of* Dr Adriana Dubbeldam, Belgium. Available at: www. radiopedia.org.)

incidence may be because these mothers are more likely to harbor uropathogens transmitted to the infant that then result in an ascending UTI.

CLINICAL CORRELATIONS

Full-term infants with UTIs often present with fever (≥38°C), poor feeding, vomiting, diarrhea, and lethargy (**Table 2**).[12,32] The clinical manifestations in premature infants are similar. In addition, greater than 50% of premature infants with UTI present with

Table 2
Common symptoms and signs associated with neonatal UTI

Signs and Symptoms	Percentage	References
Fever >38.5°C	77–85	12,32
Poor feeding	48–90	12,32
Tachypnea or grunting	36–45	12,33
Lethargy	26–30	12,33
Jaundice	6–18	12,36
Diarrhea	13	12
Vomiting	8–9	12,32
Failure to thrive	7	12

respiratory symptoms such as apnea, hypoxia, or tachypnea.[33] A fever greater than 39°C is more likely among infants with a serious bacterial illness such as a UTI compared with infants with a viral illness.[3,12,34]

Neonatal UTIs have been associated with jaundice[12,31]; 6% to 18% of full-term or preterm infants presenting with prolonged or worsening jaundice were found to have UTIs.[35–38] Onset of jaundice after 8 days of life in particular has been associated with UTI.[37,39] Twenty-eight of 30 infants with UTI-induced jaundice had indirect hyperbilirubinemia, and about half of them had renal cortical changes on DMSA scan.[39] In another cohort,[37] most of the infants presenting with a UTI after 8 days of life had direct hyperbilirubinemia. The American Academy of Pediatrics recommends that infants with elevated direct bilirubin levels be screened for UTIs.[40] However, those with elevated unconjugated bilirubin levels should not be excluded, especially if other concerning clinical features are present. A urinalysis may not be sufficient to exclude UTI in infants with jaundice, and a urine culture should be obtained.[41] E coli is the most commonly isolated pathogen in UTIs associated with jaundice.[37,38,41,42]

Infants with Urinary Tract Infection Are at Risk for Concomitant Bacteremia and Meningitis

Several studies have examined the concordance between UTI, bacteremia, and cerebrospinal fluid (CSF) pleocytosis/culture positivity. In a cohort of 163 infants less than 1 month of age with a UTI only 2 had meningitis.[43] Another study from the United States reported that 44 of 100 patients had concomitant positive blood and urine culture; E coli was isolated in all cases.[5] A study from India reported a 6.3% concordance between blood and urine cultures.[10] Concordance between urine, blood, and CSF cultures is higher in infants less than 26 weeks' gestation and those with candiduria.[19,21]

DIAGNOSIS
Blood Cell Indices and Inflammatory Markers Are not Specific Indicators of Urinary Tract Infections

Laboratory values such as white blood cell (WBC) count, erythrocyte sedimentation rate, and C-reactive protein are not significantly different among infants with and without UTIs.[5,44]

Urethral Catheterization is the Preferred Method for Sample Collection

Urine culture is typically obtained through 3 different methods in infants: urinary catheterization, suprapubic aspiration, or sterile bag collection. The sterile bag collection method has a contamination rate as high as 46% compared with about 9% to 12% for the other methods and, when possible, should be avoided.[45,46] Although contamination rates for suprapubic aspiration are slightly lower than those for urethral catheterization,[45] it does require a more advanced skill set and has lower parental acceptance rate, making the latter the preferred method by most providers. Although definitions vary, some investigators have defined a positive urine culture as growth of a known bacterial pathogen from a catheterized specimen at a level of (1) $\geq$50,000 colony-forming units (cfu)/mL or (2) $\geq$10,000 cfu/mL in association with a positive dipstick test or urinalysis.[3,5,47]

Pyuria Is Defined as White Blood Cell Count of $\geq10/mm^3$

The standard method of detecting pyuria, defined as at least 5 WBCs per high-powered field, is useful in predicting less than half of the UTIs in infants.[48] However, a method (often termed the *enhanced* method) initially described by Dukes,[49] in which WBCs are counted using a hemocytometer in uncentrifuged urine and reported as cells per cubic millimeter has been shown to be reproducible and more closely related to a positive urine culture. A pediatric study including young infants showed that a WBC count of $\geq 10/mm^3$ had a sensitivity of 91% and a specificity of 96% for predicting a positive culture of $\geq 50,000$ cfu/mL.[50] A more recent study, also including young infants, compared the enhanced method with automated urinalysis and found similar sensitivity and specificity for detecting pyuria associated with a bacterial culture of $\geq 50,000$ cfu/mL.[51] For bacteriuria, the same study found that the enhanced method using a manual Gram stain for organisms was about 10% more sensitive and specific than the automated analysis.

Urine Nitrites and Leukocyte Esterase Are Unreliable Parameters in Infants

Other commonly examined urinalysis parameters include nitrites and leukocyte esterase. The nitrite test indicates the presence of nitrate reductase, produced by some but not all uropathogens, which converts endogenous nitrates to nitrites. Leukocyte esterase is released by WBCs and indicates the presence of pyuria. In a systematic review of several studies, nitrites and leukocyte esterase were shown to have good sensitivity and specificity for detection of UTI in older children but were less reliable in infants.[52] This is likely related to frequent micturition in infants which does not allow for sufficient concentrations of these substrates to develop. However, a more recent study of infants between 1 and 90 days of age showed that when microscopy is added to the urine dipstick the negative predictive value is 99.2%, but would result on average in 8 false positives for every missed episode of true UTI.[53]

TREATMENT
Local Patterns of Antibiotic Resistance Should Determine Choice of Empiric Therapy

Empiric therapy for neonatal UTI and sepsis are similar because of common etiology. Traditionally parental antibiotics such as ampicillin and gentamicin are started once appropriate cultures are obtained. Within the US, the incidence of ampicillin resistance in neonatal *E. coli* isolates has been reported to be as high as 75% and gentamicin resistance as high as 12%–17%.[54,55] In spite of approximately 90% resistance against ampicillin among the *E. coli* isolates from a neonatal ward, Taheri and colleagues[56] reported that clinical response was obtained in 50% of the patients, suggesting that that there is a discordance between *in vitro* and *in vivo* activity of these drugs. This may be because the urinary concentration of ampicillin is much higher than the plasma level since it is excreted through the kidneys which may allow it to overcome the minimum inhibitory concentration of certain pathogens.[57]

Peripartum Use of Maternal Antibiotics Increases the Risk of Resistant Clones in Infants

Use of maternal peripartum exposure antibiotics increases the risk of neonatal UTI and bloodstream infections with β-lactamase producing *E coli*: 82% versus 36% in infants of treated and untreated mothers, respectively.[13] Common scenarios for maternal antibiotic exposure include preterm premature rupture of membranes (PPROM)[58,59] and intrapartum prophylaxis.[13,60]

Treatment of Candiduria

The presence of candiduria in a neonate indicates hematogenous spread and systemic disease. Treatment of systemic candidiasis is reviewed elsewhere in this issue by Kelly and colleagues and Wade and colleagues.

Neonatal Urinary Tract Infection can be Treated with a Combination of Parental and Oral Therapy

Data regarding the length of duration of treatment and the transition from parenteral to oral therapy in the infant are lacking. In the extremely premature infant, bioavailability of most antibiotics is not known; therefore, intravenous therapy is typically preferred. Documentation of negative blood and CSF cultures in both extremely premature and older infants provides optimal care. In older infants, Benador and colleagues[61] found that the risk of renal scarring was no different between infants that received 3 days of parental therapy followed by 7 days of oral therapy compared with 10 days of oral therapy. In older and more mature infants with negative blood and CSF cultures, 3 to 4 days of parental therapy followed by transition to oral medications to complete a 7- to 14-day course of treatment can be used.[62]

Renal Imaging Usually Includes a Renal Ultrasound Scan During the Acute Infection and a Voiding Cystourethrogram to Identify Vesicoureteral Reflux Approximately 2 to 4 Weeks After Resolution of Infection

Most practitioners recommend a RUS after an episode of UTI in the neonatal period to rule out congenital abnormalities. A VCUG is usually delayed for 2 to 4 weeks after successful treatment to assess for vesicoureteral reflux. Grade III or higher VUR is significantly associated with a higher risk of renal cortical damage; a DMSA scan should be considered to assess for renal scarring.[28]

In a study of 100 infants with UTI, 47% had an abnormal RUS.[5] However, the incidence of abnormalities was much lower in premature infants (4%).[63] Siomou and colleagues[64] prospectively evaluated 72 infants with an RUS and DMSA scan within 72 hours of diagnosis. Approximately 71% of the kidneys with grade III or more VUR on RUS were found to have normal early DMSA scans, 7% had evidence of permanent renal damage at the 6-month follow-up, all of which had an abnormal early DMSA scan. Therefore, an acute DMSA scan may be helpful in identifying the risk of renal scarring, but it does not reliably diagnose VUR.

The Risk of Recurrence Is Highest in First 6 Months After an Episode of Urinary Tract Infection

A long-term follow-up of 71 infants with UTI showed a recurrence rate of 28%.[65] Recurrence in premature infants was slightly more common than in full-term infants, but the difference was not significant. Most of the episodes of recurrence (65%) occur in the first 6 months after the initial UTI, and 75% occur in patients without any renal abnormalities.

Prophylactic Antibiotics Are Not Effective in Reducing Renal Scarring, but Do Increase the Risk of Recurrence with a Resistant Strain

Evidence regarding the efficacy of prophylactic therapy to prevent recurrences after the first episode of UTI is lacking for the neonatal population. Even for older infants, several small trials have found that antimicrobial prophylaxis may not be effective in preventing renal scarring.[66,67] Other more recent studies found that although the prophylaxis may decrease the risk of recurrence, its effect on renal scarring is not significant, and recurrent episodes are more likely to be caused by a more resistant strain.[68,69]

SUMMARY

UTI is common in infants. It may indicate an underlying renal disorder, but most cases occur in the absence of any abnormalities. UTIs are rare in the first 3 days of life.

Uncircumcised boys are at the highest risk for neonatal UTI. Diagnosis is by a urine culture in association with a positive dipstick test or urinalysis. Ampicillin and gentamicin are the traditional empiric therapies; however, local antibiotic resistance patterns and maternal use of antibiotics before delivery should be considered. The risk of recurrence is highest in the first 6 months after an episode of UTI. Use of prophylaxis is controversial because, although it may reduce the risk of recurrence, it is unclear if there is any effect on renal scarring, and use of prophylaxis increases the risk of infection with a resistant strain if recurrence occurs.

Best practices box

What is the current practice?

Urinary Tract Infections in Neonate

Best Practice/Guideline/Care Path Objective(s)

- Early recognition of UTIs in neonates
- Initiation of appropriate empiric therapy
- Reduction in long-term renal sequelae

What changes in current practice are likely to improve outcomes?

- Recognition of enhanced risk for bacteremia and meningitis in neonates with UTI
- Empiric treatment of UTI based on prior maternal use of antibiotics during pregnancy and local antibiotic susceptibility profiles among uropathogens
- Cautious use of prophylactic antibiotics to prevent recurrent UTI and knowledge of the risk for emergence of resistant organisms

Major Recommendations

- Obtain urine specimen for bacterial culture by urethral catheterization; other urine parameters can be misleading in infants (grade 1A).
- Empiric therapy should include coverage against common uropathogens such as *E coli* and *Klebsiella* spp
  - Ampicillin and gentamicin are the most commonly used empiric regimen (grade 1A).
- Infants with prolonged or late-onset jaundice should be evaluated for a UTI (grade 1B).
- Infants with UTI should be evaluated for concomitant bacteremia and meningitis (grade 1B).
- Renal ultrasound scan should be done immediately after an episode of neonatal UTI, followed by a VCUG 2 to 4 weeks later to rule out anatomic abnormalities (grade 1B).
- Prophylactic antibiotics do not reduce the risk of scarring and can increase the risk of recurrent UTI with resistant organisms (grade 1B).

Summary statement

UTI in infants may indicate an underlying renal disorder; therefore, appropriate diagnosis and prompt initiation of therapy are essential to reduce long-term renal scarring.

Data from Refs.[5,19,43,46,69,72]

REFERENCES

1. Shaikh N, Morone NE, Bost JE, et al. Prevalence of urinary tract infection in childhood: a meta-analysis. Pediatr Infect Dis J 2008;27:302–8.

2. Ismaili K, Lolin K, Damry N, et al. Febrile urinary tract infections in 0- to 3-month-old infants: a prospective follow-up study. J Pediatr 2011;158:91–4.
3. Zorc JJ, Levine DA, Platt SL, et al. Clinical and demographic factors associated with urinary tract infection in young febrile infants. Pediatrics 2005;116:644–8.
4. Lin DS, Huang SH, Lin CC, et al. Urinary tract infection in febrile infants younger than eight weeks of Age. Pediatrics 2000;105:E20.
5. Bonadio W, Maida G. Urinary tract infection in outpatient febrile infants younger than 30 days of age: a 10-year evaluation. Pediatr Infect Dis J 2014;33:342–4.
6. Morley EJ, Lapoint JM, Roy LW, et al. Rates of positive blood, urine, and cerebrospinal fluid cultures in children younger than 60 days during the vaccination era. Pediatr Emerg Care 2012;28:125–30.
7. Visser VE, Hall RT. Urine culture in the evaluation of suspected neonatal sepsis. J Pediatr 1979;94:635–8.
8. Tamim MM, Alesseh H, Aziz H. Analysis of the efficacy of urine culture as part of sepsis evaluation in the premature infant. Pediatr Infect Dis J 2003;22:805–8.
9. Riskin A, Toropine A, Bader D, et al. Is it justified to include urine cultures in early (<72 hours) neonatal sepsis evaluations of term and late preterm infants? Am J Perinatol 2013;30:499–504.
10. Samayam P, Ravi Chander B. Study of urinary tract infection and bacteriuria in neonatal sepsis. Indian J Pediatr 2012;79:1033–6.
11. Wang SF, Huang FY, Chiu NC, et al. Urinary tract infection in infants less than 2 months of age. Zhonghua Min Guo Xiao Er Ke Yi Xue Hui Za Zhi 1994;35:294–300.
12. Kanellopoulos TA, Salakos C, Spiliopoulou I, et al. First urinary tract infection in neonates, infants and young children: a comparative study. Pediatr Nephrol 2006;21:1131–7.
13. Didier C, Streicher MP, Chognot D, et al. Late-onset neonatal infections: incidences and pathogens in the era of antenatal antibiotics. Eur J Pediatr 2012;171:681–7.
14. Watt K, Waddle E, Jhaveri R. Changing epidemiology of serious bacterial infections in febrile infants without localizing signs. PLoS One 2010;5:e12448.
15. Lo DS, Shieh HH, Ragazzi SL, et al. Community-acquired urinary tract infection: age and gender-dependent etiology. J Bras Nefrol 2013;35:93–8.
16. Bitsori M, Maraki S, Raissaki M, et al. Community-acquired enterococcal urinary tract infections. Pediatr Nephrol 2005;20:1583–6.
17. Zurina Z, Rohani A, Neela V, et al. Late onset group b beta-hemolytic *streptococcus* infection in a neonate manifesting as a urinary tract infection: a rare clinical presentation. Southeast Asian J Trop Med Public Health 2012;43:1470–3.
18. Hassoun A, Stankovic C, Rogers A, et al. Listeria and enterococcal infections in neonates 28 days of age and younger: is empiric parenteral ampicillin still indicated? Pediatr Emerg Care 2014;30:240–3.
19. Downey LC, Benjamin DK Jr, Clark RH, et al. Urinary tract infection concordance with positive blood and cerebrospinal fluid cultures in the neonatal intensive care unit. J Perinatol 2013;33:302–6.
20. Jean-Baptiste N, Benjamin DK Jr, Cohen-Wolkowiez M, et al. *Coagulase-negative* staphylococcal infections in the neonatal intensive care unit. Infect Control Hosp Epidemiol 2011;32:679–86.
21. Phillips JR, Karlowicz MG. Prevalence of *Candida* species in hospital-acquired urinary tract infections in a neonatal intensive care unit. Pediatr Infect Dis J 1997;16:190–4.
22. Airede AI. Urinary-tract infections in African neonates. J Infect 1992;25:55.

23. Eliakim A, Dolfin T, Korzets Z, et al. Urinary tract infection in premature infants: the role of imaging studies and prophylactic therapy. J Perinatol 1997;17:304.
24. Shim YH, Lee JW, Lee SJ. The risk factors of recurrent urinary tract infection in infants with normal urinary systems. Pediatr Nephrol 2009;24:309–12.
25. Laway MA, Wani ML, Patnaik R, et al. Does circumcision alter the periurethral uropathogenic bacterial flora. Afr J Paediatr Surg 2012;9:109–12.
26. Cleper R, Krause I, Eisenstein B, et al. Prevalence of vesicoureteral reflux in neonatal urinary tract infection. Clin Pediatr (Phila) 2004;43:619–25.
27. Jantunen ME, Siitonen A, Ala-Houhala M, et al. Predictive factors associated with significant urinary tract abnormalities in infants with pyelonephritis. Pediatr Infect Dis J 2001;20:597–601.
28. Goldman M, Lahat E, Strauss S, et al. Imaging after urinary tract infection in male neonates. Pediatrics 2000;105:1232–5.
29. Sastre JB, Aparicio AR, Cotallo GD, et al. Urinary tract infection in the newborn: clinical and radio imaging studies. Pediatr Nephrol 2007;22:1735–41.
30. Khalesi N, Khosravi N, Jalali A, et al. Evaluation of maternal urinary tract infection as a potential risk factor for neonatal urinary tract infection. J Family Reprod Health 2014;8:59–62.
31. Milas V, Puseljić S, Stimac M, et al. Urinary tract infection (UTI) in newborns: risk factors, identification and prevention of consequences. Coll Antropol 2013;37:871–6.
32. Littlewood JM. 66 infants with urinary tract infection in first month of life. Arch Dis Child 1972;47:218–26.
33. Levy I, Comarsca J, Davidovits M, et al. Urinary tract infection in preterm infants: the protective role of breastfeeding. Pediatr Nephrol 2009;24:527–31.
34. Levine DA, Platt SL, Dayan PS, et al. Risk of serious bacterial infection in young febrile infants with respiratory syncytial virus infections. Pediatrics 2004;113: 1728–34.
35. Shahian M, Rashtian P, Kalani M. Unexplained neonatal jaundice as an early diagnostic sign of urinary tract infection. Int J Infect Dis 2012;16:e487–90.
36. Pashapour N, Nikibahksh AA, Golmohammadlou S. Urinary tract infection in term neonates with prolonged jaundice. Urol J 2007;4:91–4.
37. Garcia FJ, Nager AL. Jaundice as an early diagnostic sign of urinary tract infection in infancy. Pediatrics 2002;109:846–51.
38. Mutlu M, Cayır Y, Aslan Y. Urinary tract infections in neonates with jaundice in their first two weeks of life. World J Pediatr 2014;10:164–7.
39. Xinias I, Demertzidou V, Mavroudi A, et al. Bilirubin levels predict renal cortical changes in jaundiced neonates with urinary tract infection. World J Pediatr 2009; 5:42–5.
40. American Academy of Pediatrics Subcommittee on Hyperbilirubinemia. Management of hyperbilirubinemia in the newborn infant 35 or more weeks of gestation. Pediatrics 2004;114:297–316.
41. Fang SB, Lee HC, Yeung CY, et al. Urinary tract infections in young infants with prolonged jaundice. Acta Paediatr Taiwan 2005;46:356–60.
42. Chen HT, Jeng MJ, Soong WJ, et al. Hyperbilirubinemia with urinary tract infection in infants younger than eight weeks old. J Chin Med Assoc 2011;74:159–63.
43. Tebruegge M, Pantazidou A, Clifford V, et al. The age-related risk of co-existing meningitis in children with urinary tract infection. PLoS One 2011;6:e26576.
44. Foglia EE, Lorch SA. Clinical predictors of urinary tract infection in the neonatal intensive care unit. J Neonatal Perinatal Med 2012;5:327–33.
45. Karacan C, Erkek N, Senel S, et al. Evaluation of urine collection methods for the diagnosis of urinary tract infection in children. Med Princ Pract 2010;19:188–91.

46. Tosif S, Baker A, Oakley E, et al. Contamination rates of different urine collection methods for the diagnosis of urinary tract infections in young children: an observational cohort study. J Paediatr Child Health 2012;48:659–64.

47. Hoberman A, Wald ER. Urinary tract infections in young febrile children. Pediatr Infect Dis J 1997;16:11–7.

48. Crain EF, Gershel JC. Urinary tract infections in febrile infants younger than 8 weeks of age. Pediatrics 1990;86:363–7.

49. Dukes C. The examination of urine for pus. Br Med J 1928;1:391–3.

50. Hoberman A, Wald ER, Reynolds EA, et al. Pyuria and bacteriuria in urine specimens obtained by catheter from young children with fever. J Pediatr 1994;124:513–9.

51. Shah AP, Cobb BT, Lower DR, et al. Enhanced versus automated urinalysis for screening of urinary tract infections in children in the emergency department. Pediatr Infect Dis J 2014;33:272–5.

52. Mori R, Yonemoto N, Fitzgerald A, et al. Diagnostic performance of urine dipstick testing in children with suspected UTI: a systematic review of relationship with age and comparison with microscopy. Acta Paediatr 2010;99:581–4.

53. Glissmeyer EW, Korgenski EK, Wilkes J, et al. Dipstick screening for urinary tract infection in febrile infants. Pediatrics 2014;133(5):e1121–7.

54. Hasvold J, Bradford L, Nelson C, et al. Gentamicin resistance among Escherichia coli strains isolated in neonatal sepsis. J Neonatal Perinatal Med 2013; 6:173–7.

55. Shakir SM, Goldbeck JM, Robison D, et al. Genotypic and Phenotypic Characterization of Invasive Neonatal Escherichia coli Clinical Isolates. Am J Perinatol 2014;31:975–82.

56. Taheri PA, Navabi B, Shariat M. Neonatal urinary tract infection: clinical response to empirical therapy versus in vitro susceptibility at Bahrami Children's Hospital-Neonatal Ward: 2001–2010. Acta Med Iran 2012;50:348–52.

57. Williamson JC, Craft DW, Butts JD, et al. In vitro assessment of urinary isolates of ampicillin-resistant enterococci. Ann Pharmacother 2002;36:246–50.

58. Laugel V, Kuhn P, Beladdale J, et al. Effects of antenatal antibiotics on the incidence and bacteriological profile of early-onset neonatal sepsis. A retrospective study over five years. Biol Neonate 2003;84:24–30.

59. Kuhn P, Dheu C, Bolender C, et al. Incidence and distribution of pathogens in early-onset neonatal sepsis in the era of antenatal antibiotics. Paediatr Perinat Epidemiol 2010;24:479–87.

60. Glasgow TS, Young PC, Wallin J, et al. Association of intrapartum antibiotic exposure and late-onset serious bacterial infections in infants. Pediatrics 2005;116: 696–702.

61. Benador D, Neuhaus TJ, Papazyan JP, et al. Randomised controlled trial of three day versus 10 day intravenous antibiotics in acute pyelonephritis: effect on renal scarring. Arch Dis Child 2001;84:241–6.

62. Cherry J, Demmler-Harrison GJ, Kaplan SL, et al. Feigin and Cherry's textbook of pediatric infectious diseases. Philadelphia: Elsevier Saunders; 2013.

63. Nowell L, Moran C, Smith PB, et al. Prevalence of renal anomalies after urinary tract infections in hospitalized infants less than 2 months of age. J Perinatol 2010;30:281–5.

64. Siomou E, Giapros V, Fotopoulos A, et al. Implications of 99mTc-DMSA scintigraphy performed during urinary tract infection in neonates. Pediatrics 2009; 124:881–7.

65. Biyikli NK, Alpay H, Ozek E, et al. Neonatal urinary tract infections: analysis of the patients and recurrences. Pediatr Int 2004;46:21–5.

66. Garin EH, Olavarria F, Garcia Nieto V, et al. Clinical significance of primary vesicoureteral reflux and urinary antibiotic prophylaxis after acute pyelonephritis: a multicenter, randomized, controlled study. Pediatrics 2006;117:626–32.
67. Hayashi Y, Kojima Y, Kamisawa H, et al. Is antibiotic prophylaxis effective in preventing urinary tract infections in patients with vesicoureteral reflux? Expert Rev Anti Infect Ther 2010;8:51–8.
68. Williams GJ, Wei L, Lee A, et al. Long-term antibiotics for preventing recurrent urinary tract infection in children. Cochrane Database Syst Rev 2006;(19):CD001534.
69. RIVUR Trial Investigators, Hoberman A, Greenfield SP, et al. Antimicrobial prophylaxis for children with vesicoureteral reflux. N Engl J Med 2014;370:2367–76.
70. Harris MC, Deuber C, Polin RA, et al. Investigation of apparent false-positive urine latex particle agglutination tests for the detection of group B *streptococcus* antigen. J Clin Microbiol 1989;27:2214–7.
71. Benjamin DK Jr, Stoll BJ, Gantz MG, et al. Neonatal candidiasis: epidemiology, risk factors, and clinical judgment. Pediatrics 2010;26:e865–73.
72. Cantey JB, Wozniak PS, Sánchez PJ. Prospective surveillance of antibiotic use in the neonatal intensive care unit: results from the SCOUT study. Pediatr Infect Dis J 2014. [Epub ahead of print].

Bacterial Meningitis in Infants

Lawrence C. Ku, MD[a], Kim A. Boggess, MD[b], Michael Cohen-Wolkowiez, MD, PhD[a],*

KEYWORDS

- Neonatal bacterial meningitis • Very low birth weight • Lumbar puncture
- Cerebrospinal fluid • Antibiotics • Vaccine

KEY POINTS

- Neonatal bacterial meningitis is uncommon but is associated with high mortality and morbidity.
- Group B *Streptococcus* (GBS) is the most common cause of neonatal meningitis.
- *Escherichia coli* has recently become the most common pathogen isolated from very low birth weight infants with meningitis.
- Infants with culture-proven meningitis can have negative blood cultures and normal cerebrospinal fluid parameters.
- All infants showing signs of infection and with suspected early-onset or late-onset sepsis should undergo a lumbar puncture.
- A GBS vaccine for the prevention of neonatal GBS disease including meningitis is currently under development.

Funding support: Dr Ku receives research support from the National Institute of Child Health and Human Development (5T32GM086330-03 [Principal Investigators: Brouwer, Benjamin, Watkins]). Dr Boggess receives research support from the National Institute of Child Health and Human Development (5T32HD040672-13 [Principal Investigator: Boggess]; 5K12HD001441 [Principal Investigator: Orringer]; 1R01HD064729-01A1 [Principal Investigator: Tita]), the National Center for Advancing Translational Sciences of the National Institutes of Health (1UL1TR001111), and Research Point Corporation, Inc. Dr Cohen-Wolkowiez receives support for research from the National Center for Advancing Translational Sciences of the National Institutes of Health (UL1TR001117), the Food and Drug Administration (1U01FD004858-01), the Biomedical Advanced Research and Development Authority (BARDA) (HHSO100201300009C), the nonprofit organization Thrasher Research Fund (www.thrasherresearch.org), and from industry for drug development in adults and children (www.dcri.duke.edu/research/coi.jsp).

[a] Department of Pediatrics, Duke Clinical Research Institute, Box 17969, Durham, NC 27715, USA; [b] Department of Obstetrics & Gynecology, University of North Carolina School of Medicine, CB 7570, Chapel Hill, NC 27599-7570, USA
* Corresponding author.
E-mail address: michael.cohenwolkowiez@duke.edu

INTRODUCTION

Bacterial meningitis is a serious infection associated with high mortality and morbidity in the neonatal population. Prompt diagnosis and treatment are essential to achieving good outcomes in affected infants. Although overall incidence and mortality have declined over the last several decades, morbidity associated with neonatal meningitis remains virtually unchanged.[1,2] Prevention strategies, adjunctive therapies, and improved diagnostic strategies have been the focus of recent research seeking to improve the outcomes.[3]

DESCRIPTION OF THE DISEASE

Meningitis is the acute inflammation of the meninges, subarachnoid space, and brain vasculature resulting from infection.[4] Neonatal meningitis is categorized as early and late onset, which is defined by the presence of signs of infection and organism isolation from cerebrospinal fluid (CSF) cultures at less than or equal to 72 hours and greater than 72 hours of life, respectively.[3,5–7]

EPIDEMIOLOGY

The incidence of neonatal meningitis varies by geographic location (**Fig. 1**).[8–10] Compared with older age groups, the incidence of meningitis is highest during the neonatal period.[9,16]

Developed Countries

The incidence of culture-proven neonatal meningitis is estimated at 0.3 per 1000 live births in developed countries.[2,10,16] However, this number is likely an underestimation of the true incidence. For infants in the intensive care nursery who are evaluated for sepsis, 30% to 50% do not have a lumbar puncture (LP) performed.[6,17] When an LP is performed, more than 75% of the time it occurs after the initiation of antibiotics, possibly biasing CSF culture results.[6,17,18]

In developed countries, mortality from neonatal meningitis ranges from 10% to 15%.[2,8] In a prospective study including 444 cases of confirmed meningitis from 2001 to 2007, mortality in premature infants compared with term infants was more

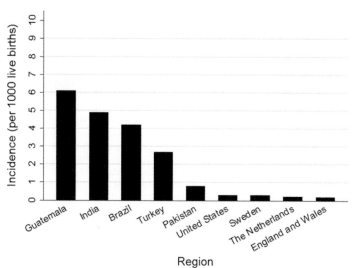

Fig. 1. Incidence of neonatal meningitis across the world. (*Data from* Refs.[2,11–15])

than 2-fold higher (26% vs 10%, $P<.01$).[8] Up to 50% of infants with a history of meningitis are neurologically impaired, with 25% having severe disability.[2,8,19] With advances in medical practices, the incidence and mortality associated with meningitis have declined over the past 40 years; however, morbidity remains unchanged.[19]

Developing Countries

In developing countries, the reported incidence of neonatal meningitis is much higher at 0.8 to 6.1 per 1000 live births, with a mortality of 40% to 58%.[9,11] True values may be higher because of underreporting in regions with limited resources, diagnostic testing, and access to health care.[9]

CAUSE

The types and distribution of organisms commonly observed in neonatal meningitis depend on postnatal age, location, and gestational age. The distribution of organisms seen in neonatal meningitis is similar to that of neonatal sepsis (**Table 1**).[1,6,16]

Early-onset Meningitis

Despite the institution of maternal intrapartum prophylaxis, group B *Streptococcus* (GBS) has remained the most common cause of neonatal sepsis and meningitis since the early 1980s, responsible for greater than 40% of all early-onset infections.[2,6,20] *Escherichia coli* is the second most common pathogen and is isolated in 30% of all early-onset infections.[6] Since the 1990s, *E coli* has emerged as the most common cause of early-onset sepsis and meningitis among very low birth weight (VLBW; ie, <1500 g birth weight) infants.[21–24]

Late-onset Meningitis

Late-onset meningitis is predominantly seen in premature infants, and the incidence is directly related to decreasing birth gestational age and weight.[25] Surveillance of 6956 VLBW infants from 1998 to 2000 found coagulase-negative staphylococci (48%) and *Staphylococcus aureus* (8%) to be the first and second most common pathogens, respectively.[7] *E coli* (5%) and *Klebsiella* (4%) spp were the most common gram-negative causes of late-onset infections.[5,7] Although GBS (2%) was less common in this cohort, other studies found that infants were more likely to have confirmed meningitis with late-onset GBS sepsis compared with early-onset GBS sepsis (**Table 2**).[7,26,27]

Table 1
Common pathogens of meningitis and commonly used empiric antibiotics

Type	Major Pathogens	Empiric Antibiotics
Early onset	Group B *Streptococcus* *Escherichia coli* *Listeria monocytogenes* *Streptococcus pneumoniae*	Ampicillin Gentamicin Cefotaxime
Late onset	Coagulase-negative *Staphylococcus* *Staphylococcus aureus* *E coli* *Klebsiella* spp *Enterococcus* spp *Enterobacter* spp *Pseudomonas* spp Group B *Streptococcus*	Vancomycin Gentamicin Cefotaxime Ampicillin

			Proportion of Infants with Late-onset GBS Sepsis Complicated by Meningitis, n (%)	Proportion of Infants with Early-onset GBS Sepsis Complicated by Meningitis, n (%)	
Table 2 **Infants with late-onset versus early-onset GBS sepsis complicated by meningitis**					
N (Ref.)	**Years**	**Study Population**			***P***
347[26]	2001–2003	GA 23–43 wk PNA ≤90 d Confirmed GBS sepsis	84 of 136 (62)	33 of 206 (16)	<.001
179[27]	1997–2004	GA 31–40 wk Confirmed GBS sepsis	13 of 24 (54)	22 of 155 (14)	<.01

Abbreviations: GA, gestational age; PNA, postnatal age.

PATHOGENESIS

Although several mechanisms in the development of neonatal meningitis have been described, primary bloodstream infection with secondary hematogenous distribution to the central nervous system (CNS) is the most common (**Box 1**).[16] For this reason, the epidemiology and microbiology of neonatal meningitis are similar to those of neonatal sepsis.[1]

Early-onset Infection

Organisms present in the maternal genitourinary tract ascend from the vagina and can infect the amniotic fluid through disruptions in the amniotic membranes, which the infant then aspirates.[28] Organisms can also colonize exposed neonatal skin and mucosa during passage through the birth canal and invade through barrier disruptions.[1] Organisms such as *Listeria monocytogenes* can also be transmitted transplacentally.[16] In rare cases, hematogenous transmission of GBS from maternal bacteremia has been reported as a cause of early-onset GBS infections in infants.[29]

Late-onset Infection

Organisms can be acquired from the colonized mother, as seen with GBS.[30,31] Poor hand hygiene among caregivers and hospital staff can result in the transfer of organisms between infected and uninfected infants.[32] Foreign, invasive devices such as ventricular reservoirs, ventricular shunts, endotracheal tubes, venous or arterial catheters, urinary catheters, and feeding tubes can also introduce pathogens to the infant.[16] Exposure to prolonged courses of empiric antibiotics for suspected infections can also result in increased risk for late-onset infections.[33] Among 365 VLBW infants

---

Box 1
Mechanisms for development of neonatal meningitis

1. Primary bloodstream infection with secondary hematogenous spread to CNS
2. Presence of an infectious focus with secondary bloodstream infection and hematogenous spread (eg, osteomyelitis)
3. Presence of an infectious focus with direct extension into the CNS (eg, sinus infection)
4. Primary CNS infection resulting from disruptions caused by head trauma, neurosurgery, or congenital defects (eg, myelomeningocele)

less than or equal to 32 weeks' gestational age, infants exposed to empiric antibiotics for greater than or equal to 5 days had increased odds of developing late-onset sepsis (odds ratio, 2.45; 95% confidence interval, 1.28–4.67).[34]

Infection of the Central Nervous System

After attaching to the endothelium of the cerebral microvasculature and choroid plexus, bacteria can enter the CSF by several mechanisms (**Box 2**).[1,4,35] Inflammatory mediators are then released into the CSF in response to the presence of bacterial products, resulting in meningitis and increased permeability of the blood-brain barrier.[1,31]

RISK FACTORS

Risk factors for the development of neonatal meningitis are similar to those for neonatal sepsis (**Box 3**).[5,10,36] Immaturity of the neonatal immune system, impaired phagocytic ability of neutrophils and monocytes, and diminishing maternal antibodies all contribute to increased risk of infections in both term and preterm infants.[4,24] Because most maternal immunoglobulins do not cross the placenta before 32 weeks' gestation, infants born extremely preterm are at significantly higher risk for infections.[10] However, early initiation of breastfeeding may be protective against infections because of transfer of immunoglobulin A.[37]

CLINICAL PRESENTATION

The clinical signs of neonatal meningitis can be subtle and nonspecific (**Box 4**).[16,19,38] Meningitic signs such as convulsions, irritability, bulging fontanel, and nuchal rigidity are often late findings that are associated with poor outcomes.[2,10,38]

Exposure to intrapartum antibiotic prophylaxis (IAP) against GBS has led to concerns that the signs of neonatal infections could be delayed or masked. Several studies have determined no significant difference in the clinical presentation of early-onset GBS disease between infected infants with and without prior exposure to IAP.[20] Signs of early-onset sepsis manifested in 90% of infected infants within the first 24 hours of life.[20]

DIAGNOSIS

To confirm the diagnosis of neonatal meningitis, an LP is needed to collect CSF. Positive growth on the CSF culture provides identification of the organism and enables refinement of therapy.[2,39] The LP is frequently deferred during the septic work-up because of concerns of exacerbating clinical deterioration in the sick infant.[39–41]

Performing or Deferring the Lumbar Puncture

Because the LP is an invasive procedure with risks, it is difficult to determine which infant should receive one as part of the septic work-up.[40,41] Among infants with positive blood cultures, up to 30% have a concurrent positive CSF culture.[42] However, in

---

Box 2
Bacterial mechanisms for entry into the CSF

1. Transcellular movement across the endothelial cell (eg, GBS, *E coli*)

2. Paracellular movement by disruption of intercellular tight junctions

3. Transport across the blood-brain barrier and blood-CSF barriers within phagocytes (eg, *L monocytogenes*)

Box 3
Risk factors for neonatal meningitis

1. Prematurity
2. Maternal rectovaginal GBS colonization
3. Chorioamnionitis or maternal fever
4. Premature rupture of membranes
5. Prolonged rupture of membranes (>18 hours)
6. Invasive fetal monitoring
7. VLBW (<1500 g)
8. Prolonged hospitalization
9. Presence of external devices (eg, reservoirs, shunts, catheters)

---

infants with confirmed meningitis, 15% to 38% have a negative blood culture.[27,43–45] In rare cases, the blood and CSF cultures can be discordant.[44] Approaches in which only infants with confirmed bacteremia are evaluated for meningitis result in missed diagnoses of meningitis.

The incidence of meningitis among asymptomatic infants with risk factors is very low (<1%).[46,47] When clinical signs can be attributed to noninfectious causes, such as respiratory distress syndrome or transient tachypnea of the newborn, clinical judgment is required in deciding when to perform an LP.[43] Among 238 infants admitted for respiratory distress without other symptoms, 17 of 238 (7%) infants had a positive blood culture, and none had meningitis.[48]

The current recommendation is to perform an LP on all clinically stable infants suspected to have early-onset or late-onset sepsis and who are showing signs of

---

Box 4
Clinical signs of neonatal meningitis

1. Fever or hypothermia
2. Irritability or lethargy
3. Hypotonia
4. Feeding intolerance or vomiting
5. Respiratory distress
6. Apnea
7. Bradycardia
8. Hypotension
9. Poor perfusion
10. Seizures
11. Bulging anterior fontanel
12. Nuchal rigidity
13. Jaundice
14. Hypoglycemia or hyperglycemia
15. Diarrhea

---

infection.[20,39,43] Whenever possible, the LP should be performed before the administration of antibiotics.

Interpreting Cerebrospinal Fluid Parameters

Infants are often exposed to intrapartum or empiric antibiotics before receiving an LP, which can result in falsely negative CSF cultures in those with meningitis.[18] In these cases, CSF parameters are used to help determine the likelihood of meningitis.

CSF indexes vary according to age, with normal values in infants poorly defined.[16,44,45] Common practice in infants states that a CSF leukocyte count greater than or equal to 20/mm^3 suggests bacterial meningitis.[16] A study involving 1064 infants showed that infants less than 28 days old without bacterial meningitis had a median CSF leukocyte count of 3/mm^3 and 95th percentile value of 19/mm^3.[49] However, in a study evaluating 9111 infants at greater than or equal to 34 weeks' gestational age, the use of 20/mm^3 as a cutoff resulted in a missed diagnosis in 13% of infants with confirmed meningitis.[44] Several infants with confirmed meningitis had normal CSF parameters without bacteremia. CSF protein and glucose were considered poor predictors of meningitis because of considerable overlap of values between infants with and without confirmed meningitis. A study of 4632 infants of less than 34 weeks' gestational age reached similar conclusions in the preterm population.[45] There is great difficulty in predicting the diagnosis of meningitis solely based on CSF parameters, so CSF culture continues to be the gold standard for diagnosis.

Ancillary Tests

The polymerase chain reaction (PCR) has been explored as a diagnostic tool for meningitis. In addition to improved sensitivity and specificity, PCR also allows quicker detection of pathogens compared with traditional cultures.[50] A real-time PCR assay designed to detect multiple pathogens including *Streptococcus pneumoniae, E coli,* GBS, *S aureus,* and *L monocytogenes* had an overall higher detection rate of any CSF pathogen compared with traditional cultures (72% vs 48%).[51] Among patients exposed to antibiotics before collection of CSF, PCR had a higher detection rate compared with culturing (58% vs 29%).[51] Further testing is needed before PCR can be used routinely in the diagnosis of bacterial meningitis.[52]

Other tests used to aid in clinical decision making include the complete blood count with differential and C-reactive protein. Studies examining the usefulness of these tests in the diagnosis of neonatal bacterial meningitis are limited (**Table 3**).

Repeating the Lumbar Puncture

The need for a repeat LP during treatment in an infant with confirmed meningitis has been debated. Some experts recommend routinely repeating an LP in all patients at 48 hours, whereas others suggest repeating an LP only if clinical conditions are not improved by 24 to 72 hours after beginning therapy.[56–59]

In a retrospective study of 14,018 infants, 221 infants were identified as having culture-positive meningitis, with 118 infants (53%) receiving 2 or more LPs during the treatment course.[56] Among infants with available mortality data receiving 2 or more LPs, 6 of 23 (26%) infants with repeat positive cultures died compared, with 6 of 81 (7%) infants with repeat negative cultures ($P = .02$). No significant difference in mortality was seen among the 81 (7%) infants with a repeat negative culture compared with the 90 (12%) infants with meningitis with no repeat LP ($P = .32$). A survey of 109 pediatricians and neonatologists across the northwest England found that 89 (82%) practitioners did not routinely repeat the LP in infants with bacterial meningitis unless clinically indicated.[57]

Table 3
Available studies on biomarkers for neonatal meningitis

Biomarker	N (Ref.)	Study Population	Notable Findings
Complete blood count differential ratio $\left(\dfrac{\%\ \text{lymphocytes} + \%\ \text{monocytes}}{\%\ \text{polymorphonuclear leukocytes} + \%\ \text{band forms}}\right)$	72[53]	Term PNA <4 wk	Complete blood count differential ratio <1.5 as cutoff for predicting bacterial meningitis, test achieved the following: Sensitivity = 100% Specificity = 67% Positive predictive value = 47% Negative predictive value = 100%
	40[54]	Term PNA <28 d	Used same cutoff values as previous study on different cohort achieved the following: Sensitivity = 70% Specificity = 54% Positive predictive value = 39% Negative predictive value = 81%
Peripheral white blood cell count	8312[44]	GA ≥34 wk PNA 0–150 d	Use as predictor for bacterial meningitis had positive likelihood ratio <1.0 Neither sensitive nor specific
C-reactive protein, CSF	23[55]	GA 28–41 wk PNA 0–6 wk	1 of 7 infants without infection, 0 of 5 infants with sepsis without meningitis, and 2 of 11 infants with meningitis had C-reactive protein >1 mg/dL Levels do not distinguish between infants with meningitis and those with no confirmed infection

TREATMENT
Antimicrobial Therapy

Prompt initiation of antibiotics is critical. Delays in treatment are associated with increased mortality and morbidity.[60] Empiric antimicrobials used in suspected meningitis require adequate CSF penetration and sensitivity against the most probable pathogens.[10,60] On identification of the pathogen and its susceptibilities, antimicrobial coverage should be adjusted accordingly (**Table 4**).

Duration of Antimicrobial Therapy

For uncomplicated meningitis, the minimum recommended treatment durations are the following[10,61,64]:

- Fourteen days for GBS, *L monocytogenes*, and *S pneumoniae*
- Twenty-one days for *Pseudomonas* and gram-negative enteric bacteria such as *E coli*

Longer treatment courses are recommended for infants with meningitis with delayed clinical improvement after beginning therapy or with complications such as brain abscesses, ventriculitis, or brain infarctions.[62]

Table 4
Common antibiotics used to treat neonatal meningitis

Antibiotic (Ref.)	Susceptible Bacteria	Notes
Penicillin G[61]	GBS	Monotherapy acceptable if GBS confirmed by culture and clinical improvement is observed
Ampicillin[2,6,62,63]	GBS *L monocytogenes* *Enterococcus* sp	17%–78% of *E coli* isolates resistant Poor CNS penetration Requires higher doses for meningitis
Gentamicin[2,62,64]	*E coli* *Klebsiella* sp *Enterobacter* sp *Pseudomonas* sp *Citrobacter* sp *Serratia* sp	Poor CNS penetration Synergistic effect with ampicillin in treatment of *L monocytogenes* *Pseudomonas* sp may require combination therapy with a second agent Requires therapeutic drug monitoring
Cefotaxime[24,62,64]	*E coli* *Klebsiella* sp *Enterobacter* sp *Citrobacter* sp *Serratia* sp	Good CNS penetration Used instead of gentamicin in cases of suspected or confirmed meningitis Not active against *L monocytogenes* or *Enterococcus* sp
Meropenem[64,65]	*E coli* *Klebsiella* sp *Enterobacter* sp *Citrobacter* sp *Serratia* sp *Pseudomonas* sp	Good CNS penetration Limit use to multidrug-resistant organisms (eg, extended-spectrum β-lactamase–producing organisms)
Vancomycin[62,66]	Coagulase-negative staphylococci *S aureus* *Enterococcus* sp	Variable CNS penetration Effective against methicillin-resistant *S aureus* Requires therapeutic drug monitoring
Nafcillin[66,67]	Methicillin-sensitive *S aureus*	Good CNS penetration Superior to vancomycin for treatment of methicillin-sensitive *S aureus*

Adjunctive Therapy

In an effort to improve outcomes in infants with meningitis, several adjunctive therapies have been explored, including the use of intraventricular antibiotics, dexamethasone, intravenous immunoglobulins, granulocyte or granulocyte macrophage colony-stimulating factor, and oral glycerol.[2] At present, none of the proposed adjunctive therapies are used in routine practice.

LONG-TERM OUTCOMES

Survivors of neonatal meningitis are at considerable risk for long-term neurologic impairment.[68,69] A prospective study that followed 1717 survivors of neonatal meningitis to 5 years of age found that children who had neonatal meningitis were 10 times more likely to have moderate or severe disability than those who never had meningitis.[68] Certain characteristics can help identify infected infants at the highest risk for a poor outcome (**Box 5**).[70,71]

PREVENTING NEONATAL MENINGITIS
Intrapartum Antibiotic Prophylaxis

Since the adoption of IAP use in 1996 and universal antenatal screening for GBS colonization in 2002, the incidence of early-onset GBS infections has decreased significantly, from 1.8 cases per 1000 live births in 1990 to 0.26 cases per 1000 live births in 2010.[72] The incidence of late-onset GBS disease remains unaffected by IAP use.[30,72]

IAP use has also been implicated in the increased proportion of non-GBS early-onset infections seen in VLBW infants. Since the late 1990s, E coli has surpassed GBS as the predominant pathogen observed in early-onset infections among VLBW infants.[6,21–23] This finding likely reflects the success of IAP in reducing the incidence of early-onset GBS infections rather than an increase in the incidence of non-GBS infections.[73] This change in proportion of non-GBS early-onset infections has not been observed in term infants.[6]

Reports from single-center studies have associated frequent use of ampicillin for IAP with an increase in ampicillin-resistant E coli infections, particularly in premature infants.[22,74] However, rates of ampicillin-resistant E coli have also increased in the general community.[20] Furthermore, a multicenter trial involving 389 infants with confirmed early-onset sepsis found that, between infants exposed and not exposed to IAP, frequencies of ampicillin-resistant E coli infections were not significantly different.[6] Although GBS has become increasingly resistant to clindamycin and erythromycin, sensitivity to ampicillin remains unchanged.[75]

Group B Streptococcus Vaccine

Vaccines against GBS can reduce the number of missed opportunities for screening and IAP administration caused by false-negative screens, precipitous deliveries, or

---

Box 5
Predictors of poor neurologic outcomes in survivors of bacterial meningitis

1. Seizures lasting more than 72 hours

2. Presence of coma

3. Hypotension requiring inotropic support

4. White blood cell count less than or equal to $5000 \times 10^9/L$

5. Abnormal electroencephalogram findings

Table 5
GBS vaccine clinical trials

ClinicalTrials.gov Identifier (Ref.)	Phase	Objectives	Vaccine	Subjects	N	Design	Study Period
NCT00645346[77]	I	Safety, tolerability, and immunogenicity	GBS glycoconjugate	Healthy nonpregnant women aged 18–40 y	130	Randomized, single center, single blind, placebo controlled	2008–2009
NCT01193920[78]	Ib/II	Safety and immunogenicity	Trivalent GBS	Healthy nonpregnant and pregnant women aged 18–40 y	380	Randomized, single center, single blind, placebo controlled	2010–2012
NCT01446289[79]	II	Immune response; amount of vaccine-induced antibody transferred to infant	Trivalent GBS	Healthy pregnant women aged 18–40 y	86	Randomized, multicenter, single blind, placebo controlled	2011–2013
NCT02046148[80]	II	Safety and immunogenicity; placental transfer of GBS antibodies; levels of GBS antibodies in infants; levels of GBS antibodies in breast milk	Trivalent GBS	Healthy pregnant women aged 18–40 y	75	Randomized, multicenter, double blind, placebo controlled	2014–2015

extremely preterm births.[6,72] Maternal immunity to the most common serotypes of GBS can be transferred passively to the infant and protect against early-onset and late-onset infections.[76] A trivalent GBS vaccine has shown promise in phase I and II trials, with another phase II trial currently recruiting participants (**Table 5**).[76]

SUMMARY

Neonatal meningitis is a serious disease that requires a high index of suspicion, prompt diagnosis, and rapid treatment. Although the incidence and mortality have declined with improved neonatal intensive care practices and universal adoption of preventative screening and prophylaxis programs, the associated morbidity remains unchanged. Performing an LP to collect CSF is critical to confirming the diagnosis, determining the causative pathogen, and refining antimicrobial therapy. Through better diagnostic practices and development of vaccines, there is hope that the burden of this dangerous disease may be further reduced.

Best practices box

What is the current practice?

Neonatal bacterial meningitis

Best practice/guideline/care path objectives

- Promptly diagnose with performance of LP
- Begin antibiotics without delay
- Reduce mortality and prevent long-term neurodevelopmental impairment

What changes in current practice are likely to improve outcomes?

- Collection of CSF in all stable, symptomatic infants suspected of early-onset or late-onset infections with additional signs beyond respiratory distress
- Increased vigilance in identifying and treating mothers with GBS colonization
- Introduction of an effective GBS vaccine in the prevention of neonatal GBS disease

Major recommendations

- Perform a LP on all clinically stable infants with suspected sepsis and meningitis (grade 1B)
- Begin empiric antibiotics in all cases of suspected sepsis and meningitis (grade 1A)
  - For suspected early-onset meningitis, consider ampicillin and gentamicin or cefotaxime in infants
  - For suspected late-onset meningitis, consider vancomycin in addition to ampicillin and gentamicin or cefotaxime
- Repeat the LP in infants who fail to show clinical improvement 24 to 48 hours after initiation of antibiotics (grade 1B)
- Repeat LPs are unnecessary in infants who show rapid clinical improvement after initiation of antibiotics and at end of successful therapy (grade 1B)
- All infants with a history of bacterial meningitis should be followed long term for development of neurologic sequelae (grade 1A)

Summary statement

A high index of suspicion, prompt diagnosis, and rapid initiation of antibiotics are essential to reducing mortality and morbidity associated with neonatal bacterial meningitis.

Data from Refs.[2,10,20]

REFERENCES

1. Polin RA, Harris MC. Neonatal bacterial meningitis. Semin Neonatol 2001;6:157–72.
2. Heath PT, Okike IO, Oeser C. Neonatal meningitis: can we do better? Adv Exp Med Biol 2011;719:11–24.
3. Shane AL, Stoll BJ. Recent developments and current issues in the epidemiology, diagnosis, and management of bacterial and fungal neonatal sepsis. Am J Perinatol 2013;30:131–41.
4. Barichello T, Fagundes GD, Generoso JS, et al. Pathophysiology of neonatal acute bacterial meningitis. J Med Microbiol 2013;62:1781–9.
5. Cohen-Wolkowiez M, Moran C, Benjamin DK, et al. Early and late onset sepsis in late preterm infants. Pediatr Infect Dis J 2009;28:1052–6.
6. Stoll BJ, Hansen NI, Sanchez PJ, et al. Early onset neonatal sepsis: the burden of group B Streptococcal and *E. coli* disease continues. Pediatrics 2011;127:817–26.
7. Stoll BJ, Hansen N, Fanaroff AA, et al. Late-onset sepsis in very low birth weight neonates: the experience of the NICHD Neonatal Research Network. Pediatrics 2002;110:285–91.
8. Gaschignard J, Levy C, Romain O, et al. Neonatal bacterial meningitis: 444 cases in 7 years. Pediatr Infect Dis J 2011;30:212–7.
9. Furyk JS, Swann O, Molyneux E. Systematic review: neonatal meningitis in the developing world. Trop Med Int Health 2011;16:672–9.
10. Heath PT, Okike IO. Neonatal bacterial meningitis: an update. Paediatr Child Health 2010;20:526–30.
11. Thaver D, Zaidi AK. Burden of neonatal infections in developing countries: a review of evidence from community-based studies. Pediatr Infect Dis J 2009;28:S3–9.
12. Okike IO, Johnson AP, Henderson KL, et al. Incidence, aetiology and outcome of bacterial meningitis in infants aged <90 days in the UK and Republic of Ireland: prospective, enhanced, national population-based surveillance. Clin Infect Dis 2014;59(10):e150–7.
13. Mulder CJ, Zanen HC. A study of 280 cases of neonatal meningitis in The Netherlands. J Infect 1984;9:177–84.
14. Kavuncuoglu S, Gursoy S, Turel O, et al. Neonatal bacterial meningitis in Turkey: epidemiology, risk factors, and prognosis. J Infect Dev Ctries 2013;7:73–81.
15. Persson E, Trollfors B, Brandberg LL, et al. Septicaemia and meningitis in neonates and during early infancy in the Goteborg area of Sweden. Acta Paediatr 2002;91:1087–92.
16. Edwards M. Postnatal bacterial infections. In: Martin RJ, Fanaroff AA, Walsh MC, editors. Fanaroff and Martin's neonatal-perinatal medicine: diseases of the fetus and infant. 9th edition. Philadelphia: Saunders/Elsevier; 2011. p. 793–830.
17. May M, Daley AJ, Donath S, et al. Early onset neonatal meningitis in Australia and New Zealand, 1992-2002. Arch Dis Child Fetal Neonatal Ed 2005;90:F324–7.
18. Kanegaye JT, Soliemanzadeh P, Bradley JS. Lumbar puncture in pediatric bacterial meningitis: defining the time interval for recovery of cerebrospinal fluid pathogens after parenteral antibiotic pretreatment. Pediatrics 2001;108:1169–74.
19. Galiza EP, Heath PT. Improving the outcome of neonatal meningitis. Curr Opin Infect Dis 2009;22:229–34.
20. Verani JR, McGee L, Schrag SJ. Prevention of perinatal group B streptococcal disease–revised guidelines from CDC, 2010. MMWR Recomm Rep 2010;59:1–36.

21. Stoll BJ, Hansen NI, Higgins RD, et al. Very low birth weight preterm infants with early onset neonatal sepsis: the predominance of gram-negative infections continues in the National Institute of Child Health and Human Development Neonatal Research Network, 2002-2003. Pediatr Infect Dis J 2005;24:635–9.

22. Bizzarro MJ, Dembry LM, Baltimore RS, et al. Changing patterns in neonatal *Escherichia coli* sepsis and ampicillin resistance in the era of intrapartum antibiotic prophylaxis. Pediatrics 2008;121:689–96.

23. Stoll BJ, Hansen N, Fanaroff AA, et al. Changes in pathogens causing early-onset sepsis in very-low-birth-weight infants. N Engl J Med 2002;347:240–7.

24. Camacho-Gonzalez A, Spearman PW, Stoll BJ. Neonatal infectious diseases: evaluation of neonatal sepsis. Pediatr Clin North Am 2013;60:367–89.

25. Fanaroff AA, Korones SB, Wright LL, et al. Incidence, presenting features, risk factors and significance of late onset septicemia in very low birth weight infants. The National Institute of Child Health and Human Development Neonatal Research Network. Pediatr Infect Dis J 1998;17:593–8.

26. Fluegge K, Siedler A, Heinrich B, et al. Incidence and clinical presentation of invasive neonatal group B streptococcal infections in Germany. Pediatrics 2006;117:e1139–45.

27. Ansong AK, Smith PB, Benjamin DK, et al. Group B streptococcal meningitis: cerebrospinal fluid parameters in the era of intrapartum antibiotic prophylaxis. Early Hum Dev 2009;85:S5–7.

28. Polin RA, Committee on Fetus and Newborn. Management of neonates with suspected or proven early-onset bacterial sepsis. Pediatrics 2012;129:1006–15.

29. Ferrieri P, Wallen LD. Neonatal bacterial sepsis. In: Gleason CA, Devaskar SU, editors. Avery's diseases of the newborn. 9th edition. Philadelphia: Saunders/Elsevier; 2012. p. 538–50.

30. Berardi A, Rossi C, Lugli L, et al. Group B streptococcus late-onset disease: 2003-2010. Pediatrics 2013;131:e361–8.

31. Pong A, Bradley JS. Bacterial meningitis and the newborn infant. Infect Dis Clin North Am 1999;13:711–33, viii.

32. Ng PC, Wong HL, Lyon DJ, et al. Combined use of alcohol hand rub and gloves reduces the incidence of late onset infection in very low birthweight infants. Arch Dis Child Fetal Neonatal Ed 2004;89:F336–40.

33. Cotten CM, Smith PB. Duration of empirical antibiotic therapy for infants suspected of early-onset sepsis. Curr Opin Pediatr 2013;25:167–71.

34. Kuppala VS, Meinzen-Derr J, Morrow AL, et al. Prolonged initial empirical antibiotic treatment is associated with adverse outcomes in premature infants. J Pediatr 2011;159:720–5.

35. Kim KS. Acute bacterial meningitis in infants and children. Lancet Infect Dis 2010;10:32–42.

36. Mukhopadhyay S, Puopolo KM. Risk assessment in neonatal early onset sepsis. Semin Perinatol 2012;36:408–15.

37. Debes AK, Kohli A, Walker N, et al. Time to initiation of breastfeeding and neonatal mortality and morbidity: a systematic review. BMC Public Health 2013;13(Suppl 3):S19.

38. Nizet V, Klein J. Bacterial sepsis and meningitis. In: Remington J, Klein J, Wilson C, et al, editors. Infectious diseases of the fetus and newborn infant. 7th edition. Philadelphia: Saunders/Elsevier; 2011. p. 222–75.

39. Stoll BJ, Hansen N, Fanaroff AA, et al. To tap or not to tap: high likelihood of meningitis without sepsis among very low birth weight infants. Pediatrics 2004;113:1181–6.

40. Speidel BD. Adverse effects of routine procedures on preterm infants. Lancet 1978;1:864–6.
41. Weisman LE, Merenstein GB, Steenbarger JR. The effect of lumbar puncture position in sick neonates. Am J Dis Child 1983;137:1077–9.
42. Visser VE, Hall RT. Lumbar puncture in the evaluation of suspected neonatal sepsis. J Pediatr 1980;96:1063–7.
43. Committee on Infectious Diseases, Committee on Fetus and Newborn, Baker CJ, et al. Policy statement. Recommendations for the prevention of perinatal group B streptococcal (GBS) disease. Pediatrics 2011;128:611–6.
44. Garges HP, Moody MA, Cotten CM, et al. Neonatal meningitis: what is the correlation among cerebrospinal fluid cultures, blood cultures, and cerebrospinal fluid parameters? Pediatrics 2006;117:1094–100.
45. Smith PB, Garges HP, Cotton CM, et al. Meningitis in preterm neonates: importance of cerebrospinal fluid parameters. Am J Perinatol 2008;25:421–6.
46. Johnson CE, Whitwell JK, Pethe K, et al. Term newborns who are at risk for sepsis: are lumbar punctures necessary? Pediatrics 1997;99:E10.
47. Fielkow S, Reuter S, Gotoff SP. Cerebrospinal fluid examination in symptom-free infants with risk factors for infection. J Pediatr 1991;119:971–3.
48. Eldadah M, Frenkel LD, Hiatt IM, et al. Evaluation of routine lumbar punctures in newborn infants with respiratory distress syndrome. Pediatr Infect Dis J 1987;6: 243–6.
49. Kestenbaum LA, Ebberson J, Zorc JJ, et al. Defining cerebrospinal fluid white blood cell count reference values in neonates and young infants. Pediatrics 2010;125:257–64.
50. Backman A, Lantz P, Radstrom P, et al. Evaluation of an extended diagnostic PCR assay for detection and verification of the common causes of bacterial meningitis in CSF and other biological samples. Mol Cell Probes 1999;13: 49–60.
51. Chiba N, Murayama SY, Morozumi M, et al. Rapid detection of eight causative pathogens for the diagnosis of bacterial meningitis by real-time PCR. J Infect Chemother 2009;15:92–8.
52. Liu CL, Ai HW, Wang WP, et al. Comparison of 16S rRNA gene PCR and blood culture for diagnosis of neonatal sepsis. Arch Pediatr 2014;21:162–9.
53. Bonadio WA, Smith DS. CBC differential profile in distinguishing etiology of neonatal meningitis. Pediatr Emerg Care 1989;5:94–6.
54. Metrou M, Crain EF. The complete blood count differential ratio in the assessment of febrile infants with meningitis. Pediatr Infect Dis J 1991;10:334–5.
55. Philip AG, Baker CJ. Cerebrospinal-fluid C-reactive protein in neonatal meningitis. J Pediatr 1983;102:715–7.
56. Greenberg RG, Benjamin DK Jr, Cohen-Wolkowiez M, et al. Repeat lumbar punctures in infants with meningitis in the neonatal intensive care unit. J Perinatol 2011; 31:425–9.
57. Agarwal R, Emmerson AJ. Should repeat lumbar punctures be routinely done in neonates with bacterial meningitis? Results of a survey into clinical practice. Arch Dis Child 2001;84:451–2.
58. Heath PT, Nik Yusoff NK, Baker CJ. Neonatal meningitis. Arch Dis Child Fetal Neonatal Ed 2003;88:F173–8.
59. Klein JO, Feigin RD, McCracken GH Jr. Report of the task force on diagnosis and management of meningitis. Pediatrics 1986;78:959–82.
60. Weisfelt M, de Gans J, van de Beek D. Bacterial meningitis: a review of effective pharmacotherapy. Expert Opin Pharmacother 2007;8:1493–504.

61. American Academy of Pediatrics. Group B streptococcal infections. In: Pickering LK, Baker CJ, Kimberlin DW, et al, editors. Red book: 2012 report of the committee on infectious disease. 29th edition. Elk Grove Village (IL): American Academy of Pediatrics; 2012. p. 680–5.

62. Stockmann C, Spigarelli MG, Campbell SC, et al. Considerations in the pharmacologic treatment and prevention of neonatal sepsis. Paediatr Drugs 2014;16:67–81.

63. Tadesse DA, Zhao S, Tong E, et al. Antimicrobial drug resistance in *Escherichia coli* from humans and food animals, United States, 1950-2002. Emerg Infect Dis 2012;18:741–9.

64. American Academy of Pediatrics. *Escherichia coli* and other gram-negative bacilli. In: Pickering LK, Baker CJ, Kimberlin DW, et al, editors. Red book: 2012 report of the committee on infectious disease. 29th edition. Elk Grove (IL): American Academy of Pediatrics; 2012. p. 321–4.

65. Smith PB, Cohen-Wolkowiez M, Castro LM, et al. Population pharmacokinetics of meropenem in plasma and cerebrospinal fluid of infants with suspected or complicated intra-abdominal infections. Pediatr Infect Dis J 2011;30:844–9.

66. American Academy of Pediatrics. Staphylococcal infections. In: Pickering LK, Baker CJ, Kimberlin DW, et al, editors. Red book: 2012 report of the committee on infectious disease. 29th edition. Elk Grove (IL): American Academy of Pediatrics; 2012. p. 653–68.

67. Frame PT, Watanakunakorn C, McLaurin RL, et al. Penetration of nafcillin, methicillin, and cefazolin into human-brain tissue. Neurosurgery 1983;12:142–7.

68. Bedford H, de Louvois J, Halket S, et al. Meningitis in infancy in England and Wales: follow up at age 5 years. BMJ 2001;323:533–6.

69. Bassler D, Stoll BJ, Schmidt B, et al. Using a count of neonatal morbidities to predict poor outcome in extremely low birth weight infants: added role of neonatal infection. Pediatrics 2009;123:313–8.

70. Klinger G, Chin CN, Beyene J, et al. Predicting the outcome of neonatal bacterial meningitis. Pediatrics 2000;106:477–82.

71. Klinger G, Chin CN, Otsubo H, et al. Prognostic value of EEG in neonatal bacterial meningitis. Pediatr Neurol 2001;24:28–31.

72. Schrag SJ, Verani JR. Intrapartum antibiotic prophylaxis for the prevention of perinatal group B streptococcal disease: experience in the United States and implications for a potential group B streptococcal vaccine. Vaccine 2013; 31(Suppl 4):D20–6.

73. Puopolo KM, Eichenwald EC. No change in the incidence of ampicillin-resistant, neonatal, early-onset sepsis over 18 years. Pediatrics 2010;125:e1031–8.

74. Alarcon A, Pena P, Salas S, et al. Neonatal early onset *Escherichia coli* sepsis: trends in incidence and antimicrobial resistance in the era of intrapartum antimicrobial prophylaxis. Pediatr Infect Dis J 2004;23:295–9.

75. Castor ML, Whitney CG, Como-Sabetti K, et al. Antibiotic resistance patterns in invasive group B streptococcal isolates. Infect Dis Obstet Gynecol 2008;2008: 727505.

76. Oster G, Edelsberg J, Hennegan K, et al. Prevention of group B streptococcal disease in the first 3 months of life: would routine maternal immunization during pregnancy be cost-effective? Vaccine 2014;32(37):4778–85.

77. Novartis Vaccines. A phase I, randomized, single-blind, controlled, single center study to evaluate the safety and immunogenicity of a dose range of glycoconjugate antigen vaccine of group B *Streptococcus* in healthy women 18-40 years of age. Bethesda (MD): National Library of Medicine (US); 2000. Available at: https://clinicaltrials.gov/ct2/show/NCT00645346. Accessed July 28, 2014.

78. Novartis Vaccines. Safety and immunogenicity of a group B *Streptococcus* vaccine in non pregnant and pregnant women 18-40 years of age. Bethesda (MD): National Library of Medicine (US); 2000. Available at: https://clinicaltrials.gov/ct2/show/NCT01193920. Accessed July 28, 2014.
79. Novartis Vaccines. Immune response induced by a vaccine against group B *Streptococcus* and safety in pregnant women and their offsprings. Bethesda (MD): National Library of Medicine (US); 2000. Available at: https://clinicaltrials.gov/ct2/show/NCT01446289. Accessed July 28, 2014.
80. Novartis Vaccines. Safety and immunogenicity of a trivalent group B *Streptococcus* vaccine in healthy pregnant women. Bethesda (MD): National Library of Medicine (US); 2000. Available at: https://clinicaltrials.gov/ct2/show/NCT02046148. Accessed July 28, 2014.

Neonatal Herpes Simplex Virus Infection

Epidemiology and Treatment

Scott H. James, MD[a], David W. Kimberlin, MD[b],*

KEYWORDS

- Herpes simplex virus • Genital herpes • Pregnancy • Mother-to-child transmission
- Neonatal herpes • Polymerase chain reaction • Antiviral therapy

KEY POINTS

- Both herpes simplex virus types 1 (HSV-1) and 2 (HSV-2) can cause genital infections, although in recent years HSV-1 has become the predominant cause of genital herpes.
- Despite the relatively high HSV-1 and HSV-2 seroprevalence rates, neonatal HSV infection remains rare.
- Recurrent HSV genital lesions pose a lower risk for transmission to exposed infants than primary HSV genital lesions.
- Neonatal HSV infection is categorized as skin, eye, and/or mouth (SEM), disseminated, or central nervous system (CNS) disease; these categories are predictive of morbidity and mortality.
- Efforts to prevent vertical transmission and use of appropriate antiviral therapy are necessary to help reduce neonatal HSV disease burden.

INTRODUCTION

HSV genital infections are common in adolescents and adults worldwide. Although less common, HSV infections that are transmitted from pregnant women to their infants can cause substantial morbidity and mortality in the infants. There are 2 distinct types of HSV, HSV-1 and HSV-2, both of which can be responsible for neonatal disease. Advances in diagnostic capabilities and antiviral treatment options have led to improved clinical outcomes in infected infants, but significant morbidity and mortality remain in infants with invasive HSV disease, particularly those with CNS (morbidity) or disseminated (mortality) involvement. This review offers a description of the pathogen

Disclosures: None.
[a] University of Alabama at Birmingham, Children's Harbor Building 308, 1600 7th Avenue South, Birmingham, AL 35233-1711, USA; [b] Department of Pediatrics, University of Alabama at Birmingham, Children's Harbor Building 303, 1600 7th Avenue South, Birmingham, AL 35233-1711, USA
* Corresponding author.
E-mail address: dkimberlin@peds.uab.edu

http://dx.doi.org/10.1016/j.clp.2014.10.005
0095-5108/15/$ – see front matter
perinatology.theclinics.com

and the epidemiology of maternal and neonatal infection, as well as an overview of clinical features associated with mother-to-child transmission (MTCT), methods of preventing transmission, and, finally, current treatment considerations for neonatal HSV infections.

DESCRIPTION OF THE PATHOGEN

HSV-1 and HSV-2 are members of the alpha herpes virus subfamily of the family Herpesviridae. HSV virions consist of a core containing a single linear, double-stranded DNA molecule approximately 152 kilo base pairs in length; an icosahedral capsid made up of 162 capsomeres surrounded by an amorphous, tightly adherent tegument; and a lipid bilayer envelope containing viral glycoprotein spikes surrounding the capsid-tegument complex. These glycoprotein spikes mediate attachment and entry into host cells and are responsible for evoking the host response.[1]

HSV DNA consists of 2 covalently linked components, designated simply as long (L) and short (S), each consisting of unique regions (U_L and U_S) flanked by inverted repeats.[2] The genomes of HSV-1 and HSV-2 share approximately 50% homology, resulting in significant cross-reactivity between antigenically related glycoproteins of both HSV types.[3] Type-specific glycoproteins, such as glycoprotein G, do occur (gG-1 and gG-2 for HSV-1 and HSV-2, respectively), allowing for differentiation of the 2 virus types via antigen-specific antibody response. HSV type differentiation can also be achieved by restriction endonuclease fingerprinting and DNA sequencing.[4,5]

HSV infection is characterized by short reproductive cycles, host cell destruction during active replication, and the virus' ability to establish lifelong latency in sensory neural ganglia.[6] Within an HSV-infected cell, key steps in viral replication include cell surface attachment, entry of the viral genome into the nucleus, transcription, DNA synthesis, capsid assembly, DNA packaging, and envelopment as new virions pass through the trans-Golgi network.

EPIDEMIOLOGY

Humans are the only known natural reservoir of HSV, and seroprevalence studies indicate that HSV-1 and HSV-2 infections are common worldwide, in both developed and undeveloped countries.[7] Acquisition of HSV results in lifelong infection, with periodic clinical or subclinical viral reactivation. Prevalence of HSV antibodies increases with age, although earlier acquisition of infection is seen with HSV-1 as compared to HSV-2, and in people of lower socioeconomic status for both HSV-1 and HSV-2.[8,9] More than 90% of adults have acquired HSV-1 infection by their fifth decade of life, although only a minority develop clinically apparent disease at the time of acquisition.[10]

Previous studies indicated an increasing seroprevalence of HSV-2 in developed countries,[11,12] but more recent seroepidemiologic studies performed as a part of the National Health and Nutrition Examination Surveys (NHANES) have indicated otherwise. Specifically, while the seroprevalences of HSV-1 and HSV-2 in the United States were approximately 58% and 17%, respectively, in persons aged 14 to 49 years during the period 1999 to 2004, a follow-up study from 2005 to 2010 showed that HSV-1 seroprevalence had decreased to 54%, whereas HSV-2 seroprevalence had not significantly changed (nearly 16%).[13,14] Further analysis of HSV-1 seroprevalence within this larger study population shows that the largest decline in HSV-1 seropositivity occurred in the 14- to 19-year-old group.

HSV-1 and HSV-2 can both cause genital infection, with HSV-1 being more historically associated with orolabial lesions and HSV-2 being the more common cause of genital lesions. More recently, however, HSV-1 has become the predominant virus causing genital herpes, responsible for up to 80% of genital herpes in some populations of young women.[15,16] When considered alongside the decreasing HSV-1 seroprevalence in adolescents and young adults, these trends mean that an increasing number of young persons are without protective HSV-1 antibodies at the time of their sexual debut.[17] Risk factors for acquiring HSV genital infection include: female gender, lower family income, minority ethnic group, longer duration of sexual activity, prior history of other genital infections, and number of sexual partners.[18]

Between 20% and 30% of pregnant women are seropositive for HSV-2.[19,20] In pregnant women who report a prior history of genital herpes, 75% have at least 1 recurrence during pregnancy.[21,22] Women lacking antibodies to both HSV-2 and HSV-1 have a nearly 4% chance of acquiring HSV-1 or HSV-2 during the course of their pregnancy, whereas women with only HSV-1 antibodies have a 2% chance of also acquiring HSV-2 during pregnancy.[23] As with nonpregnant women, as many as two-thirds of pregnant women who acquire genital HSV infection have asymptomatic or subclinical infections and are not appropriately diagnosed. This is consistent with studies showing that 60% to 80% of women who have vertically transmitted HSV to their infants do not report a prior history of genital herpes.[24–26]

Despite the relatively high seroprevalence of HSV-1 and HSV-2, neonatal HSV infection remains rare, occurring in about 1 in 3200 deliveries in the United States.[27] Most neonatal HSV infections in many parts of the world are now caused by HSV-1, which is consistent with the increasing proportion of HSV-1 genital infections.[28,29]

TERMINOLOGY OF MATERNAL GENITAL HERPES INFECTION

When a person with no prior presence of antibody to HSV-1 or HSV-2 acquires either of these viruses in the genital tract, a first-episode primary infection results. If a person with preexisting antibody to HSV-1 acquires an HSV-2 infection (or vice versa), it results in a first-episode nonprimary infection. Viral reactivation from latency and ensuing antegrade translocation of virus from sensory neural ganglia to skin and mucosal surfaces produces a recurrent infection.

Correct identification of a primary or nonprimary first-episode genital HSV infection during pregnancy can be challenging because, similar to nonpregnant women, most of these genital infections are either asymptomatic or are so clinically subtle that they are misdiagnosed. As such, it is not surprising that nearly 80% of women who vertically transmit HSV to their newborn have no known history of genital HSV lesions.[26]

CLINICAL FEATURES OF MATERNAL HERPES SIMPLEX VIRUS INFECTION

Primary or first-episode HSV genital infections in pregnant and nonpregnant women are commonly asymptomatic. Genital HSV infections can also present symptomatically with lesions on the vulva, labia, vaginal introitus, or cervix. Cutaneous lesions typically present as painful erythematous papules that quickly progress to vesicular lesions filled with clear fluid, often developing in clusters. These fragile vesicles usually burst, but if they do not, pustules may develop because of an influx of inflammatory cells. After rupturing, lesions transition into shallow ulcers on an erythematous base. Mucosal lesions typically have no vesicles and progress directly to ulcerations. These ulcers are painful, gray or white, approximately 1 to 4 mm in diameter, and crust over as the healing process begins. The total healing process can last as little as 8 to 10 days or as long as 21 days. A more severe illness with systemic involvement can also occur during primary or first-episode HSV infections, but this is rare in immunocompetent hosts.

Similar to primary or first-episode HSV genital infections, viral reactivation from latency may also be symptomatic or asymptomatic. Recurrent infections are clinically indistinguishable from primary or first-episode HSV genital infections; the determination must rely on a combination of virologic (viral culture or polymerase chain reaction [PCR]) and serologic data (**Table 1**). Viral shedding from the genital mucosa occurs with both symptomatic and asymptomatic reactivation. Regardless of the reported history of HSV infection, up to 0.4% of pregnant women will shed HSV from the genital tract during the time of delivery.[30] Among pregnant women with a history of recurrent genital HSV infections, the rate of shedding has been reported as high as 1.4%.[31] Given the high prevalence of genital HSV infection, these rates of viral shedding suggest that caring for newborns who have been perinatally exposed to HSV is not uncommon.

RISK OF MOTHER-TO-CHILD TRANSMISSION OF HERPES SIMPLEX VIRUS

Recurrent genital lesions pose less of a risk for transmission to an exposed infant than primary or nonprimary first-episode infections, likely because of the presence of protective maternal antibodies. In the largest study evaluating the effect of maternal infection status on neonatal transmission, Brown and colleagues[27] demonstrated an increased transmission risk of 57% in infants born to women with first-episode primary genital infections, a 25% risk in infants born to women with first-episode

Table 1
Maternal infection classification by genital HSV viral type and maternal serology

Classification of Maternal Infection	PCR/Culture Result from Genital Lesion	Maternal HSV-1 and HSV-2 IgG Antibody Status
Documented first-episode primary infection	Positive, either virus	Both negative
Documented first-episode nonprimary infection	Positive for HSV-1	Positive for HSV-2 *and* negative for HSV-1
	Positive for HSV-2	Positive for HSV-1 *and* negative for HSV-2
Assume first-episode (primary or nonprimary) infection	Positive for HSV-1 *or* HSV-2 Negative *or* not available[a]	Not Available Negative for HSV-1 and/or HSV-2, *or* not available
Recurrent infection	Positive for HSV-1 Positive for HSV-2	Positive for HSV-1 Positive for HSV-2

To be used for women without a clinical history of genital herpes.
Abbreviation: IgG, immunoglobulin G.
[a] When a genital lesion is strongly suspicious for HSV, clinical judgment should supersede the virologic test results for the conservative purposes of this neonatal management algorithm. Conversely, if, in retrospect, the genital lesion was not likely to be caused by HSV and the result of PCR test/culture result is negative, departure from the evaluation and management in this conservative algorithm may be warranted.
Adapted from Kimberlin DW, Baley J, Committee on Infectious Diseases, Committee on Fetus and Newborn. Guidance on management of asymptomatic neonates born to women with active genital herpes lesions. Pediatrics 2013;131(2):384.

nonprimary infection, and a 2% risk increase in those born to women with recurrent genital herpes.

In addition to stratifying risk of transmission in primary versus recurrent maternal infection, this landmark study also identified several other statistically significant factors associated with increased risk of MTCT of HSV, including vaginal delivery (vs cesarean delivery), disruption of the infant's cutaneous barrier by the use of a fetal scalp electrode or other invasive instrumentation, and infection with HSV-1 (vs HSV-2). Other factors that influence the vertical transmission of HSV are detection of HSV-1 or HSV-2 from the cervix or external genitalia via viral culture or PCR at the time of labor and prolonged duration of rupture of membranes.[27,32]

CLINICAL FEATURES OF NEONATAL HERPES SIMPLEX VIRUS INFECTION

Neonatal HSV infection can be acquired during 1 of the following 3 distinct time periods:

1. In utero (5%)
2. Peripartum (85%)
3. Postpartum (10%)

In utero (congenital) HSV transmission has been found to occur with both primary and recurrent maternal HSV infections,[33] with recurrent infections carrying a lower risk. In utero transmission of HSV is rare, having an estimated transmission rate of 1 in 300,000 deliveries in the United States.[34] This mode of transmission presents as a distinct clinical entity characterized by a triad of clinical manifestations present at birth:

1. Cutaneous findings (active lesions, scarring, aplasia cutis, hyperpigmentation or hypopigmentation)
2. Neurologic findings (microcephaly, intracranial calcifications, hydranencephaly)
3. Ocular findings (chorioretinitis, microphthalmia, optic atrophy).

This triad describes the classic findings of congenital HSV infection. More subtle presentations can also occur.

Peripartum neonatal transmission of HSV can occur when there is shedding of the virus from the genital tract around the time of delivery, whereas postpartum (postnatal) acquired HSV infection can also occur as a result of direct contact with HSV-infected persons, usually from an orolabial or cutaneous source. Peripartum and postpartum acquired HSV infections cause the same range of neonatal disease, with no appreciable difference in the severity of disease on average.

Neonatal HSV infection acquired during the peripartum or postpartum period can be categorized as follows:

1. SEM disease
2. CNS disease
3. Disseminated disease

SEM disease accounts for approximately 45% of neonatal HSV infections. By definition, SEM disease does not involve the CNS or other organ systems. CNS disease makes up about 30% of neonatal HSV infections. These infants may have mucocutaneous involvement, but they do not have evidence of any other organ system involvement. Disseminated disease accounts for the remaining 25% of neonatal HSV infections. Disseminated HSV infection may involve multiple organ systems including the liver, lungs, adrenals, gastrointestinal tract, and the skin, eyes, or mouth.[35]

Approximately two-thirds of infants with disseminated HSV infection also have CNS involvement. Combined, nearly 50% of infants with neonatal HSV infection have CNS involvement, whether in isolation (CNS disease) or as a part of disseminated disease. The presentation of SEM and disseminated disease typically occurs earlier than that of CNS disease (on average, 9–11 days after birth vs 16–17 days).[36]

The clinical presentation of neonatal HSV CNS disease commonly involves nonspecific symptoms such as lethargy, irritability, poor oral intake, and temperature instability. Cutaneous lesions can be a diagnostic clue, but as many as 35% of infants with HSV CNS disease do not have a vesicular rash identified, so the absence of a rash does not rule out neonatal HSV infection.[35] Other symptoms more indicative of underlying encephalitis can also be present, including a bulging fontanelle and focal or generalized seizures. Retrograde axonal transport can result in focal CNS involvement, whereas hematogenous spread to the CNS is more commonly associated with diffuse brain involvement.

Disseminated neonatal HSV infections may present with a septic appearance, including respiratory failure, hepatic failure, and disseminated intravascular coagulopathy. When present, vesicular skin lesions are a key component in recognizing the clinical presentation of HSV disease, but as with CNS disease, cutaneous findings are not always present. Up to 40% of infants with disseminated disease never develop a vesicular rash during the course of their illness.

PREVENTION OF MOTHER-TO-CHILD TRANSMISSION OF HERPES SIMPLEX VIRUS INFECTION

Most MTCTs of HSV infections occur as a result of exposure to virus shed from the genital tract as the infant passes through the birth canal. One challenge with prevention of this is that routine antepartum screening for HSV, whether by history, physical examination, or virologic testing, does not predict those women who are shedding HSV at delivery.[31] Therefore, the most common strategies for preventing HSV transmission seek to reduce neonatal exposure to active genital lesions.

In women with active genital lesions, whether primary or recurrent, or with prodromal symptoms that may indicate an impending genital outbreak, the American College of Obstetricians and Gynecologists (ACOG) recommends cesarean delivery.[18] This practice reduces the infant's risk of acquiring HSV, although it does not completely eliminate it.[27] For maximum risk reduction, cesarean delivery should be performed before the rupture of membranes. If rupture has already occurred and genital lesions are present, cesarean delivery is still recommended. Cesarean delivery is not advised for women with a history of recurrent genital herpes but with no active lesions or prodromal symptoms at the time of delivery.

Another preventative strategy for women with active recurrent genital HSV lesions is the use of antiviral suppressive therapy with oral acyclovir or valacyclovir. This practice has been associated with decreased genital lesions at the time of delivery, decreased viral detection by viral culture or PCR at delivery, and subsequently a reduced need for cesarean delivery because of active HSV lesions.[37] Despite these benefits, antiviral suppressive therapy has not yet been studied well enough to definitively show that this practice prevents neonatal HSV disease. Nevertheless, ACOG recommends that women with active recurrent genital herpes be offered suppressive antiviral therapy commencing at 36 weeks' gestation.[18] A recent multicenter case series reporting neonatal HSV infection in 8 infants whose mothers received antiviral suppressive therapy should serve as a reminder that suppressive therapy does not completely eliminate the risk of perinatal transmission.[38]

For asymptomatic infants born to women with active herpetic genital lesions, guidance has been proposed to help determine the risk of HSV transmission and to optimize intervention for the infant.[39] This 2-part algorithm (**Figs. 1** and **2**), developed jointly by the American Academy of Pediatrics' Committee on Infectious Diseases and Committee on Fetus and Newborn, provides guidance regarding risk stratification, diagnostic workup, and appropriate antiviral therapy (including the use of preemptive antiviral therapy in certain high-risk situations) in asymptomatic infants.

TREATMENT OF NEONATAL HERPES SIMPLEX VIRUS INFECTION

Most neonatal HSV infections resulted in significant morbidity or mortality before the era of antiviral therapy. Infants with disseminated HSV disease had 85% mortality by the age of 1 year. Of those who survived, only 50% had a normal neurodevelopmental outcome. Infants with CNS disease had a comparably lower mortality rate (50%) by the age of 1 year, but only 33% of survivors had normal neurodevelopmental outcomes.[40]

The early era of antiviral therapy for neonatal HSV infection was marked by improved mortality with vidarabine as well as with acyclovir dosed at 30 mg/kg/d. The 1-year mortality for disseminated disease improved to 50% with vidarabine and to 61% with acyclovir, 30 mg/kg/d, whereas the 1-year mortality for CNS disease dropped to 14% for both vidarabine and this dose of acyclovir.[41] More recently, the use of 60 mg/kg/d of acyclovir in 3 divided doses has improved the 1-year mortality rates to 29% and 4% for disseminated and CNS diseases, respectively.[42] Furthermore, this 60 mg/kg/d dosing of acyclovir was shown to improve neurodevelopmental outcomes in infants with disseminated disease (83% of survivors demonstrating normal neurodevelopmental outcomes), but it did not improve outcomes in infants with CNS disease (31% of survivors having normal neurodevelopmental outcomes).

While improved neurodevelopmental outcomes in infants surviving CNS disease were not achieved with 60 mg/kg/d dosing of intravenous acyclovir, improved outcomes have been demonstrated with oral suppressive acyclovir therapy given for 6 months following the completion of a standard parenteral acyclovir treatment course. Infants with CNS disease who received suppressive acyclovir therapy at a dose of 300 mg/m^2/dose administered orally 3 times a day had better neurodevelopmental outcomes compared with infants who received placebo, and infants with CNS and SEM disease had less-frequent recurrences of skin lesions while receiving the suppressive therapy.[43]

It is currently recommended that all infants with HSV disease be treated with intravenous acyclovir, 60 mg/kg/d in 3 divided daily doses.[42] Disseminated and CNS disease should be treated for a minimum duration of 21 days, whereas infants with SEM disease should receive 14 days' treatment. The absolute neutrophil count (ANC) should be followed twice weekly while on parenteral acyclovir therapy. All infants with CNS involvement should have a repeat lumbar puncture at the end of therapy to document a negative result of HSV cerebrospinal fluid (CSF) PCR. If this repeat PCR shows positive result at the end of therapy, acyclovir should be continued until PCR negativity is achieved. On completion of the course of parenteral acyclovir, suppressive oral acyclovir (300 mg/m^2/dose by mouth 3 times a day) should be administered for 6 months. ANCs should be followed at 2 and 4 weeks and then monthly during this period of antiviral suppression.

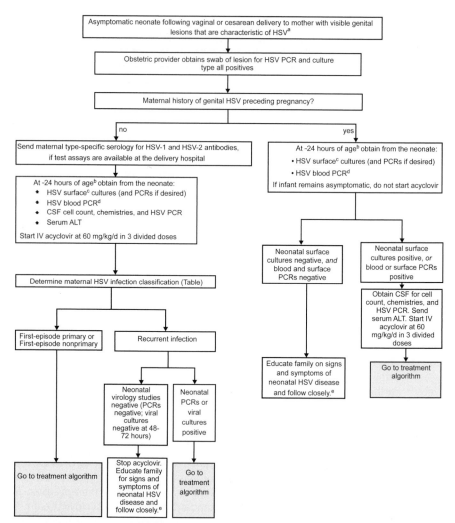

Fig. 1. Algorithm for the evaluation of asymptomatic neonates after vaginal or cesarean delivery to women with active genital HSV lesions. ALT, alanine aminotransferase; CSF, cerebrospinal fluid. [a] This algorithm should be applied only in facilities in which access to PCR and type-specific serologic testing is readily available and turnaround time for test results is appropriately short. In situations in which this is not possible, the approach detailed in the algorithm will have limited, and perhaps no, applicability. [b] Evaluation and treatment is indicated before 24 hours of age if the infant develops signs and symptoms of neonatal HSV disease. In addition, immediate evaluation and treatment may be considered if: there is prolonged rupture of membrane (>4–6 hours) and the infant is preterm (=37 weeks' gestation). [c] Conjunctivae, mouth, nasopharynx, and rectum, and scalp electrode site, if present. [d] HSV blood PCR assay is not used for assignment of disease classification. [e] Discharge after 48 hours of negative HSV cultures (and negative PCRs) is acceptable if other discharge criteria have been met, there is ready access to medical care, and a person who is able to comply fully with instructions for home observation will be present. If any of these conditions is not met, the infant should be observed in the hospital until HSV cultures are finalized as negative or are negative for HSV for 96 hours after being set up in cell culture, whichever is shorter. (*Adapted from* Kimberlin DW, Baley J, Committee on Infectious Diseases, Committee on Fetus and Newborn. Guidance on management of asymptomatic infants born to women with active genital herpes lesions. Pediatrics 2013;131(2):385; with permission.)

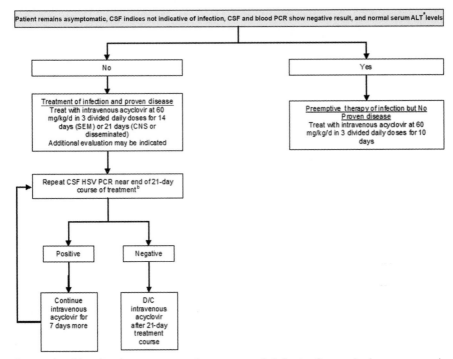

Fig. 2. Algorithm for the *treatment* of asymptomatic infants after vaginal or cesarean delivery to women with active genital lesions. ALT, alanine aminotransferase; CSF, cerebrospinal fluid; D/C, discontinue. [a] Serum ALT values in neonates may be elevated because of noninfectious causes (delivery-related perfusion, etc). For this algorithm, ALT values more than 2 times the upper limit of normal may be considered to suggest neonatal disseminated HSV disease for HSV-exposed neonates. [b] If evidence of CNS disease at beginning of therapy. (*Adapted from* Kimberlin DW, Baley J, Committee on Infectious Diseases, Committee on Fetus and Newborn. Guidance on management of asymptomatic infants born to women with active genital herpes lesions. Pediatrics 2013;131(2):386; with permission.)

SUMMARY

HSV-1 and HSV-2 are highly prevalent viruses capable of establishing lifelong infection that is punctuated by episodic reactivation. Genital HSV infection in women of childbearing age represents a significant risk for MTCT of HSV. Although neonatal exposure to HSV around the time of delivery is not uncommon, neonatal infections remain uncommon. Primary and first-episode genital HSV infections pose the greatest risk for MTCT.

Neonatal HSV infection is categorized as SEM, disseminated, or CNS disease, and these groupings are predictive of morbidity and mortality. The advent of parenteral acyclovir as antiviral therapy for neonatal HSV infection has led to significant overall improvement in disease outcomes, but long-term neurodevelopmental outcomes in CNS disease remain unacceptably poor. Further studies are needed to improve the clinician's ability to identify infants at increased risk for HSV infection and prevent MTCT, as well as to develop novel antiviral agents with increased efficacy in infants with HSV infection.

Best practices

What is the current practice?

Neonatal HSV infection

Best practice/guideline/care path objective

- Recognition and diagnosis of infants with suspected neonatal HSV infection as quickly as possible
- Begin empirical intravenous acyclovir promptly
- Reduce mortality and minimize long-term neurodevelopmental impairment

What changes in current practice are likely to improve outcomes?

- Increased vigilance in identifying and promptly treating infants with suspected neonatal HSV infection
- Enhanced diagnostic capability for detecting women who are asymptomatically shedding HSV at the time of delivery
- Improved treatment and vaccine strategies aimed at preventing maternal transmission of HSV

Major recommendations

- Perform diagnostic evaluation on infants with suspected neonatal HSV infection, including:
  - HSV culture on swab specimens from the mouth, nasopharynx, conjunctivae, and anus (surface cultures) obtained at least 12 to 24 hours after birth
  - HSV culture from any skin vesicle present (with or without PCR as well)
  - HSV PCR on CSF and whole blood
  - Serum alanine aminotransferase levels
- Begin empirical intravenous acyclovir at a dose of 60 mg/kg/d in 3 divided daily doses in suspected cases of neonatal HSV disease
- If result of diagnostic evaluation is positive, continue intravenous acyclovir for:
  - 14 days in SEM disease
  - At least 21 days in CNS disease or disseminated disease
- In CNS disease, repeat HSV PCR on CSF near the end of the 21-day course of treatment to ensure viral clearance
- After completion of parenteral therapy for CNS, disseminated, or SEM disease, administer a suppressive course of oral acyclovir at a dose of 300 mg/m^2/dose 3 times a day for 6 months
- Monitor ANC at the second and fourth week of suppressive therapy and then monthly throughout the remainder of the treatment period

Summary statement

A high index of suspicion and then prompt recognition and initiation of intravenous acyclovir are important in reducing mortality and morbidity associated with neonatal HSV infection.

Data from Pickering LK, editor. Red Book: 2012 Report of the Committee on Infectious Diseases. 29th edition. Elk Grove Village (IL): American Academy of Pediatrics; 2012; and Kimberlin DW, Whitley RJ, Wan W, et al. Oral acyclovir suppression and neurodevelopment after neonatal herpes. N Engl J Med 2011;365(14):1284–92.

REFERENCES

1. Akhtar J, Shukla D. Viral entry mechanisms: cellular and viral mediators of herpes simplex virus entry. FEBS J 2009;276(24):7228–36.
2. Roizman B, Knipe DM, Whitley RJ. Herpes simplex viruses. In: Knipe DM, Howley PM, editors. Fields virology. 5th edition. Philadelphia: Lippincott, Williams, & Wilkins; 2007. p. 2501–601.
3. Roizman B. The structure and isomerization of herpes simplex virus genomes. Cell 1979;16(3):481–94.
4. Buchman TG, Roizman B, Adams G, et al. Restriction endonuclease finger-printing of herpes simplex virus DNA: a novel epidemiological tool applied to a nosocomial outbreak. J Infect Dis 1978;138(4):488–98.
5. Umene K, Kawana T. Divergence of reiterated sequences in a series of genital isolates of herpes simplex virus type 1 from individual patients. J Gen Virol 2003;84(Pt 4):917–23.
6. Whitley RJ. Herpes simplex virus. In: Scheld MW, Whitley RJ, Marra CM, editors. Infections in the central nervous system. 3rd edition. Philadelphia: Lippincott Williams & Wilkins; 2004. p. 123–44.
7. Smith JS, Robinson NJ. Age-specific prevalence of infection with herpes simplex virus types 2 and 1: a global review. J Infect Dis 2002;186(Suppl 1):S3–28.
8. Nahmias AJ, Lee FK, Beckman-Nahmias S. Sero-epidemiological and sociological patterns of herpes simplex virus infection in the world. Scand J Infect Dis Suppl 1990;69:19–36.
9. Tunback P, Bergstrom T, Andersson AS, et al. Prevalence of herpes simplex virus antibodies in childhood and adolescence: a cross-sectional study. Scand J Infect Dis 2003;35(8):498–502.
10. Corey L. Herpes simplex virus. In: Mandell GL, Bennett JE, Dolin R, editors. Mandell, Douglas, and Bennett's principles and practice of infectious diseases. 6th edition. Philadelphia: Elsevier Churchill Livingstone; 2005. p. 1762–80.
11. Corey L, Wald A, Celum CL, et al. The effects of herpes simplex virus-2 on HIV-1 acquisition and transmission: a review of two overlapping epidemics. J Acquir Immune Defic Syndr 2004;35(5):435–45.
12. Fleming DT, McQuillan GM, Johnson RE, et al. Herpes simplex virus type 2 in the United States, 1976 to 1994. N Engl J Med 1997;337(16):1105–11.
13. Xu F, Sternberg MR, Kottiri BJ, et al. Trends in herpes simplex virus type 1 and type 2 seroprevalence in the United States. JAMA 2006;296(8):964–73.
14. Bradley H, Markowitz LE, Gibson T, et al. Seroprevalence of herpes simplex virus types 1 and 2–United States, 1999-2010. J Infect Dis 2014;209(3):325–33.
15. Bernstein DI, Bellamy AR, Hook EW 3rd, et al. Epidemiology, clinical presentation, and antibody response to primary infection with herpes simplex virus type 1 and type 2 in young women. Clin Infect Dis 2013;56(3):344–51.
16. Roberts CM, Pfister JR, Spear SJ. Increasing proportion of herpes simplex virus type 1 as a cause of genital herpes infection in college students. Sex Transm Dis 2003;30(10):797–800.
17. Kimberlin DW. The scarlet H. J Infect Dis 2013;209(3):315–7.
18. ACOG Committee on Practice Bulletins. ACOG Practice Bulletin. Clinical management guidelines for obstetrician-gynecologists. No. 82 June 2007. Management of herpes in pregnancy. Obstet Gynecol 2007;109(6):1489–98.
19. Kulhanjian JA, Soroush V, Au DS, et al. Identification of women at unsuspected risk of primary infection with herpes simplex virus type 2 during pregnancy. N Engl J Med 1992;326(14):916–20.

20. Kucera P, Gerber S, Marques-Vidal P, et al. Seroepidemiology of herpes simplex virus type 1 and 2 in pregnant women in Switzerland: an obstetric clinic based study. Eur J Obstet Gynecol Reprod Biol 2012;160(1):13–7.

21. Sheffield JS, Hill JB, Hollier LM, et al. Valacyclovir prophylaxis to prevent recurrent herpes at delivery: a randomized clinical trial. Obstet Gynecol 2006; 108(1):141–7.

22. Watts DH, Brown ZA, Money D, et al. A double-blind, randomized, placebo-controlled trial of acyclovir in late pregnancy for the reduction of herpes simplex virus shedding and cesarean delivery. Am J Obstet Gynecol 2003;188(3):836–43.

23. Brown ZA, Selke S, Zeh J, et al. The acquisition of herpes simplex virus during pregnancy. N Engl J Med 1997;337(8):509–15.

24. Yeager AS, Arvin AM. Reasons for the absence of a history of recurrent genital infections in mothers of neonates infected with herpes simplex virus. Pediatrics 1984;73(2):188–93.

25. Whitley RJ, Nahmias AJ, Visintine AM, et al. The natural history of herpes simplex virus infection of mother and newborn. Pediatrics 1980;66(4):489–94.

26. Whitley RJ, Corey L, Arvin A, et al. Changing presentation of herpes simplex virus infection in neonates. J Infect Dis 1988;158(1):109–16.

27. Brown ZA, Wald A, Morrow RA, et al. Effect of serologic status and cesarean delivery on transmission rates of herpes simplex virus from mother to infant. JAMA 2003;289(2):203–9.

28. Kropp RY, Wong T, Cormier L, et al. Neonatal herpes simplex virus infections in Canada: results of a 3-year national prospective study. Pediatrics 2006;117(6):1955–62.

29. Jones CA, Raynes-Greenow C, Issacs D. Population-based surveillance of neonatal HSV infection in Australia (1997-2011). Clin Infect Dis 2014;59(4):525–31.

30. Brown ZA, Benedetti J, Ashley R, et al. Neonatal herpes simplex virus infection in relation to asymptomatic maternal infection at the time of labor. N Engl J Med 1991;324(18):1247–52.

31. Arvin AM, Hensleigh PA, Prober CG, et al. Failure of antepartum maternal cultures to predict the infant's risk of exposure to herpes simplex virus at delivery. N Engl J Med 1986;315(13):796–800.

32. Pinninti SG, Kimberlin DW. Maternal and neonatal herpes simplex virus infections. Am J Perinatol 2013;30(2):113–9.

33. Hutto C, Arvin A, Jacobs R, et al. Intrauterine herpes simplex virus infections. J Pediatr 1987;110(1):97–101.

34. Baldwin S, Whitley RJ. Intrauterine herpes simplex virus infection. Teratology 1989;39(1):1–10.

35. Kimberlin DW, Lin CY, Jacobs RF, et al. Natural history of neonatal herpes simplex virus infections in the acyclovir era. Pediatrics 2001;108(2):223–9.

36. Whitley RJ, Roizman B. Herpes simplex viruses. In: Richman DD, Whitley RJ, Hayden FG, editors. Clinical virology. 2nd edition. Washington, DC: ASM Press; 2004. p. 375–401.

37. Sheffield JS, Hollier LM, Hill JB, et al. Acyclovir prophylaxis to prevent herpes simplex virus recurrence at delivery: a systematic review. Obstet Gynecol 2003;102:1396–403.

38. Pinninti SG, Angara R, Feja KN, et al. Neonatal herpes disease following maternal antenatal antiviral suppressive therapy: a multicenter case series. J Pediatr 2012; 161(1):134–8.e1-e3.

39. Kimberlin DW, Baley J, Committee on Infectious Diseases, Committee on Fetus and Newborn. Guidance on management of asymptomatic neonates born to women with active genital herpes lesions. Pediatrics 2013;131(2):383–6.

40. Whitley RJ, Nahmias AJ, Soong SJ, et al. Vidarabine therapy of neonatal herpes simplex virus infection. Pediatrics 1980;66(4):495–501.
41. Whitley R, Arvin A, Prober C, et al. A controlled trial comparing vidarabine with acyclovir in neonatal herpes simplex virus infection. N Engl J Med 1991;324(7): 444–9.
42. Kimberlin DW, Lin CY, Jacobs RF, et al. Safety and efficacy of high-dose intravenous acyclovir in the management of neonatal herpes simplex virus infections. Pediatrics 2001;108(2):230–8.
43. Kimberlin DW, Whitley RJ, Wan W, et al. Oral acyclovir suppression and neurodevelopment after neonatal herpes. N Engl J Med 2011;365(14):1284–92.

Perinatal Cytomegalovirus and Varicella Zoster Virus Infections

Epidemiology, Prevention, and Treatment

Kristy M. Bialas, PhD[a], Geeta K. Swamy, MD[b],
Sallie R. Permar, MD, PhD[c],*

KEYWORDS

- Cytomegalovirus (CMV) • Varicella zoster virus (VZV) • Birth defects
- Neurologic impairment

KEY POINTS

- Congenital cytomegalovirus (CMV) infection is the leading infectious cause of hearing loss and neurologic deficits, affecting up to 1% of all pregnancies worldwide.
- Perinatal varicella zoster virus infections are rare and primarily preventable through combined active and passive maternal/infant immunization.
- Long-term antiviral treatment of infants with congenital CMV infection and associated neurologic sequelae is effective in improving hearing and developmental outcome.
- Development of active and passive maternal CMV vaccine strategies is a top priority in pediatric health.

INTRODUCTION

Human cytomegalovirus (CMV) is a ubiquitous pathogen, with a 45% to 100% adult seroprevalence rate worldwide.[1] In addition, CMV is the most common cause of congenital infection, affecting 0.5% to 2% of all live-born infants.[2] Although most affected infants are asymptomatic at birth, 10% to 15% show signs of CMV-associated sequelae,

Funded by National Institutes of Health; grant number DP2HD075699.
a Human Vaccine Institute, Duke University Medical Center, Duke University School of Medicine, Box 103020, Durham, NC 27710, USA; b Division of Maternal-Fetal Medicine, Department of Obstetrics and Gynecology, Duke University Medical Center, Duke University, 2608 Erwin Road, Suite 210, Durham, NC 27705, USA; c Department of Pediatrics, Human Vaccine Institute, Duke University Medical Center, Duke University School of Medicine, Box 103020, Durham, NC 27710, USA
* Corresponding author.
E-mail address: sallie.permar@duke.edu

Clin Perinatol 42 (2015) 61–75
http://dx.doi.org/10.1016/j.clp.2014.10.006
perinatology.theclinics.com

including thrombocytopenia, hepatitis, chorioretinitis, sensorineural hearing loss (SNHL), intrauterine growth restriction, and mental retardation (**Box 1**).[3,4] An additional 5% to 15% of asymptomatic infants infected with CMV develop late-onset sequelae, most commonly SNHL, within the first 2 years of life.[3] Congenital CMV accounts for 25% of all cases of childhood deafness and results in more long-term pediatric disabilities in US children than any other common causes of birth defects, including Down syndrome and spina bifida (**Fig. 1**).[4] Several maternal factors (**Table 1**) are known to increase the incidence and severity of congenital CMV disease, of which maternal CMV immune status plays an important role. In cases of primary maternal infection with no preexisting immunity, 40% of women transmit CMV *in utero* compared with only 1% to 2% of CMV-seropositive women.[5] Furthermore, neurologic deficits are more common following primary maternal CMV infection, and result in the most severe fetal disease outcomes.[5]

Also at risk for developing severe CMV-associated sequelae are premature infants who acquire CMV postnatally through exposure via breast milk or blood transfusions. Although breast milk transmission of CMV is asymptomatic in full-term infants, postnatal acquisition in very low birth weight premature infants can be associated with a sepsis-like illness with sequelae including pneumonitis, enteritis, thrombocytopenia, and hepatitis.[6,7] Although transfusion-associated postnatal CMV infection of premature infants has nearly been eliminated by the use of leukoreduced and CMV-seronegative blood products, encouragement of breast milk feeding to improve health outcomes for premature infants has increased the need to address breast milk transmission of CMV in neonatal intensive care settings.[8] However, it remains unclear whether postnatal CMV infection of premature infants results in long-term deficits.

Box 1
Clinical manifestations of CMV and varicella zoster virus (VZV) infection in neonates. Infants born with congenital CMV or VZV infection can display a wide range of sequelae, many of which can result in permanent developmental and neurologic impairment

Clinical manifestations

Congenital CMV

- Petechiae
- Jaundice
- Hepatosplenomegaly
- Microcephaly
- Chorioretinitis
- Intrauterine growth restriction
- Cognitive deficits
- SNHL

Congenital VZV

- Ocular defects
- Limb abnormalities
- Microcephaly
- Seizures
- Intrauterine growth restriction
- Cognitive deficits

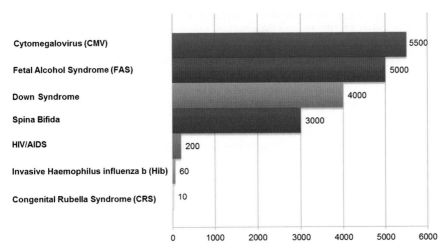

Fig. 1. Annual number of US children born with long-term pediatric disabilities. Congenital CMV infection in the United States causes more long-term pediatric disabilities than other common causes of birth defects, including fetal alcohol syndrome, Down syndrome, spina bifida, human immunodeficiency virus, haemophilus and congenital rubella syndrome. AIDS, acquired immunodeficiency syndrome. (*Adapted from* Cannon MJ, Davis KF. Washing our hands of the congenital cytomegalovirus disease epidemic. BMC Public Health 2005;5(70):2.)

Varicella zoster virus (VZV), like CMV, is a member of the herpes virus family and can lead to adverse pregnancy and infant outcomes when transmitted following acute maternal infection during pregnancy. Although preexisting VZV immunity has remained high in pregnant women both before and after the advent of VZV vaccination, immunity to VZV is routinely documented during early pregnancy. Infants with the highest risk of acquiring VZV are born to women with acute infection appearing between 5 days before and 2 days following delivery, because the infant is exposed to VZV at birth in the setting of limited or no placental VZV-specific immunoglobulin (Ig) G transfer. VZV, rarely, can be transmitted *in utero* during a primary maternal infection, and if this occurs in the first 20 weeks of pregnancy, fetal demise, intrauterine growth restriction, hydrops, limb deformities, microcephaly, and other neurologic defects can result from the congenital infection (congenital varicella syndrome).[9]

PREVALENCE/INCIDENCE

An estimated 0.7% of all live-born infants are born with congenital CMV infection. Between 10% and 15% of congenitally infected infants display symptoms at birth[10]

Table 1	
Maternal risk factors associated with mother-to-child transmission	
CMV	**VZV**
Young age	VZV immune status
Nonwhite race	Acute infection at time of delivery
Single marital status	—
CMV immune status	—

Abbreviation: VZV, varicella zoster virus.

and half of these symptomatic infants infected with CMV have long-term sequelae, often SNHL, mental retardation, and microcephaly.[2] Furthermore, 10% of infants who are asymptomatic at birth develop CMV-associated SNHL early in life and approximately 5% are reported to have additional cognitive defects, making it a leading cause of pediatric long-term disability in US children (see **Fig. 1**).[10]

The incidence of birth defects and pediatric neurologic abnormalities attributable to congenital VZV infection is considerably lower than that of CMV, because the US maternal CMV seroprevalence is approximately 50% compared with greater than 90% for VZV, leaving more women at risk of acute CMV infection during pregnancy. Moreover, the rate of congenital transmission of CMV following acute primary maternal infection is approximately 40%, compared with less than 2% following acute maternal infection with VZV.[9,11]

WORLDWIDE/REGIONAL INCIDENCE AND MORTALITIES

The incidence of congenital CMV transmission is greatly affected by CMV seroprevalence in women of childbearing age. In populations of low socioeconomic status (SES), CMV prevalence in pregnant women can reach as high as 80% to 100%.[1] Because approximately two-thirds of congenital CMV transmissions occur in CMV-seropositive women, the incidence of congenital CMV infection is high in populations of low SES and high CMV seroprevalence, averaging 1.2% compared with the worldwide incidence rate of 0.7%.[10] In the United States, where CMV seroprevalence is close to 50% in women of childbearing age, there is an increase in the number of primary maternal CMV infections during pregnancy, and, as a result, more severe infant outcomes.[12] Mortality in infants caused by congenital CMV infection ranges from 100 to 200 in the United States each year.[13]

CLINICAL CORRELATION
Maternal Interventions for the Prevention/Treatment of Congenital Cytomegalovirus and Perinatal Varicella Zoster Virus Infections

Routine prenatal CMV screening is not currently recommended given the lack of a proven effective intervention to prevent congenital CMV.[14,15] Furthermore, differentiating primary infection from reinfection or reactivation is difficult because of the poor reliability of IgM antibody assays. With a sensitivity ranging from 50% to 90% and a high rate of false positivity, IgM is detectable in less than 30% of women with a primary infection.[16–18] In addition, IgM can be detectable during reactivation or reinfection and can persist for many months following a primary infection.[18,19] Maternal immunity shown by IgG positivity alone does not eliminate the potential for congenital CMV because two-thirds of cases result from reinfection with a new CMV strain or reactivation of latent virus.[20] The addition of IgG avidity, a measure of antibody maturity, significantly improves the ability to identify primary infection.[21] The detection of IgM and IgG combined with low IgG avidity suggests a primary CMV infection occurring in the past 2 to 4 months.[16,22]

In addition to vaccine development (discussed later), there is ongoing research to determine the potential effectiveness of CMV-specific hyperimmune globulin (HIG) in congenital CMV treatment (**Table 2**). Nigro and colleagues[23] initially showed some promise for the possible efficacy of CMV HIG in treating congenital infection, although this was a cohort study. Revello and colleagues[24] recently completed a trial of 124 pregnant women with documented primary CMV infection randomized to receive serial CMV HIG infusions or placebo. Thirty percent of the CMV HIG

Table 2
Prospective studies of CMV HIG to prevent congenital CMV

Study, Location	Phase	Randomized	Binding	Placebo	Subject #	Study Group	Study Notes
Nigro et al, 2005,[23] Italy	I	No	No	No	45 84	Treatment group Prevention group	Treatment group: women with CMV+ amniotic fluid who were offered CMV HIG at 200 U/kg; 31 of 45 woman received CMV HIG Prevention group: women with a recent primary infection before 21 wk of gestation or who declined amniocentesis and were offered monthly CMV HIG at 100 U/kg; 37 of 84 women received CMV HIG In multivariate analysis, CMV HIG was associated with lower rates of congenital CMV Difficult to interpret in noncontrolled study design
Revello et al, 2014,[24] Italy	II	Yes	Yes	Yes	61 63	Treatment control	All participants received CMV HIG or placebo every 4 wk until 36 wk or CMV+ amniotic fluid 30% (18 of 61) of cases of congenital CMV in treatment group vs 44% (27 of 62) of cases in control group (*P* = .13) Among 95 infants with birth data available, there was a higher incidence of preterm birth in the treatment group: 15% (7 of 48) vs 2% (1 of 47) Lack of statistical significance likely caused by the study being underpowered
Biotest AG,[25] Europe	III	Yes	Yes	Yes	Unknown	Treatment control	Study participants have primary CMV infections Interim analysis in 2011 showed a trend in efficacy comparing treatment with control group Currently enrolling
NIH-NICHD,[26] United States	III	Yes	Yes	Yes	Planned n = 800	Treatment control	Study participants have primary CMV infection based on CMV IgM+, IgG+, IgG avidity <50%, before 24 wk gestation Randomized to receive CMV HIG or placebo every 4 wk At present enrolling

Abbreviations: CMV+, CMV positive; NIH, National Institutes of Health; NICHD, National Institute of Child Health and Human Development.

group delivered infants with congenital CMV compared with 44% in the placebo group, which was encouraging but not statistically significant, likely because of inadequate power. It is hoped that 2 ongoing large-scale randomized trials of CMV HIG to prevent congenital CMV will provide definitive evidence of its potential efficacy.[25,26]

In lieu of vaccination or effective antenatal treatment, prevention or reduction in congenital CMV must focus on educating all women of childbearing potential on preventive strategies. There are several risk factors for infection, including low SES; history of sexually transmitted infections, including human papillomavirus/abnormal cervical cytology; and very young maternal age (<15 years). Women at higher risk for primary infection include child care workers and those with young children in the home. In one study, 11% of seronegative child care workers seroconverted within the first year of employment.[27] Yeager and colleagues[28] showed that more than half of all family members of young children seroconvert within a year, and increasing parity was shown to be an independent risk factor for CMV seroconversion.[29] All women of childbearing potential, regardless of the presence or absence of risk factors, should be counseled that their personal risk of CMV acquisition can be significantly reduced with proper hygiene and behavioral practices.

Regarding VZV, prior history of infection is 97% to 99% predictive of seropositivity, which confers long-term immunity.[30] Thus, routine prenatal VZV screening based on reported history combined with serology during early pregnancy is recommended.[30] Women who are VZV-seronegative should be vaccinated postpartum. Such a strategy is supported by cost-effectiveness and cost-benefit analyses, given that the associated morbidity and mortality are high and there is potential for prophylaxis/treatment to prevent congenital infection.[31,32] If nonimmune, pregnant women should be advised to avoid contact with infected individuals until they are noninfectious.[30] If a susceptible pregnant woman has exposure to an individual infected with chickenpox, varicella immunoglobulin (VZIG) should be administered within 96 hours of exposure to prevent infection and reduce infant morbidity and mortality.[33] Although unproved through randomized clinical trials, prevention of maternal VZV infection theoretically should prevent congenital VZV. Nonpregnant women of childbearing potential should have documentation of prior history of chickenpox in their medical records with preconception vaccination if no such history exists or if documented IgG negative.

Infant Interventions for the Prevention/Treatment of Congenital Cytomegalovirus and Perinatal Varicella Zoster Virus Infections

Maternal VZV-specific IgG is highly effective in protecting infants against neonatal and congenital VZV infection. There are a few settings in which postexposure prophylaxis with VZIG is recommended for infants who are deficient in maternal VZV-specific IgG. One such scenario is primary maternal infection near the time of delivery, which can lead to severe disease in the newborn, and up to 30% mortality.[34] VZIG should similarly be administered to infants born to nonimmune mothers and all premature infants born at less than 28 weeks of gestational age who are postnatally exposed to an individual with acute VZV infection, because both of these settings leave the infant without maternal antibody protection. If infection occurs in an infant who is deficient in VZV-specific maternal IgG, antiviral treatment with high-dose acyclovir should be initiated.[35]

There are currently no well-established methods to prevent congenital CMV transmission (discussed earlier). However, because CMV-associated neurologic complications continue to develop throughout the first 2 years of life in congenitally infected infants, antiviral suppression of CMV replication may prevent or ameliorate some of these sequelae. The Collaborative Antiviral Study Group performed a clinical trial in infants congenitally infected with CMV with CMV-associated disease in the central nervous system with 6 weeks of intravenous ganciclovir (6 mg/kg every 12 hours), an antiviral that specifically targets the CMV phosphotransferase UL97, compared with no treatment.[36] This study showed clear improvement in hearing outcome for the infants treated with ganciclovir, although neutropenia, a known side effect of this drug, occurred in two-thirds of the infants treated with ganciclovir. Although the clinical improvements with ganciclovir treatment were promising, this long-term intravenous treatment was challenging to implement in infected infants who typically do not require long-term hospitalization. Thus, the same group performed a pharmacokinetic study comparing intravenous ganciclovir with the oral ganciclovir prodrug valganciclovir in neonates. Oral valganciclovir administration achieved similar plasma levels of the active drug and had a similar side effect profile to that of intravenous ganciclovir, thus providing a practical oral option for treatment of congenital CMV disease.[37] In a comparison of infant hearing and developmental outcomes after 6 weeks versus 6 months of oral valganciclovir treatment,[38] oral valganciclovir treatment until 6 months of age led to improved hearing and developmental outcomes for children infected with CMV. Moreover, the incidence of neutropenia was similar in the placebo-treated and valganciclovir-treated groups between 6 weeks and 6 months of treatment, suggesting that the neutropenia in valganciclovir-treated infants may be at least partly attributable to the viral infection. Thus, infants congenitally infected with CMV showing CMV-associated neurologic sequelae should receive valganciclovir treatment and be followed closely for suppression of viremia and hematologic abnormalities. However, because 10% to 15% of congenitally infected infants who are asymptomatic at birth develop CMV-associated neurologic sequelae (namely hearing loss) before 2 years of age, more work is needed to determine whether asymptomatic infants would benefit from this antiviral treatment. Furthermore, it is not known whether premature infants who experience symptomatic postnatal CMV infection via breast milk feeding benefit from antiviral treatment.

Infant Cytomegalovirus Diagnostics

The advent of a safe, oral option for effective CMV antiviral treatment of congenitally infected infants, combined with the high burden of congenital CMV as a major contributor to pediatric disabilities, has made it more critical to institute standard, routine CMV testing so that all congenitally infected infants may be evaluated for potential antiviral treatment that could affect their future cognitive abilities. Because infant serologic assessments are affected by issues including the presence of maternal IgG and the poor performance and predictive capacity of CMV-specific IgM, detection of the virus is a more practical approach. The current standard of diagnosing congenital CMV infection in infants is a CMV culture from the urine or saliva, including rapid virus detection in culture via immunohistochemistry. However, this diagnostic technique is labor intensive and challenging in laboratories with limited tissue culture facilities. Boppana and colleagues[39] have made considerable progress in developing a high-throughput saliva or urine quantitative real-time polymerase chain reaction (PCR) assay that is highly sensitive and specific for CMV detection compared with the gold standard of urine CMV culture.[40] Although implementation of CMV PCR of dried blood spots would have been a convenient way to integrate this testing into the standard newborn screening program, this assay has low sensitivity.[41] However, the saliva real-time PCR has been validated on dried saliva spots, facilitating batched sample

Table 3
Phase 1 and 2 clinical CMV vaccine trials targeting women of childbearing age

Platform	Phase	Randomized	Blinding	Placebo	Subject #	Study Group	Study Notes	Reference
Live-attenuated Towne	I	No	No	No	10	Seronegative (pediatric nurses of childbearing age)	Symptoms limited to local tenderness, mild fever, and increased LDH levels No virus isolated from subjects CMV-specific antibody responses elicited in all woman; declined over 12 mo Lymphoproliferative responses present in 9 of 9 subjects	43
Live-attenuated Towne	I	Yes	Partial	Yes	42 38	Seropositive/seronegative (women of childbearing age with toddlers attending day care)	Symptoms limited to mild soreness at injection site All 19 vaccinees produced CMV-specific antibodies 10-fold to 20-fold lower than naturally seropositive immune sera Lymphoproliferative responses present in all 19 vaccines Eight of 19 vaccinees and 9 of 19 women treated with placebo-acquired CMV within 1 y Only 3 of 42 seropositive, nonvaccinated women acquired CMV in the same time period	44
Live-attenuated Towne	I	Yes	No	No	63	Seropositive (women of childbearing age)	Local reactions occurred in 1 of 3 of women Women were given 1, 2, or 4 doses of Towne with or without an 8-wk booster Women receiving multiple doses had higher geometric mean antibody titers than women administered a single dose	45

Subunit gB/MF59 or alum adjuvant	I	Yes	Double	Yes	150	Seropositive (women of childbearing age)	Vaccine administered IM at 0, 1 and 6 mo with MF59 or alum Neutralizing antibodies were elicited following initial dose but did not increase with additional boosting gB-specific CD4+ T-cell proliferative responses were significantly higher in vaccinated subjects MF59 adjuvant was proved more immunogenic than alum in this study	[46]
Subunit gB/MF59 adjuvant	II	Yes	Double	Yes	464	Seronegative (predominantly African American)	Three doses were administered at 0, 1, and 6 mo After 42 mo 18 of 225 vaccinees and 31 of 216 women treated with placebo tested positive for HCMV infection Reported vaccine efficacy, 50% Of 81 infants born to vaccinated women, 1 had confirmed HCMV infection with no sequelae or late-onset symptoms 3–5 y later Of 97 infants born to women treated with placebo, 3 had confirmed HCMV infection; 1 of 3 had severe sequelae at birth and 2 of 3 were asymptomatic 3–5 y later	[47]

Abbreviations: HCMV, human CMV; IM, intramuscularly; LDH, lactate dehydrogenase.

analysis.[39] Therefore, because large-scale infant CMV testing is feasible, and treatment of congenitally infected infants has proved to benefit their long-term outcome, the implementation of universal screening for congenital CMV infection is now a top priority for improving pediatric health.

PROSPECTS AND PRIORITIES FOR MATERNAL CYTOMEGALOVIRUS VACCINE RESEARCH

The large number of infants severely affected by congenital CMV transmission, and the substantial economic burden associated with long-term treatment and care of children with CMV-associated disabilities, has prompted the Institute of Medicine to recognize the development of a maternal vaccine to be of the highest priority.[42] However, despite continuous vaccination efforts for the prevention of CMV infection for nearly 40 years, clinical trials still remain at the earliest stages. The important successes and failures of previous vaccination attempts that inform the new directions for current and future CMV vaccine research are summarized below and in **Table 3**.

Live-attenuated Cytomegalovirus Vaccines

Vaccination against CMV infection began in the early 1970s with 2 live-attenuated vaccine candidates, AD169 and the well-characterized Towne strain, both of which underwent extensive passaging in human fibroblasts before being tested in humans.[48,49] Symptoms following vaccination with either strain were mild, restricted to the site of injection, and did not result in virus shedding or latency in any of the groups tested, therefore proving to be safe and well tolerated.[43–45,48–50] Furthermore, it was discovered that, among the different routes evaluated, subcutaneous vaccination was the most effective at inducing the production of CMV-specific neutralizing antibodies and lymphoproliferative cellular responses.[48,49,51,52] Vaccine efficacy of the live-attenuated Towne strain was analyzed in 2 high-risk populations: seronegative renal transplant candidates receiving seropositive donor organs, and seronegative women of childbearing age with young children attending day care. Multiple independent studies in renal transplant recipients reported that vaccination with the Towne strain before transplantation did not alter the rate of CMV infection compared with nonvaccinated individuals; however, vaccination did reduce the severity of disease following primary CMV infection by 84% to 100% according to a preestablished scoring system.[53] Vaccination with the Towne strain in seronegative women with children attending day care also failed to protect the women from acquiring CMV, but child-to-mother transmission was rarely detected in naturally seropositive women.[44] This last observation suggested that the Towne vaccine was incapable of eliciting wild-type immunity, a common problem in most live-attenuated clinical vaccine trials. To address this issue, recent efforts have been made to elicit a stronger and longer-lasting immune response to CMV with the Towne vaccine that include the addition of an interleukin-12 adjuvant and the creation of several Towne chimeric viruses encoding portions of the genome found in other nonattenuated strains, neither of which have been successful at achieving wild-type immunity.[51,52]

Cytomegalovirus Subunit Vaccines

Most subunit vaccines to date have focused primarily on the surface glycoprotein, gB. The gB protein is directly involved in the attachment and entry of CMV into fibroblasts, and is a major target of neutralizing antibodies present in seropositive plasma. In the first human gB vaccine trial, soluble gB was administered to seronegative adults with either a squalene and water emulsion adjuvant MF59, or aluminum hydroxide.[54] The recipients were given varying doses of the vaccine in 3 different regimens. Mild discomfort at the site of injection was common, but no serious side effects were reported in any of the treatment groups. Scheduled immunizations at 0, 1, and 6 months elicited the highest neutralizing antibody response between 2 and 6 months after the final dose, and was strongest when combined with MF59. Moreover, the level of neutralizing antibodies induced after the third dose of the gB/MF59 vaccine was above that of naturally infected, seropositive individuals. Consistent with this finding, children receiving the same gB/MF59 vaccine regimen at 0, 1, and 6 months were also shown to produce neutralizing antibody titers that exceeded those seen in naturally immune sera.[55] In a cohort of CMV-seropositive women, the gB/MF59 vaccine was also capable of boosting antibody and CD4 T-cell immune responses.[46] Data from these studies, and its proven safety in transplant recipients, prompted the first and only phase 2, placebo-controlled, randomized, double-blinded trial in seronegative women.[47] More than 400 women were vaccinated with the gB/MF59 vaccine or placebo within 1 year of giving birth, and thus were at high risk for acquiring primary infection. After 42 months, 18 of 225 vaccinated women and 31 of 234 women treated with placebo had experienced a CMV infection, yielding a vaccine efficacy of 50%. Among the women in this study, 81 vaccinees and 97 placebo recipients became pregnant. Only 1 of 81 infants born to vaccinated women had confirmed CMV infection and was nonsymptomatic. Three infants were born with CMV infection in the placebo-treated group, 1 of whom presented severe sequelae at birth, whereas the other 2 remained asymptomatic. Although the numbers in this study are too small to evaluate the efficacy of the gB/MF59 vaccine on preventing mother-to-child transmission of CMV in seronegative women, the results are promising and encourage a future phase 3 trial.

With the present knowledge that CMV contains multiple glycoprotein complexes on the surface of virions involved in cell entry, it is unlikely that production of neutralizing antibodies to a single glycoprotein will provide broad protection against all CMV isolates. Therefore, recent emphasis has been placed on the development of a vaccine that elicits neutralizing antibodies to a second glycoprotein complex consisting of gH, gL, UL128, UL130, and UL131 (important for epithelial cell tropism).[56] These studies are still in early preclinical evaluation. Future vaccine platforms that include both the gB protein and pentameric complex as targets will be key to determining the immune responses required for protection against maternal infection and congenital transmission of a range of CMV variants. Additional vaccine strategies currently underway include CMV vector and DNA vaccines designed to elicit both neutralizing antibody and cell-mediated immune responses.[57–60]

SUMMARY/DISCUSSION

Although effective interventions to prevent perinatal VZV infection exist, strategies to prevent congenital CMV infection are urgently needed to reduce the high pediatric health and economic burden of this common congenital infection. Long-term antiviral treatment can improve hearing and developmental outcomes for infants congenitally infected with CMV, but do not prevent the lifelong neurologic impairment. The development of active and passive vaccine strategies for impeding maternal CMV acquisition and placental transmission is key to eliminating this common and potentially preventable cause of pediatric disabilities.

Best practices box

What is the current practice?

Congenital CMV infection:

- Screen infants for congenital CMV infection who show signs of congenital infection (including microcephaly, petechial rash, hepatosplenomegaly, hepatitis, thrombocytopenia, and failing the newborn hearing screen)
- Antiviral treatment of infants infected with CMV with neurologic involvement

What changes in current practice are likely to improve outcomes?

- Establishment of the impact of passive CMV hyperimmune globulin on congenital CMV transmission
- Implementation of standard congenital CMV screening at birth using infant dried saliva spots
- Research on the effect of antiviral treatment in congenitally CMV-infected, premature, and asymptomatic term infants
- Implementation of standard CMV serologic screening and hygiene/behavioral CMV avoidance education for all mothers during pregnancy

Major recommendations:

- Screen infants showing signs consistent with congenital CMV infection with urine or saliva human CMV culture or dried saliva spot PCR

REFERENCES

1. Cannon M, Shmid D, Hyde T. Review of cytomegalovirus seroprevalence and demographic characteristics associated with infection. Rev Med Virol 2010;20(4): 202–13.
2. Kenneson A, Cannon M. Review and meta-analysis of the epidemiology of congenital cytomegalovirus (CMV) infection. Rev Med Virol 2007;17(4):254–77.
3. Britt W. Cytomegalovirus. In: Morton CC, Nance WE, editors. Infectious disease of the fetus and newborn infant. Philadelphia: Elsevier Saunders; 2011. p. 706.
4. Cannon MJ, Davis KF. Washing our hands of the congenital cytomegalovirus disease epidemic. BMC Public Health 2005;5:70–7.
5. Yow M, Williamson D, Leeds L, et al. Epidemiologic characteristics of cytomegalovirus infection in mothers and their infants. Am J Obstet Gynecol 1988;158(5): 1189–95.
6. Lombardi G, Garofoli F, Manzoni P, et al. Breast milk-acquired cytomegalovirus infection in very low birth weight infants. J Matern Fetal Neonatal Med 2012; 25(S3):57–62.
7. Hamprecht K, Maschmann J, Jahn G, et al. Cytomegalovirus transmission to preterm infants during lactation. J Clin Virol 2008;41(3):198–205.
8. Bhatia J. Human milk and the premature infant. Ann Nutr Metab 2013;62(S3): 8–14.
9. Pastuszak AL, Levy M, Schick B, et al. Outcome after maternal varicella infection in the first 20 weeks of pregnancy. N Engl J Med 1994;330:901–5.
10. Dollard SC, Grosse SD, Ross DS. New estimates of the prevalence of neurological and sensory sequelae and mortality associated with congenital cytomegalovirus infection. Rev Med Virol 2007;17(5):355–63.

11. Enders G, Miller E, Cradock-Watson J, et al. Consequences of varicella and herpes zoster in pregnancy: prospective study of 1739 cases. Lancet 1994; 343(8912):1548–51.

12. Plosa EJ, Esbenshade JC, Fuller MP, et al. Cytomegalovirus infection. Pediatr Rev 2012;33(4):156–63.

13. Ross SA, Boppana SB. Congenital cytomegalovirus infection: outcome and diagnosis. Semin Pediatr Infect Dis 2005;16(1):44–9.

14. Grangeot-Keros L, Simon B, Audibert F, et al. Should we routinely screen for cytomegalovirus antibody during pregnancy? Intervirology 1998;41(4–5):158–62.

15. CDC. Cytomegalovirus (CMV) and congenital CMV infection - clinical diagnosis & treatment. Available at: http://www.cdc.gov/cmv/clinical/diagnosis-treatment. html. Accessed June 25, 2014.

16. Lazzarotto T, Guerra B, Lanari M, et al. New advances in the diagnosis of congenital cytomegalovirus infection. J Clin Virol 2008;41(3):192–7.

17. Guerra B, Simonazzi G, Banfi A, et al. Impact of diagnostic and confirmatory tests and prenatal counseling on the rate of pregnancy termination among women with positive cytomegalovirus immunoglobulin M antibody titers. Am J Obstet Gynecol 2007;196(3):221.e1–6.

18. Stagno S, Tinker MK, Elrod C, et al. Immunoglobulin M antibodies detected by enzyme-linked immunosorbent assay and radioimmunoassay in the diagnosis of cytomegalovirus infections in pregnant women and newborn infants. J Clin Microbiol 1985;21(6):930–5.

19. Hagay ZJ, Biran G, Ornoy A, et al. Congenital cytomegalovirus infection: a longstanding problem still seeking a solution. Am J Obstet Gynecol 1996;174(1 Pt 1): 241–5.

20. Wang C, Zhang X, Bialek S, et al. Attribution of congenital cytomegalovirus infection to primary versus non-primary maternal infection. Clin Infect Dis 2011;52(2): e11–3.

21. Lazzarotto T, Spezzacatena P, Pradelli P, et al. Avidity of immunoglobulin G directed against human cytomegalovirus during primary and secondary infections in immunocompetent and immunocompromised subjects. Clin Diagn Lab Immunol 1997;4(4):469–73.

22. CDC. Cytomegalovirus (CMV) and congenital CMV infection - interpretation of laboratory tests. Available at: http://www.cdc.gov/cmv/clinical/lab-tests.html. Accessed June 25, 2014.

23. Nigro G, Adler SP, La Torre R, et al. Passive immunization during pregnancy for congenital cytomegalovirus infection. N Engl J Med 2005;353(13):1350–62.

24. Revello MG, Lazzarotto T, Guerra B, et al. A randomized trial of hyperimmune globulin to prevent congenital cytomegalovirus. N Engl J Med 2014;370(14): 1316–26.

25. Biotest AG. Interim analysis of the Cytotect(R) phase III trial in congenital cytomegalovirus (CMV) infection shows clear indication of efficacy. Available at: http://www.biotest.com/ww/en/pub/investor_relations/news/newsdetails.cfm? newsID=1025191. Accessed July 30, 2014.

26. NIH. A randomized trial to prevent congenital cytomegalovirus (CMV). Available at: http://clinicaltrials.gov/show/NCT01376778. Accessed June 25, 2014.

27. Pass RF, August AM, Dworsky M, et al. Cytomegalovirus infection in a day-care center. N Engl J Med 1982;307(8):477–9.

28. Yeager AS. Transmission of cytomegalovirus to mothers by infected infants: another reason to prevent transfusion-acquired infections. Pediatr Infect Dis 1983;2(4):295–7.

29. Tookey PA, Ades AE, Peckham CS. Cytomegalovirus prevalence in pregnant women: the influence of parity. Arch Dis Child 1992;67(Spec No 7):779–83.
30. Marin M, Guris D, Chaves SS, et al. Prevention of varicella: recommendations of the Advisory Committee on Immunization Practices (ACIP). MMWR Recomm Rep 2007;56(RR-4):1–40.
31. Pinot de Moira A, Edmunds WJ, Breuer J. The cost-effectiveness of antenatal varicella screening with post-partum vaccination of susceptibles. Vaccine 2006; 24(9):1298–307.
32. Rouse DJ, Gardner M, Allen SJ, et al. Management of the presumed susceptible varicella (chickenpox)-exposed gravida: a cost-effectiveness/cost-benefit analysis. Obstet Gynecol 1996;87(6):932–6.
33. Ogilvie MM. Antiviral prophylaxis and treatment in chickenpox. A review prepared for the UK Advisory Group on Chickenpox on behalf of the British Society for the Study of Infection. J Infect 1998;36(Suppl 1):31–8.
34. Brunell PA. Fetal and neonatal varicella-zoster infections. Semin Perinatol 1983; 7(1):47–56.
35. Marin M, Bialek SR, Seward JF. Updated recommendations for use of VariZIG-United States, 2013. MMWR Morb Mortal Wkly Rep 2013;62(28):574–6.
36. Kimberlin D, Lin CY, Sanches PJ, et al. Effect of ganciclovir therapy on hearing in symptomatic congenital cytomegalovirus disease involving the central nervous system: a randomized, controlled trial. J Pediatr 2003;143(1):16–25.
37. Kimberlin DW, Acosta EP, Sanchez PJ, et al. Pharmacokinetic and pharmacodynamic assessment of oral valganciclovir in the treatment of symptomatic congenital cytomegalovirus disease. J Infect Dis 2008;197(6):836–45.
38. Kimberlin DW, Jester P, Sanchez PJ, et al. Six months versus six weeks of oral valganciclovir for infants with symptomatic congenital cytomegalovirus (CMV) disease with and without central nervous system (CNS) involvement: Results of a Phase III, randomized, double-blind, placebo-controlled, multinational study. In: Infectious Diseases Society of America meeting. 2013. Available at: https://idsa.confex.com/idsa/2013/webprogram/Paper43178.html. Accessed June 25, 2014.
39. Boppana SB, Ross SA, Shimamura M, et al. Saliva polymerase-chain-reaction assay for cytomegalovirus screening in newborns. N Engl J Med 2011;362(22):2111–8.
40. Ross SA, Ahmed A, Palmer AL, et al. Detection of congenital cytomegalovirus infection by real-time polymerase chain reaction of saliva or urine specimens. J Infect Dis 2014;210:1415–8.
41. Boppana SB, Ross SA, Novak Z, et al. Dried blood spot real-time polymerase chain reaction assays to screen newborns for congenital cytomegalovirus infection. JAMA 2010;303(14):1375–82.
42. Arvin AM, Fast P, Myer M, et al. Vaccine development to prevent cytomegalovirus disease: report from the National Vaccine Advisory Committee. Clin Infect Dis 2004;39(2):233–9.
43. Fleisher GR, Starr SE, Friedman HM, et al. Vaccination of pediatric nurses with live attenuated cytomegalovirus. Am J Dis Child 1982;136(4):294–6.
44. Adler SP, Starr SE, Plotkin SA, et al. Immunity induced by primary human cytomegalovirus infection protects against secondary infection among women of childbearing age. J Infect Dis 1995;171(1):26–32.
45. Adler SP, Hempfling SH, Starr SE, et al. Safety and immunogenicity of the Towne strain cytomegalovirus vaccine. Pediatr Infect Dis J 1998;17(3):200–6.
46. Sabbaj S, Pass RF, Goepfert PA, et al. Glycoprotein B vaccine is capable of boosting both antibody and CD4 T-cell responses to cytomegalovirus in chronically infected women. J Infect Dis 2011;203(11):1534–41.

47. Pass RF, Zhang C, Evans A, et al. Vaccine prevention of maternal cytomegalovirus infection. N Engl J Med 2009;360(12):1191–9.
48. Elek SD, Stern H. Development of a vaccine against mental retardation caused by cytomegalovirus infection in utero. Lancet 1974;303(7845):1–5.
49. Plotkin SA, Farquhar J, Hornberger E. Clinical trials of immunization with the Towne strain of human cytomegalovirus. J Infect Dis 1976;134(5):470–5.
50. Glazer JP, Friedman HM, Grossman RA, et al. Live cytomegalovirus vaccination of renal transplant candidates. Ann Intern Med 1979;91(5):676–83.
51. Gonczol E, Ianacone J, Furlini G, et al. Humoral immune response to cytomegalovirus Towne vaccine strain and to Toledo low-passage strain. J Infect Dis 1989; 159(5):851–9.
52. Starr SE, Glazer JP, Friedman HM, et al. Specific cellular and humoral immunity after immunization with live Towne strain cytomegalovirus vaccine. J Infect Dis 1981;143(4):585–9.
53. Plotkin SA. Vaccination against cytomegalovirus, the changeling demon. Pediatr Infect Dis J 1999;18(4):313–25.
54. Pass RF, Duliege AM, Boppana S, et al. A subunit cytomegalovirus vaccine based on recombinant envelope glycoprotein b and a new adjuvant. J Infect Dis 1999;180(4):970–5.
55. Mitchell DK, Holmes SJ, Burke RL, et al. Immunogenicity of a recombinant cytomegalovirus gB vaccine in seronegative toddlers. Pediatr Infect Dis J 2002;21(2): 133–8.
56. Rychman BJ, Chase MC, Johnson DC. HCMV gH/gL/UL128-131 interferes with virus entry into epithelial cells: evidence for cell type-specific receptors. Proc Natl Acad Sci U S A 2008;105(37):14118–23.
57. Adler SP, Plotkin SA, Gonczol E, et al. A canarypox vector expressing cytomegalovirus (CMV) glycoprotein B primes for antibody responses to a live attenuated CMV vaccine (Towne). J Infect Dis 1999;180(3):843–6.
58. Bernstein DI, Reap EA, Katen K, et al. Randomized, double-blind, phase I trial of an alphavirus replicon vaccine for cytomegalovirus in CMV seronegative adult volunteers. Vaccine 2010;28(2):484–93.
59. Wloch MK, Smith LR, Boutsaboualoy S, et al. Safety and immunogenicity of a bivalent cytomegalovirus DNA vaccine in healthy adult subjects. J Infect Dis 2008;197(12):1634–42.
60. Kharfan-Dabaja MA, Boeckh M, Wilck MB, et al. A novel therapeutic cytomegalovirus DNA vaccine in allogeneic haemopoietic stem-cell transplantation: a randomised, double-blind, placebo-controlled, phase 2 trial. Lancet Infect Dis 2012; 12(4):290–9.

TORCH Infections

Natalie Neu, MD, MPH[a],*, Jennifer Duchon, MDCM, MPH[b],
Philip Zachariah, MD[b]

KEYWORDS

- TORCH • Toxoplasmosis • *Treponema pallidum* • Rubella • Parvovirus • HIV
- Hepatitis B • Hepatitis C

KEY POINTS

- The TORCH pneumonic typically comprises toxoplasmosis, *Treponema pallidum*, rubella, cytomegalovirus, herpesvirus, hepatitis B virus, hepatitis C virus, human immunodeficiency virus and other viruses, including varicella, parvovirus B19.
- These infections are well-described causes of stillbirth and may account for up to half of all perinatal deaths globally.
- The burden is especially great in developing countries.
- Stigmata of disease may be seen at birth, in the early neonatal period, or later.
- Treatment strategies are available for many of the TORCH infections.
- Early recognition, including maternal prenatal screening and treatment when available, are key aspects in management of TORCH infections.

INTRODUCTION

Congenital infection is a well-described cause of stillbirths, as well as perinatal morbidity. TORCH infections classically comprise toxoplasmosis, *Treponema pallidum*, rubella, cytomegalovirus (CMV), herpes simplex virus (HSV), hepatitis viruses, human immunodeficiency virus (HIV), and other infections, such as varicella and parvovirus B19. The epidemiology of these infections varies, and in low-income and middle-income countries, where the burden of disease is greatest, TORCH infections are major contributors to prenatal and infant morbidity and mortality (**Table 1**).[1–14] Transmission of the pathogens may occur prenatally, perinatally, and postnatally, through, respectively, transplacental passage of organisms, from contact with blood and vaginal secretions, or from exposure to breast milk for CMV, HIV, and HSV. Evidence of infection may be seen at birth, in infancy, or not even until years later,

Disclosure statement: the authors have nothing to disclose.
[a] Division of Pediatric Infectious Disease, Columbia University Medical Center, 622 West 168th Street, PH-468, New York, NY 10032, USA; [b] Division of Pediatric Infectious Disease, New York-Presbyterian Morgan Stanley Children's Hospital, 622 West 168th Street, PH-471, New York, NY 10032, USA
* Corresponding author.
E-mail address: nn45@columbia.edu

Table 1
Worldwide prevalence estimates of selected TORCH infections

	Worldwide Prevalence	US Prevalence of Congenitally Acquired Disease in the United States	Seropositivity in Women of Childbearing Age[a]	
			Low Prevalence (%)	High Prevalence (%)
Toxoplasmosis	201,000[b]	10–33/100,000 live births	11 (Europe)	77 (South America)
Treponema pallidum	36.4 million	7.8/100,000 live births	0.67 (North America)	10 (Central Africa)
CMV	Unavailable	800/1000,000 live births	30–50 (United States)	>90 (South America)
Hepatitis B	240 million	<0.1/1000,000 US population	1.3 (North America)	8.7 (west sub-Saharan Africa)
Hepatitis C	130–150 million	<0.1/100,000 US population	1.2 (North America)	>10 (Middle East, Eastern Asia)
HIV	35.3 million	162 infants/y, 2010	0.1 (North America, Western Europe)	12 (Southern Africa)

[a] Women aged 15–49 y.
[b] Congenital toxoplasmosis.

because the fetal origins of adult disease are now increasingly recognized. The infected newborn infant may show abnormal growth, developmental anomalies, or multiple clinical and laboratory abnormalities. Many of the clinical syndromes for those viruses that present in the immediate neonatal period overlap, as shown in **Table 2**.[15] Some have classic physical stigmata, as shown in **Figs. 1** and **2**.[16,17] For many of these pathogens, treatment or prevention strategies are available; early recognition, including prenatal screening, is key, and recognized national and international standards and protocols are available to the provider. This article covers toxoplasmosis, parvovirus B19, syphilis, rubella, hepatitis B virus (HBV), hepatitis C virus (HCV), HIV; other sections are dedicated to HSV, CMV, and varicella zoster virus.

TOXOPLASMOSIS
Disease Description

The protozoa *Toxoplasma gondii* is an obligate intracellular parasite, which is ubiquitous in the environment, and whose only definitive hosts are members of the feline family. The forms of the parasite are oocysts, which contain sporozoites; these sporozoites divide and become tachyzoites; tachyzoites localize in neural and muscle tissue and develop under the pressure of the host immune system into bradyzoites, which congregate into tissue cysts. These cysts remain in skeletal and heart muscle, brain and retinal tissue, and lymph nodes. Cats acquire the infection either by consuming tissue cysts from their prey or ingesting oocysts in soil. Replication occurs in the intestine of the cat, and oocysts are formed, excreted, and sporulate to become infectious in as little as 24 hours.[18–21]

Transmission/Pathogenesis

Both animals in the wild and animals bred for human consumption may become infected from oocysts in the environment. Human infection (other than congenital) occurs by ingestion of the tissue cysts from undercooked or raw meat or oocysts from contact with cat feces or contaminated food or soil, or from transfusion of blood products or organ transplantation. Three genotypes (I, II, III) of *T gondii* have been isolated.

Table 2
Clinical findings associated with selected TORCH infections

	Hepatosplenomegaly	Cardiac Lesions	Skin Lesions	Hydrocephalus	Microcephaly	Intracranial Calcifications	Ocular Disease	Hearing Deficits
Toxoplasmosis	+	(−)	Petechiae/purpura, maculopapular rash	++	+	Diffuse intracranial calcifications	Chorioretinitis	(−)
Treponema pallidum	+	(−)	Petechiae/purpura, maculopapular rash	(−)	(−)	(−)	Chorioretinitis, glaucoma	(−)
Rubella	+	Patent ductus arteriosus, pulmonary artery stenosis, myocarditis	Petechiae/purpura	+	(−)	(−)	Chorioretinitis, cataracts, microphthalmia	++
CMV	+	+	Petechiae/purpura	(−)	++	Periventricular calcifications	Chorioretinitis	++
HSV	+	Myocarditis	Petechiae/purpura, vesicles	+	+	(−)	Chorioretinitis, cataracts	+
Parvovirus B19	+	Myocarditis	Subcutaneous edema, petechiae	(−)	(−)	(−)	Microphthalmia, retinal and corneal abnormalities	(−)

Adapted from Remington J, Klein J, Wilson C, et al, editors. Infectious diseases of the fetus and newborn infant. 7th edition. Philadelphia: Elsevier Saunders, 2011; with permission.

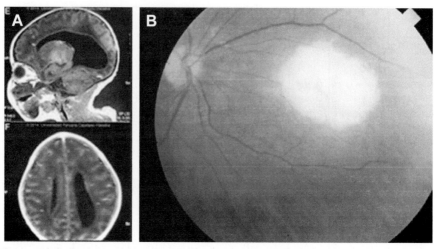

Fig. 1. Ophthalmologic and cerebral findings of congenital toxoplasmosis. (*A*) Diffuse intracerebral calcifications and hydrocephalus. (*B*) Acute retinitis.

Type II is the predominate lineage responsible for up to 80% of congenital infections in Europe and in the United States. During active parasitemia, the tachyzoite replicates rapidly and destroys infected cells, causing necrosis, which may then transform into tissue calcification.[18,22,23]

Congenital infection results most commonly from the transplacental transmission of *T gondii* after maternal primary infection during pregnancy, during a time of high parasite burden with tachyzoites. However, women infected shortly (≤3 months) before conception may also transmit *T gondii* as a result of persistent parasitemia, which continues into the pregnancy. In addition, reactivation of toxoplasmosis in immunocompromised women (ie, women with HIV) may also lead to congenital toxoplasmosis. Infection with *T gondii* leads to lifelong immunity; however, it has also been posited that women may be infected with a different genotype of *T gondii* during pregnancy.[18,20,22–24]

As shown in **Fig. 3**,[25] the risk of transmission increases with the date of maternal infection, from less than 15% at 13 weeks of gestation to greater than 70% at 36 weeks.

Epidemiology

Seroprevalence in pregnant women varies greatly among countries; the highest prevalence is noted in regions with tropical climates, where the oocysts can survive

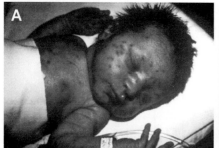
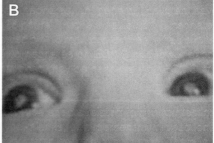

Fig. 2. Cutaneous and ophthalmologic findings of congenital rubella. (*A*) Purpuric "blueberry muffin" rash and (*B*) Cataracts. (*Courtesy of* CDC Public Health Image Library.)

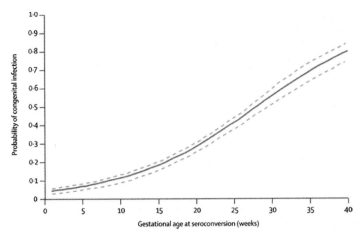

Fig. 3. Risk of MTCT of *T gondii* by gestational age at maternal seroconversion (n = 1721). Dotted lines are bounds of 95% confidence interval. (*From* SYROCOT (Systematic Review on Congenital Toxoplasmosis) study group, Thiébaut R, Leproust S, et al. Effectiveness of prenatal treatment for congenital toxoplasmosis: a meta-analysis of individual patients' data. Lancet 2007;369(9556):118; with permission.)

in soil, as well as countries with dietary customs of raw meat consumption. Seroprevalence among Brazilian, French women, and women in the United States at childbearing age is approximately 77%, 44%, and 11%, respectively. Prevalence of congenital infection ranges from 0.1 to 0.01 per 1000 live births, with concomitant decrease in both maternal prevalence and congenital infection as a result of aggressive screening approaches in certain countries.[8,18,23,26,27]

Clinical Correlation

Most (70%–90%) infants infected with *T gondii* are asymptomatic at birth; the classic diagnostic triad of symptoms (chorioretinitis, hydrocephalus, and intracranial calcifications) is rare but still remains highly suggestive. More common manifestations include[18,22]:

- Anemia
- Seizures
- Jaundice
- Splenomegaly
- Hepatomegaly
- Thrombocytopenia

The signs and symptoms of *T gondii* overlap other TORCH infections; more severe manifestations usually indicate infection earlier in gestation, whereas fetal infections occurring in the third trimester are usually subclinical at birth. Newborns who show mild or no signs and symptoms are still at high risk for development of late manifestations and sequelae of the disease.[28,29] These manifestations and sequelae include:

- Chorioretinitis
  - Approximately 20% of infants are noted to have retinal lesions at birth, but up to 90% of untreated congenitally infected infants develop chorioretinitis, into and including early adulthood[30]
- Motor and cerebellar dysfunction

- Microcephaly
- Seizures
- Intellectual disability (mental retardation)
- Sensorineural hearing loss

Discussion

Diagnosis and treatment

Prenatal There is no 1 universally endorsed screening protocol for *T gondii* in pregnant women: most providers take a risk factor–based approach,[8,25] and screen based on suspicious findings (ie, hydrocephalus, cerebral, hepatic, or splenic calcifications) on ultrasonography. Maternal screening comprises[31,32]:

- *T gondii* IgM
  - This test has a high false-positive rate and may persist for up to 2 years after acute infection
- *T gondii* IgG
  - More sensitive techniques such as IgG avidity testing allow for more accurate timing of maternal infection
- Polymerase chain reaction (PCR)
  - Amniotic fluid PCR at 18 weeks' gestation can determine fetal infection and guide medical therapy

Maternal treatment

- For maternal infection diagnosed before 18 weeks' gestation, treatment begins with spiramycin until PCR and ultrasonography results are available[25,28]
- If fetal infection is confirmed, treatment switches to pyramethamine sulfadiazine and folinic acid, and spiramycin
- No trial data exist on the efficacy of either of these therapies to reduce transmission to the fetus or reduce disease burden in congenitally infected infants; however, observational data[29] do suggest both decreased fetal infection and incidence of serious neurologic sequelae

Postnatal Infant with stigmata of congenital toxoplasmosis:

- IgG, IgM, and IgA, which is more sensitive than IgM, as well as serum (and cerebrospinal fluid [CSF], if indicated); PCR should be obtained.
  - Testing should be performed at experienced reference laboratories.
- Ophthalmologic, auditory, and neurologic examinations
- Computed tomography of the head is the preferred method of visualization of intracranial calcifications.

For infants diagnosed prenatally with toxoplasmosis, either symptomatic or asymptomatic, as well as infants diagnosed postnatally, treatment of 12 months with pyrimethamine and sulfadiazine is indicated. Folinic acid is also given to minimize pyrimethamine-associated hematologic toxicity.[8,18,28–32] Repeat testing is recommended 1 month after discontinuation of therapy. Close and sequential follow-up with serial ophthalmologic as well as auditory and neurologic examinations is the key to recognizing sequelae from this disease.

TREPONEMA PALLIDUM
Disease Description

Syphilis is a sexually transmitted infection caused by the spirochete *Treponema pallidum*. Unlike many other congenital infections, syphilis is treatable, and thus, preventing infection of the infant is possible. Infection may occur in the newborn as a result of transmission of spirochetes across the placenta during pregnancy.

Transmission/Pathogenesis

Characteristic features of congenital infection are detectable after 18 to 22 weeks' gestation, when the fetal immune response occurs. It has been postulated[33,34] that congestion of the placenta as a result of infection may cause constricted blood flow and result in severe adverse pregnancy outcomes, such as miscarriage and stillbirth. Diagnosis and treatment of syphilis in the mother during antepartum visits is critical for prevention of maternal to child transmission (MTCT) of syphilis. Recognizing the stages of maternal infection is important. The primary stage (3–6 weeks) presents as a painless, spontaneously resolving papule. The secondary stage occurs 6 to 8 weeks later, with diffuse inflammation and a disseminated rash (often on the palms and soles). The latent stage then occurs, in which women are characteristically asymptomatic. If untreated, maternal syphilis may then progress to the final or tertiary stage of the disease, which is characterized by granulomas affecting the bones and joints as well as the cardiovascular and neurologic systems. Infection of the neonate occurs when maternal infection is active, inadequately treated, or untreated.

Risk for congenital syphilis is dependent on the stage of maternal infection and the stage of infection at the time of exposure during pregnancy. One of the most important risk factors for neonatal infection is lack of maternal prenatal care, including antenatal clinic visits, screening, and treatment of syphilis.[35] Other factors that increase the risk of transmission of congenital syphilis include high nontreponemal test titers, early stages of syphilis during pregnancy, late treatment of infection (eg, short time between treatment and delivery), and lack of complete treatment.[36]

Epidemiology

MTCT of syphilis is declining but is still prevalent in the United States. The US Centers for Disease Control and Prevention (CDC) estimates that the annual rate of primary or secondary syphilis among women was 0.9 cases per 100,000, representing approximately 1500 cases in 2012.[37] The incidence of congenital syphilis was 7.8 cases per 100,000 live births for a total of 322 congenital cases reported in 2012.[38] Southern states in the United States have the highest incidence of MTCT of syphilis.[39] Global estimates of pregnant women with syphilis indicate that approximately 2 million women were infected in 2003 and 1.4 million cases in 2008.[35,40] World Health Organization (WHO) data are based on voluntary reporting by countries, which is incomplete and variable. However, from reported data, it can be concluded that maternal syphilis is a significant problem in African countries as well as countries in the Americas.

In addition, recent increases in seroprevalence have also been documented in China.[37] In 2007, WHO launched a program for the global elimination of syphilis with the goal of 50 or fewer cases of congenital syphilis per 100,000 live births. These goals were to be achieved by structured service delivery interventions, including increasing the number of women having at least 1 antenatal care visit ($\geq$95% compliance), increased testing of pregnant women ($\geq$95% compliance), and early treatment of syphilis in pregnancy ($\geq$95% compliance).[40,41]

Clinical Correlation

A recent literature review and meta-analysis on adverse outcomes of maternal syphilis infection from 1917 to 2000[42] showed that the range of adverse pregnancy outcomes ranged from 53% to 82% in untreated women versus 10% to 20% in women without syphilis. A study to estimate global impact of adverse outcomes in pregnancy based on antenatal surveillance found that 520,905 adverse outcomes occurred because of maternal syphilis. These estimates included 212,327 stillbirths, 92,764 neonatal deaths, 65,267 preterm or low birth weight infants, and 151,547 infected newborns.[35] Approximately 66% of the adverse outcomes occurred in antenatal clinic attendees who were not screened or treated.

Clinical evidence of congenital syphilis may be characterized as early manifestations (within 2 years) and late. Early findings may include hepatosplenomegaly, snuffles (nasal secretions), lymphadenopathy, mucous membrane lesions, pneumonia, osteochondritis and pseudoparalysis, maculopapular rash, edema, Coombs negative hemolytic anemia, and thrombocytopenia. Untreated infants, even those without early evidence of infection, may present with manifestations involving the central nervous system, bone and joint, teeth, eyes, and skin. **Table 3** shows both early and late sequelae of congenital syphilis.[43]

Discussion

Diagnosis and treatment
Prenatal Maternal screening

- All pregnant women should be screened for syphilis at the first prenatal visit; many advocate repeat screening at the time of delivery[44]

Maternal treatment comprises:

- Intramuscular (IM) benzathine penicillin; pregnant women with syphilis who are allergic to penicillin should be desensitized

Postnatal

- Diagnosis of congenital syphilis may be made by examination of the placenta (dark field microscopy to detect spirochetes, which is clinically and practically not available in most settings)

Table 3
Selected early and late sequelae of congenital syphilis

Organ System	Signs and Symptoms	Percent of Cases and Approximate Time of Presentation
Reticuloendothelial	Lymphadenopathy	4–8 wk
	Anemia	
	Leukopenia or leukocytosis	
	Thrombocytopenia	30%
	Hepatosplenomegaly	50%–90%
Mucocutaneous	Rhinitis	<5%; within first week of life
	Maculopapular rash on palms and soles	1–2 wk of life and lasts ≤3 mo of age
	Mucous patches	
Skeletal	Symmetric long bone lesions (upper extremity>lower extremity)	50%–95%; 6 wk–6 mo (resolve spontaneously)
	Metaphyseal and osteochondritis	
	Ostitis and dactylitis	
Neurologic	Meningitis	40%–60% abnormal CSF parameters
	Infarction and hydrocephalus	10–40 y
	Cranial nerve deafness	
Ocular	Chorioretinitis	5–20 y
	Glaucoma	

Adapted from Follett T, Clarke D. Resurgence of congenital syphilis: diagnosis and treatment. Neonatal Netw 2011;30(5):320–8.

- After evaluation of maternal testing, the infant should be tested using standard nontreponemal serologic tests, including:
  - The Venereal Disease Research Laboratory test or
  - The rapid plasma regain test
- Nontreponemal tests detect antibodies to the cardiolipin
- False-negative results may occur in congenital syphilis as a result of high titers (called the prozone effect), and thus, diluting the sample before testing is recommended
- Reactive nontreponemal tests should be confirmed with a *Treponema*-specific test, such as:
  - Fluorescent antibody absorption, microhemagglutination tests for antibodies to *T pallidum*, *T pallidum* enzyme immunoassay, or *T pallidum* particle agglutination tests.

Guidance on interpretation of maternal and infant testing, as well as the treatment guidelines endorsed by the American Academy of Pediatrics (AAP) are provided on page 695 of the AAP 2012 *Report of the Committee on Infectious Diseases*.[45]

RUBELLA
Disease Description

Congenital rubella is infection with a single-stranded positive-sense RNA virus. Transmission and infection of the mother occurs by inhalation of aerosolized particles from an infected individual.

Transmission/Pathogenesis

Congenital rubella occurs primarily after maternal infection in the first trimester (80%–100%), with decreasing risk to the fetus of congenital infection in the second trimester (10%–20%), but higher risk again at term (up to 60%). Infection with the rubella virus causes cellular damage as well as having an effect on dividing cells. The pathologic effects result in progressive necrotizing vasculitis and focal inflammatory response.[46] Infection may also result in miscarriage, stillbirth, or congenital rubella syndrome (CRS). There is a higher risk of vertical transmission (80%–90%) from a nonimmune mother with primary rubella infection in the first trimester of pregnancy, and infection during this period is associated with the most severe manifestations at birth.

Epidemiology

Indigenous rubella transmission and CRS were declared eliminated in the United States in 2004.[47] However, worldwide, it is estimated that around 110,000 infants are born with CRS every year, and WHO has targeted regional elimination of CRS by 2015.[48]

Clinical Correlation

The classic picture of CRS is a small for age infant with a constellation of anomalies, including:

- Sensorineural deafness (66%)
- Cataracts (78%)
- Cardiac defects (58%)[49]:
  - Patent ductus arteriosus
  - Pulmonary artery stenosis
  - Coarctation of aorta

- Other ocular findings:
  - Microphthalmia
  - Corneal opacity
  - Glaucoma

Features common to other perinatal infections such as the blueberry muffin rash, hepatosplenomegaly, and thrombocytopenia may also be present.

Delayed manifestations include a higher incidence of:

- Diabetes mellitus
- Hypertension
- Panencephalitis
- Behavioral disorders

Discussion

Diagnosis, prevention, and treatment
Prenatal Prevention of congenital rubella is achieved by providing rubella vaccination to all children and adolescents. Women who are of childbearing age should have evidence of immunity to rubella. If they are fond to be nonimmune, the Advisory Committee on Immunization Practices (ACIP) recommendation is for vaccination with 1 dose of measles-mumps-rubella (MMR) vaccine. Pregnant women should have serologic screening with rubella IgG if they lack evidence of rubella immunity; those who are not immune should be vaccinated with 1 dose of the MMR vaccine on completion of their pregnancies and be counseled to avoid becoming pregnant for 28 days after administration of MMR vaccine.[50]

Postnatal Case definitions and testing recommendations for suspected and probable CRS were published by the CDC in 2009.[48] Diagnosis can be based on:

- Isolation of the virus by PCR or culture
- Rubella-specific IgM, which is usually positive at birth to 3 months for congenital infection
  - This diagnosis is confirmed by stable or increasing serum concentrations of rubella-specific IgG over the first 7 to 11 months of life
  - False-positive IgM can occur
    - Avidity testing of IgG can help diagnose recent infection
- Rubella virus RNA can be also be detected by reverse transcriptase PCR in nasopharyngeal swabs, urine, CSF, and blood at birth[48]

Specific treatment of infected children is not available. All suspected cases of CRS should be reported to the CDC. All infants with CRS are considered contagious until at least 1 year of age, unless 2 cultures of clinical specimens obtained 1 month apart are negative for rubella virus after 3 months of age.[51]

PARVOVIRUS B19
Disease Description

Human parvovirus B19 is a single-stranded DNA virus in the family Parvoviridae. Parvovirus B19 is primarily transmitted by respiratory droplets, but infection from blood products as well as prenatal vertical transmission can occur.

Transmission/Pathogenesis

Approximately 35% to 55% women of childbearing age are not immune to parvovirus. The incidence of parvovirus infection in pregnancy is approximately 1% to 2%, with differential incidence occurring seasonally or during outbreak conditions. The vertical transmission rate is approximately 35%. Fetal parvovirus infection takes place via transplacental transmission 1 to 3 weeks after maternal infection, during peak maternal viremia.[52–55] Occupational exposures (ie, health care workers, childcare workers, or teachers) have historically been described as having increased risk of parvovirus seroconversion between early pregnancy and birth. However, the CDC does not recommend that pregnant women refrain from employment in these areas.[56]

Clinical Correlation

Infection with parvovirus B19 is characterized by a distinctive facial rash, described as slapped cheek, with a pruritic, laticiform macular rash on the trunk, which spreads to the extremities and may be accompanied by a polyarthritis. The rash is often preceded by a mild, nonspecific illness consisting of fever, malaise, myalgia, and headache 1 week before the exanthem. However, many women are asymptomatic during primary infection. Fetal infection may resolve spontaneously or lead to severe consequences such as nonimmune hydrops fetalis and miscarriage.

Parvovirus shows a high affinity toward erythroid progenitor cells. Cellular receptors, including the receptor of blood group P antigen are present in erythroid precursor cells. In addition, some antigenic receptors are present in endothelial cells and myocardial cells and may therefore be infected with parvovirus. Both direct toxic cell injury by the viral proteins and the induction of apoptosis contribute to cell death and the manifestations as fetal anemia and myocarditis. The risk of fetal complications is believed to be highest when infection occurs before the end of the first trimester of pregnancy. Fetal anomalies are typically evident on prenatal sonograms at 1 to 33 weeks of gestation, regardless of the gestational age at time of maternal infection.[52,53,57–59]

Fetal parvovirus infection may lead to:
- Fetal demise
- Severe anemia
- Nonimmune hydrops fetalis caused by fetal heart failure
  - High-output cardiac failure from anemia
  - Myocardial failure attributable directly to parvovirus infection
- Thrombocytopenia
- Maternal mirror syndrome
- Meningoencephalitis is rare but described[60]

Many of these conditions necessitate premature delivery. In the infant, persistent viremia with anemia caused by red cell aplasia after perinatal infection with parvovirus has been well described.[59,61,62]

Discussion

Diagnosis and treatment
Prenatal There is no endorsed routine screening protocol for parvovirus in pregnant women. Diagnosis of infection is made whether caused by maternal symptoms with the classic clinical presentation, suspicious finding (ie, hydrops fetalis) on screening ultrasonography, or known maternal exposure.[52,55,58,59]

Diagnosis of maternal infection[57]:
- Parvovirus IgM
  - Becomes detectable in serum 7 to 10 days after infection, peaks at 10 to 14 days
  - The sensitivity of IgM antibody detection between 8 and 12 weeks after maternal infection is reported as 60% to 70%

- Parvovirus B19 DNA PCR
  - Sensitivity reported up to 96%
  - B19V DNA levels may persist for longer periods after acute infection

Fetal infection

- Amniotic fluid PCR can determine fetal infection
- Monitoring for fetal hydrops and anemia is recommended for at least 12 and up to 20 weeks after exposure

Treatment

- There is no treatment of maternal infection
- Fetal treatment is targeted toward anemia and subsequent fetal hydrops, with a goal of reduction in fetal demise
  - In utero fetal transfusion has become the mainstay of treatment

Postnatal Treatment of the hydropic neonate is primarily supportive.

Persistent congenital infection manifested as red cell aplasia has increasingly been reported, because supportive care has improved and prenatal transfusion therapy is now widely used. The use of intravenous γ globulin has been extrapolated from its use in persistent symptomatic parvovirus infection in immunocompromised hosts. Case studies in infants have shown that this therapy may be adventitious in improving the need for red blood cell transfusion but that repeated infusions are often required for weeks to months after birth.[61,62]

Case series only are available to evaluate the long-term outcomes of infants with congenital parvovirus infection; it has been posited that survivors of the neonatal period may have an increased risk of neurodevelopmental impairment when compared with healthy population standards, but these finding may be confounded[63]; in general, survivors of the neonatal period have a good prognosis and neurologic outcomes.[64,65]

PERINATAL HUMAN IMMUNODEFICIENCY VIRUS INFECTION
Disease Description

HIV-1 and HIV-2 are lentiviruses that belong to the family Retroviridae. There are 3 distinct groups of the virus worldwide: M (major), O (outlier), and N (new). HIV infection is transmitted by exposure to infected body fluids, including through sexual contact, percutaneous blood exposure, mucous membrane exposure, and MTCT during pregnancy, labor, and delivery, or through breastfeeding. The pathogenesis of infection is complex and not completely understood. HIV infects dendritic cells; active replication occurs at the lymphoid tissues, with resultant primary viremia. This stage is followed by a massive loss of gut-associated lymphoid tissues, downregulation of CD8 cells, and the production of neutralizing antibodies. There are usually no clinical manifestations of HIV infection at birth.

Epidemiology

Perinatally acquired HIV-1 infection is less common in the United States as a result of earlier identification of maternal HIV infection, access to comprehensive HIV treatment programs, including combination antiretroviral therapy (cART) for pregnant women, and the avoidance of breastfeeding. The perinatal transmission rate has been reduced from 18% to 32% in the preantiretroviral era to 1% to 2% in the United States as a result of these interventions.[66] In 2011, it was estimated that there were 192 children younger than 13 years who were diagnosed with HIV in the United States.[67] Globally, WHO estimates that there are 3.2 million children younger than 15 years living with HIV. Most (>90%) of these children live in sub-Saharan Africa. Interventions instituted in resource-limited settings have reduced the estimated number of children newly infected with HIV from greater than 400,000 in 2009 to approximately 200,000 in 2013.[68] HIV-2 is endemic in some West African countries but rare in the United States and is not discussed further in this article. **Table 4**, from the *Global Update on Health Sector Response to HIV*, describes the impact of efforts to prevent MTCT of HIV.

Transmission/Pathogenesis

There are several factors that increase the risk of perinatal HIV transmission. These factors include maternal plasma viral load, maternal CD4 count, more advanced WHO clinical disease stage, breastfeeding and mastitis, and acute maternal infection.[69,70] A recent meta-analysis[71] reported that incident HIV during pregnancy and postpartum was associated with a significantly higher risk of MTCT of HIV. **Table 5** shows the timing of HIV transmission and some possible mechanisms for transmission.[72,73]

Discussion

Diagnosis and treatment

In the United States, recommendations for HIV testing in early pregnancy have been promoted by many prominent medical service groups, including the Panel on

Table 4			
The global impact of prevention of MTCT			
Year	Estimated Number of Pregnant Women Living with HIV (Range)	Estimated Mother-to-Child Transmission Rate of HIV (Range) (%)	Estimated Number of Children Newly Infected with HIV (Range)	Estimated Cumulative Number of Infections Averted by Prevention of MTCT (Range)[a]
2005	1,410,000 (1,320,000–1,520,000)	33 (31–36)	470,000 (430,000–510,000)	41,000
2006	1,390,000 (1,290,000–1,490,000)	32 (30–35)	450,000 (420,000–490,000)	73,000
2007	1,370,000 (1,270,000–1,470,000)	31 (29–33)	420,000 (390,000–460,000)	130,000
2008	1,360,000 (1,260,000–1,450,000)	29 (27–31)	400,000 (360,000–430,000)	200,000
2009[b]	1,340,000 (1,250,000–1,430,000)	26 (24–28)	350,000 (310,000–380,000)	320,000
2010	1,330,000 (1,230,000–1,420,000)	23 (21–25)	300,000 (280,000–330,000)	480,000
2011	1,310,000 (1,210,000–1,400,000)	21 (20–23)	280,000 (250,000–300,000)	660,000
2012	1,290,000 (1,190,000–1,380,000)	17 (16–19)	220,000 (200,000–250,000)	880,000
2013	1,260,000 (1,170,000–1,360,000)	16 (15–17)	200,000 (170,000–230,000)	1,120,000

[a] Compared with the counterfactual scenario in which no ARVs are provided for MTCT.
[b] Baseline year for the Global Plan.
From WHO. Global update on the health sector response to HIV, 2014. Geneva: World Health Organization, 2014; with permission.

Table 5
Mechanisms and timing of MTCT of HIV

Timing of Transmission	Rate (%)	Mechanism	Prevention
In utero	Approximately 30	Placental breakdown and microtransfusions; chorioamnionitis	Early maternal diagnosis Maternal cART
Intrapartum	Approximately 50	Contact with infant mucous membranes and >4 h rupture of amniotic membranes	cART Cesarean section Neonatal ART
Breastfeeding	Approximately 20	Contact with infant mucous membranes	No breastfeeding

Antiretroviral Therapy and Medical Management of HIV-Infected Children, the US Public Health Service, the AAP, the American College of Obstetricians and Gynecologists, and the US Preventive Services Task Force. These testing algorithms have made a significant impact on perinatal HIV as a result of early identification of maternal infection.[74–80]

Prenatal: maternal testing Opportunities for testing include:

- Early in pregnancy
- Third trimester of pregnancy
- At the time of labor or delivery
- Immediately post partum

Postnatal testing of HIV-exposed infants Diagnosis of HIV infection in infants requires the use of nucleic acid tests (NATs), including HIV DNA or HIV RNA assays. For high-risk exposures, such as maternal HIV, or when maternal HIV status is unknown, testing of the infant at birth is recommended.[75] In general, testing for the HIV-exposed infant should be:

- Within 48 hours of birth
- At 2 weeks of life
- At 4 to 6 weeks of life
- At 4 to 6 months of life

Both HIV DNA PCR and qualitative HIV RNA are sensitive for the diagnosis of perinatally acquired infection, although HIV DNA PCR may be less affected by cART. Therefore, infants who receive cART at birth should be retested with an HIV NAT to 4 weeks after cessation of cART. HIV RNA testing of infants does have the advantage of being more sensitive than HIV DNA PCR for nonsubtype B viruses, which are found around the world. An HIV-exposed infant is generally considered to be HIV-1 negative if the HIV NAT is negative at up to 4 months of age. Any infant with a positive HIV NAT should have the test repeated immediately to confirm the result.[75]

Treatment Early cART for HIV-infected infants is associated with reduced mortality and attainment of normal developmental milestones and gross motor skills when compared with infants who have cART delayed.[81,82] The reported functional cure in an HIV-infected child in Mississippi led many experts to consider early cART initiation for HIV-exposed infants. This child was treated at 30 hours of life to 18 months of age and maintained HIV viral suppression for a period.[83] However, current data now show HIV viral rebound in this child off therapy. Therefore, empirical treatment at birth and interruption of therapy after early initiation cannot be recommended.[84]

The latest guideline recommendations for infant antiretroviral (ARV) prophylaxis are shown in **Table 6** and include[85]:

- Six-week zidovudine regimen or 4-week regimen if maternal cART was given with consistent viral suppression and no concerns for lack of maternal adherence
- Zidovudine regimen started as close to birth as possible and within 6 to 12 hours of delivery
- Infants born to women who did not receive cART should receive 6 weeks of zidovudine combined with 3 doses of nevirapine in the first week of life (first dose given from birth to 8 hours, second dose given 48 hours after the first dose, and third dose given 96 hours after the second dose)

Table 6
Recommendation for prophylaxis of newborns exposed to HIV

All HIV-Exposed Infants (Initiated as Soon After Delivery as Possible)		
ZDV	**Dosing**	**Duration**
ZDV	≥35 wk gestation at birth: 4 mg/kg/dose PO twice daily, started as soon after birth as possible and preferably within 6–12 h of delivery (or, if unable to tolerate oral agents, 3 mg/kg/dose IV, beginning within 6–12 h of delivery, then every 12 h)	Birth to 4–6 wk[a]
ZDV	≥30 to <35 wk gestation at birth: 2 mg/kg/dose PO (or 1.5 mg/kg/dose IV), started as soon after birth as possible, preferably within 6–12 h of delivery, then every 12 h, advanced to 3 mg/kg/dose PO (or 2.3 mg/kg/dose IV) every 12 h at age 15 d	Birth to 6 wk
ZDV	<30 wk gestation at birth: 2 mg/kg body weight/dose PO (or 1.5 mg/kg/dose IV) started as soon after birth as possible, preferably within 6–12 h of delivery, then every 12 h, advanced to 3 mg/kg/dose PO (or 2.3 mg/kg/dose IV) every 12 h after age 4 wk	Birth to 6 wk
Additional ARV Prophylaxis Agents for HIV-Exposed Infants of Women who Received No Antepartum ARV Prophylaxis (initiated as soon after delivery as possible)		
In addition to ZDV as shown above, administer NVP	Birth weight 1.5–2 kg: 8 mg/dose PO Birth weight >2 kg: 12 mg/dose PO	3 doses in the first week of life • First dose within 48 h of birth (birth–48 h) • Second dose 48 h after first • Third dose 96 h after second

Abbreviations: IV, intravenously; NVP, nevirapine; PO, orally; ZDV, zidovudine.

[a] A 6-week course of neonatal zidovudine is generally recommended. A 4-week neonatal zidovudine chemoprophylaxis regimen may be considered when the mother has received standard ART during pregnancy with consistent viral suppression and there are no concerns related to maternal adherence.

From Panel on Treatment of HIV-Infected Pregnant Women and Prevention of Perinatal Transmission. Recommendations for use of antiretroviral drugs in pregnant HIV-1-infected women for maternal health and interventions to reduce perinatal HIV transmission in the United States. Available at: http://aidsinfo.nih.gov/contentfiles/lvguidelines/PerinatalGL.pdf. Accessed October 29, 2014.

- Consult pediatric infectious diseases specialist about options for 3-drug ARV prophylaxis regimens for extremely high-risk infants (eg, mother with high viral load, known resistant virus) (discussions before delivery are recommended)
- Infants born to mother of unknown status
  ○ Expedited HIV testing of mother or infant (rapid HIV test) should be performed, followed by:
  ○ Immediate initiation of infant ARV prophylaxis if initial test positive
  ○ If confirmatory testing of the infant's mother is negative, infant ARV prophylaxis can be discontinued
- In the United States, HIV ARV drugs other than zidovudine and nevirapine cannot be recommended in premature infants, because dosing and safety data are lacking
- Free consultation is available at the National Perinatal HIV Hotline (1-888-488-8765)

HEPATITIS B
Disease Description

HBV is a partially double-stranded circular DNA enveloped hepadnavirus. It is composed of an outer lipoprotein envelope containing the hepatitis B surface antigen (HBsAg) and an inner nucleocapsid consisting of hepatitis B core antigen (HBcAg). The genome contains 4 partially overlapping open reading frames, coding for viral surface proteins, which correspond to HBsAg, the core antigen, and the soluble antigen e (HBeAg), the viral polymerase that possesses a DNA polymerase and reverse transcriptase, a regulatory X protein essential for virus replication and activating the expression of numerous cellular and viral genes.[86–88]

The virus itself is not directly cytotoxic to hepatocytes or other cells; instead, the cellular injury seen in the disease is related to the host immune response, most commonly with HBV directed cytotoxic T cells. After infection occurs, HBV DNA and HBsAg increase exponentially in the serum. The peak of HBV DNA and HBsAg is reached before the acute disease, and both decrease after the onset of clinical symptoms. HBsAg disappears, unless a chronic carrier state is present.[88] It is now known that HBV genome may also become integrated into hepatocytes, and produce an occult HBV infection, in which the carrier is HBsAg negative, but the integrated virus is able to reactivate and replicate under certain conditions.[89]

Transmission/Pathogenesis

Most MTCT of HBV occurs at the time of delivery, with less than 2% to 4% of all transmission occurring in utero. Hypothesized prenatal modes of transmission include transplacental or inhalation or chronic ingestion of infected amniotic fluid. HBV infection caused by fetal contamination with maternal blood during procedures such as amniocentesis has been posited but not proved to occur.[90]

Perinatal transmission of HBV usually occurs from exposure to blood during labor and delivery; HBV has also been isolated in vaginal secretions. The highest rate of viral transmission occurs from mothers who are HBsAg and HBeAg positive; of women who are acutely infected during pregnancy, the risk of neonatal infection is greatest when maternal infection occurs during the third trimester. Historically, of infants who do not receive appropriate prophylaxis, only 5% to 20% who are born to HBsAg-positive but HBeAg-negative mothers become infected, as opposed to up to 90% of infants born to women who are both HBsAg and HBeAg positive.[1,86,90,91]

The biological basis for this finding is that HBeAg is produced during active viral replication and is associated with high HBV DNA levels. Maternal HBeAg can pass through the placenta because of its small size. This factor induces T-cell intolerance in the fetus to both HBeAg and HBeAg as a result of cross-reactivity between HBeAg and HBcAg. After birth, cytotoxic T-helper cell recognition and response may be shown to HBeAg and HBcAg, but not to HBsAg; this enables both acute infection with HBV and persistent HBV infection after delivery.[86,88,92]

Epidemiology

HBV is estimated to affect approximately 360 million people globally. The prevalence of HBV infections varies throughout different regions of the world, but up to half of the world's population live in regions where the prevalence of chronic HBV infection (CHB) is greater than 8%. Transmission during pregnancy or delivery is responsible for more than one-third of CHBs worldwide. **Table 1**, adapted for the Red Book, shows the prevalence of HBV as indicated by HBsAg positivity and the major source of new infections.[88,93] In these regions, most new infections occurred in early childhood or perinatally. In regions of intermediate HBV endemicity, where the prevalence of HBV infection is 2% to 7%, multiple modes of transmission (ie, perinatal, household horizontal transmission, sexual transmission, injection drug use) contribute to the burden of infection. In countries of low endemicity, such as the United States, where CHB prevalence is less than 2% and immunization readily available, the peak age of new infections is among the unimmunized in older age groups.[93]

Clinical Correlation

The risk of progressing to CHB is primarily determined by the age at the time of acute infection. Approximately 90% of infants infected perinatally or in the first year of life develop CHB. Between 25% and 50% of children infected between 1 and 5 years of age develop CHB, whereas 5% to 10% of acutely infected older children and adults develop CHB. Infants infected with HBV rarely show signs of disease at birth or in the neonatal period, and the natural history of perinatally acquired chronic HBV may be classified into the immune tolerant, immune active/clearance, inactive carrier state, and reactivation stages. Children who are infected perinatally develop mildly increased alanine aminotransferase concentrations, with detectable HBeAg and high HBV DNA concentrations ($\geq$20,000 IU/mL), with minimal or mild liver histologic abnormalities, defining the immune-tolerant phase, starting at approximately 2 to 6 months of age. Spontaneous loss of HBeAg in this stage is low, which typically lasts for many years, and children are contagious as a result of their high viral burden.[87–89]

A few infants develop clinical hepatitis within a few months of age and present with jaundice, poor feeding, and vomiting.

Infection of an infant with HBV caused by vertical transmission from an HBV-infected mother is most commonly diagnosed by the presence of HBsAg by 1 to 2 months of age.

Discussion

Diagnosis and treatment
Prenatal In the past, women were screened for HBsAg if they fell into a high-risk group based on such data as immunization status, history of exposure to blood products, intravenous drug use, and so forth. However, less than 60% of HBsAg carriers were captured using these screening criteria, and thus, it is recommended that all pregnant women be screened for HBsAg at the first prenatal visit. Additional screening at the time of delivery is recommended if any of the maternal risk factors outlined earlier are present.[94,95]

Postnatal Newborns of HBsAg-positive mothers should receive:

- Hepatitis B immunoglobulin (HBIG) and
- Single-antigen hepatitis B vaccine within 12 hours of birth
- The vaccine series should then be completed according to the standard ACIP/AAP schedule[96–99]

Follow-up:

- Testing after the hepatitis B vaccine series of infants born to HBsAg-positive mothers should then be performed at 9 to 18 months of age
- Postvaccination testing is not recommended before 9 months of age, to minimize the likelihood of detecting passively transferred anti-HBs from HBIG and to maximize the likelihood of detecting HBV disease that presents with late HBsAg positivity[14]
- Although breast milk is theoretically capable of transmitting HBV, the risk for transmission in HBsAg-positive mothers whose infants have received timely HBIG and hepatitis B vaccine is not increased by breastfeeding

---

Best Practice

- Universal screening for HBV in pregnant women (HBsAg) at first prenatal visit, regardless of risk stratification
- Repeat screening for women at high risk for HBV at delivery
  - Prophylaxis of infant
    - Maternal HBsAg positive
      - HBIG 0.5 mL IM and single-antigen hepatitis B vaccine IM within 12 hours of delivery
      - Complete vaccine series by 6 months of life
      - Follow-up testing at 9 to 18 months
    - Maternal HBsAg negative
      - Single-antigen hepatitis B vaccine IM soon after birth, before hospital discharge
      - Complete vaccine series by 6 to 18 months of life months of life[99]

HEPATITIS C
Disease Description

HCV is an enveloped, single-stranded RNA with 6 main genotypes. A hypervariable region within the structural protein E2 also leads to subtypes, or quasispecies, that show varying clinical presentation and degrees of resistance to antiviral therapy. The virus infects hepatocytes or other cells, but like HBV virus, may not be directly cytotoxic to the cells. Signs and symptoms of this disease often parallel the host immune response with HCV-directed CD8+ and then CD4+ T cells.[100–102]

Transmission/Pathogenesis

MTCT of HCV in the absence of maternal viremia is rare; however, studies of perinatal transmission of HCV have yielded conflicting results, and the timing and mechanisms of transmission from mother to infant are unclear. Infants may have positive cord or serum HCV PCR tests soon after delivery, suggesting in utero transmission. However, after 18 months of age, some of these children have negative PCR testing, recommending against using early PCR as a diagnostic tool.[101] Hypothesized mechanisms of transmission include prenatal or perinatal exposure to maternal peripheral blood mononuclear cells (PBMCs) infected with HCV and release of virus into fetal or infant circulation. Fetal and maternal HLA type, as well as HCV quasispecies, has been implicated in transmission.[103–107] Research into differential predilection for PBMCs by quasispecies may help elucidate the risk of MTCT of HCV. Other risk factors described by epidemiologic studies include female gender and coinfection with HIV, mediated through viral load and immunologic status. Mode of delivery and exposure to breast milk do not seem to be associated with infection.[103–109]

Epidemiology

HCV is one of the most common causes of chronic liver disease worldwide, with global prevalence estimated at 130 to 150 million and maternal seroprevalence at approximately 1% to 2% in developed countries. MTCT has been estimated from 4% to 8% historically, and a recent meta-analysis showed that in children born to HIV-negative women, the pooled risk of vertical HCV infection was 5.8% as opposed to a 10.8% risk of HCV vertical transmission in children born to HIV-positive women. Incidence in infants and children remains low, with a prevalence of less than 0.1 per 100,000 in the United States.[12,108,110]

Clinical Correlation

Infants infected perinatally are generally asymptomatic; although up to 80% of infants infected perinatally develop chronic HCV, most are still asymptomatic at age 5 years.

Discussion

There are no known prenatal or perinatal interventions to prevent congenital HCV. Although observational studies have suggested that invasive instrumentation or prolonged rupture of membranes may confer a higher risk of transmission, no experimental data exist to confirm these finding. Elective cesarean section is not recommended in the case of maternal HCV infection, nor is breastfeeding prohibited, although mothers with cracked or bleeding nipples are advised to abstain.

Diagnosis and treatment
Prenatal
- Routine screening of pregnant women is not advocated. However, targeted screening in high-risk women (ie, HIV positive, history of intravenous drug abuse) is recommended.[102,111]

Postnatal follow-up
- Anti-HCV IgG:
  - Persistence of maternal antibodies can be as long as 18 months, and therefore, testing is after the age of 18 months
- HCV Nucleic acid amplification test (RNA PCR):
  - May be performed at 1 to 2 months of life
  - Should be repeated after 12 months of age, because up to 30% of infants may clear their infection

Although interferon-based therapy combined with ribavirin is approved for children aged 3 years and older, neither this nor therapy with intravenous γ globulin is indicated in infancy.[102,110,111] There now exist direct acting antiviral agents, both first and second generation, which have proved efficacious in the treatment of chronic HCV in adults. Therapy in pregnant women is not indicated to prevent perinatal transmission, but this may change as these drugs become more widely used.[102,112]

SUMMARY

Infants with a suspected congenital infection should undergo a judicious review of both the maternal and perinatal history to appropriately guide the next steps in evaluation and therapy. As sensitive and specific diagnostic tools become widely available, prevalence estimates of maternal, fetal, and perinatal infection will likely increase as the burden and spectrum of these diseases become more apparent. We hope that this situation will allow for the development of more sophisticated prenatal therapeutic and preventive strategies, targeted at key moments in the disease process, with the intent of mitigating sequelae of these diseases.

Best practices

What is the current practice?

- Toxoplasmosis
- *Treponema pallidum*
- Rubella
- Parvovirus B19
- HIV
- Hepatitis B
- Hepatitis C

Best practice/guideline/care path objective(s)

What changes in current practice are likely to improve outcomes?

- Universal screening for *T pallidum*, HIV, and HBV, as well as for immunity to rubella in pregnant women at first prenatal visit, regardless of risk stratification
- Targeted screening for toxoplasmosis, parvovirus B19, and HCV in pregnant women

Major Recommendations

Toxoplasmosis: CDC recommendations for prevention of toxoplasmosis in pregnant women can be found at: http://www.cdc.gov/parasites/toxoplasmosis/prevent.html.[113]

HBV: Recommendations for screening for HBV infection in pregnancy can be found at: US Preventive Services Task Force reaffirmation recommendation statement[95]

HCV: North American Society for Pediatric Gastroenterology, Hepatology and Nutrition practice guidelines for the diagnosis and management of hepatitis C infection in infants, children, and adolescents can be found at *J Pediatr Gastroenterol Nutr* 2012; 54:838–55[111]

Clinical Algorithm(s)

T pallidum: Testing and treatment algorithm endorsed by the AAP are provided on page 695 of the AAP 2012 *Report of the Committee on Infectious Diseases*[45]

HIV: Panel on Treatment of HIV-Infected Pregnant Women and Prevention of Perinatal Transmission. *Recommendations for Use of Antiretroviral Drugs in Pregnant HIV-1-Infected Women for Maternal Health and Interventions to Reduce Perinatal HIV Transmission in the United States.* Available at: http://aidsinfo.nih.gov/contentfiles/lvguidelines/PerinatalGL.pdf. Accessed October 31 2014[85]

HBV: American Academy of Pediatrics. Hepatitis B. In: *Red Book: 2012 Report of the Committee on Infectious Disease* (29th edition), Pickering, LK. (Ed), American Academy of Pediatrics, Elk Grove Village, IL 2012. p. 384, Table 3.2.

REFERENCES

INTRODUCTION

1. Ott J, Stevens G, Wiersma S. The risk of perinatal hepatitis B virus transmission: hepatitis B e antigen (HBeAg) prevalence estimates for all world regions. BMC Infect Dis 2012;12:131.
2. Hepatitis B. Available at: http://www.who.int/mediacentre/factsheets/fs204/en/. Accessed October 30, 2014.
3. Global HIV/AIDS response. Available at: http://www.who.int/reproductivehealth/topics/rtis/GlobalData_cs_pregnancy2011.pdf?ua. Accessed October 30, 2014.
4. 2012 sexually transmitted diseases surveillance. Available at: http://www.cdc.gov/std/stats12/syphilis.htm. Accessed October 30, 2014.
5. McAuley J. Congenital toxoplasmosis. J Pediatricic Infect Dis Soc 2014;3(Suppl 1):S30–5.
6. Tudor Rares O, Remington J, McLeod R, et al. Severe congenital toxoplasmosis in the United States: clinical and serologic findings in untreated infants. Pediatr Infect Dis J 2011;30(12):1056–61.
7. Gottlieb S, Pope V, Sternberg M, et al. Prevalence of syphilis seroreactivity in the United States: data from the National Health and Nutrition Examination Surveys (NHANES) 2001-2004. Sex Transm Dis 2008;35(5):507–11.
8. Pappas G, Roussos N, Falagas M. Toxoplasmosis snapshots: global status of *Toxoplasma gondii* seroprevalence and implications for pregnancy and congenital toxoplasmosis. Int J Parasitol 2009;39(12):1385–94.
9. Vaccines and immunizations. Available at: http://www.cdc.gov/vaccines/pubs/surv-manual/chpt15-crs.html. Accessed October 30, 2014.
10. Cytomegalovirus (CMV) and congenital CMV infection. Available at: http://www.cdc.gov/cmv/trends-stats.htmll. Accessed October 30, 2014.
11. Kim R. Epidemiology of hepatitis B in the United States. Hepatology 2009;49(5 suppl):S28–34.
12. Available at: http://www.cdc.gov/hepatitis/Statistics/2012Surveillance/Commentary.htm#hepC. Accessed October 30, 2014.
13. HIV among pregnant women, infants and children. Available at: http://www.cdc.gov/hiv/risk/gender/pregnantwomen/facts/. Accessed October 30, 2014.
14. Prevalence of HIV, female (% ages 15–24). Available at: http://data.worldbank.org/indicator/SH.HIV.1524.FE.ZS. Accessed October 31, 2014.
15. Maldonado A, Nizet V, Klein J, et al. Current concepts of infections of the fetus and newborn infant. In: Remington J, Klein J, Wilson C, et al, editors. Infectious diseases of the fetus and newborn infant. 7th edition. Philadelphia: Elsevier Saunders; 2011. p. 2–23.
16. Ophthalmologic manifestations of toxoplasmosis. Available at: http://emedicine.medscape.com/article/2044905-overview. Accessed October 31, 2014.
17. Rubella (German measles, three-day measles). Available at: http://www.cdc.gov/rubella/about/photos.htm. Accessed October 31, 2014.

TOXOPLASMOSIS

18. Redbook American Academy of Pediatrics. Toxoplasmosis. In: Pickering LK, editor. Red book: 2012 report of the Committee on Infectious Disease. 29th edition. Elk Grove Village (IL): American Academy of Pediatrics; 2012. p. 720–8.
19. Toxoplasmosis. Available at: http://www.cdc.gov/dpdx/toxoplasmosis/index.html. Accessed October 30, 2014.

20. Remington J, McLeod R, Wilson C, et al. Toxoplasmosis. In: Remington J, Klein J, Wilson C, Baker C, editors. Infectious diseases of the fetus and newborn infant. 7th edition. Philadelphia: Elsevier Saunders; 2011. p. 918–1041.
21. Oz H. Maternal and congenital toxoplasmosis, currently available and novel therapies in horizon. Front Microbiol 2014;24(5):385.
22. Kieffer F, Wallon M. Congenital toxoplasmosis. Handb Clin Neurol 2013;112: 1099–101.
23. Lindsay DS, Dubey JP. *Toxoplasma gondii*: the changing paradigm of congenital toxoplasmosis. Parasitology 2011;138(14):1829–31.
24. Dubey JP, Jones JL. *Toxoplasma gondii* infection in humans and animals in the United States. Int J Parasitol 2008;38(11):1257–78.
25. SYROCOT (Systematic Review on Congenital Toxoplasmosis) study group, Thiébaut R, Leproust S, et al. Effectiveness of prenatal treatment for congenital toxoplasmosis: a meta-analysis of individual patients' data. Lancet 2007; 369(9556):115–22.
26. Torgersona P, Mastroiacovob P. The global burden of congenital toxoplasmosis: a systematic review. Bull World Health Organ 2013;91:501–8.
27. Jones J, Kruszon-Moran D, Wilson M. *Toxoplasma gondii* prevalence, United States. Emerg Infect Dis 2007;13(4):656–7.
28. Wallon M, Peyron F, Cornu C, et al. Congenital *Toxoplasma* infection: monthly prenatal screening decreases transmission rate and improves clinical outcome at age 3 years. Clin Infect Dis 2013;56(9):1223–31.
29. Kieffer F, Wallon M, Garcia P, et al. Risk factors for retinochoroiditis during the first 2 years of life in infants with treated congenital toxoplasmosis. Pediatr Infect Dis J 2008;27(1):27–32.
30. Cortina-Borja M, Tan H, Wallon M, et al. Prenatal treatment for serious neurological sequelae of congenital toxoplasmosis: an observational prospective cohort study. PLoS Med 2010;7(10). pii:e1000351.
31. Murat JB, Fricker H, Brenier-Pinchart MP, et al. Human toxoplasmosis: which biological diagnostic tests are best suited to which clinical situations? Expert Rev Anti Infect Ther 2013;11(9):943–56.
32. de Jong E, Vossen A, Walther F, et al. How to use neonatal TORCH testing. Arch Dis Child Educ Pract Ed 2013;98:93–8.

TREPONEMA PALLIDUM

33. Blencow H, Cousens S, Kamb M, et al. Lives saved tool supplement detection and treatment of syphilis in pregnancy to reduce syphilis related stillbirths and neonatal mortality. BMC Public Health 2011;11(Suppl 3):S9.
34. Berman S. Maternal syphilis: pathophysiology and treatment. Bull World Health Organ 2004;82(6):433–8.
35. Newman L, Kamb M, Hawkes S, et al. Global estimates of syphilis in pregnancy and associated adverse outcomes: analysis of multinational surveillance data. PLoS Med 2013;10(2):e1001396.
36. Qui J, Yang T, Xiao S, et al. Reported estimates of adverse pregnancy outcomes among women with and without syphilis: a systematic review and meta-analysis. PLoS One 2014;9(7):e102203.
37. Sexually transmitted disease surveillance 2012. Table 28. Available at: http://www.cdc.gov/std/stats12/Surv2012.pdf. Accessed October 29, 2014.
38. Sexually transmitted disease surveillance 2012. Table 41. Available at: http://www.cdc.gov/std/stats12/Surv2012.pdf. Accessed October 29, 2014.

39. Sexually transmitted disease surveillance 2012. Tables 42b and 43. Available at: http://www.cdc.gov/std/stats12/Surv2012.pdf. Accessed October 29, 2014.
40. The global elimination of congenital syphilis: rationale and strategy for action. Available at: http://www.who.int/reproductivehealth/publications/rtis/9789241595858/en/. Accessed October 29, 2014.
41. Global guidance on criteria and process for validation: elimination of mother-to-child transmission of HIV and syphilis. Available at: http://www.aidsdatahub.org/sites/default/files/highlight-reference/document/Global_guidance_on_criteria_and_processes_for_validation_2014.pdf. Accessed October 29, 2014.
42. Gomez G, Kamb M, Newman L, et al. Untreated maternal syphilis and adverse outcomes of pregnancy: a systematic review and meta-analysis. Bull World Health Organ 2013;91(3):217–26.
43. Follett T, Clarke D. Resurgence of congenital syphilis: diagnosis and treatment. Neonatal Netw 2011;30(5):320–8.
44. 2010 STD treatment guidelines. Available at: http://www.cdc.gov/std/treatment/2010/toc.htm. Accessed October 29, 2014.
45. American Academy of Pediatrics. Syphilis. In: Pickering LK, editor. Red book: 2012 report of the Committee on Infectious Diseases. 29th edition. Elk Grove Village (IL): American Academy of Pediatrics; 2012. p. 695.

RUBELLA

46. Banatvala JE, Brown DW. Rubella. Lancet 2004;363(9415):1127–37.
47. Rubella. Available at: http://www.who.int/mediacentre/factsheets/fs367/en/#. Accessed October 29, 2014.
48. Vaccine and immunizations: congenital rubella syndrome. Available at: http://www.cdc.gov/vaccines/pubs/surv-manual/chpt15-crs.html. Accessed October 28, 2014.
49. Given K, Lee D, Jones T, et al. Congenital rubella syndrome: ophthalmic manifestations and associated systemic disorders. Br J Ophthalmol 1993;77:358–63.
50. Morbidity and mortality weekly report (MMWR). Available at: http://www.cdc.gov/mmwr/preview/mmwrhtml/rr6204a1.htm. Accessed October 28, 2014.
51. American Academy of Pediatrics. Rubella. In: Pickering LK, editor. Red book: 2012 report of the Committee on Infectious Diseases. 29th edition. Elk Grove Village (IL): American Academy of Pediatrics; 2012. p. 629.

PARVOVIRUS B19

52. American Academy of Pediatrics. Parvovirus. In: Pickering LK, editor. Red book: 2012 report of the Committee on Infectious Disease. 29th edition. Elk Grove Village (IL): American Academy of Pediatrics; 2012. p. 539–41.
53. Adler S, Kock W. Human parvovirus infections. In: Remington J, Klein J, Wilson C, et al, editors. Infectious diseases of the fetus and newborn infant. 7th edition. Philadelphia: Elsevier Saunders; 2011. p. 834–60.
54. Young N, Brown K. Mechanisms of disease: parvovirus B19. N Engl J Med 2004; 350:586–97.
55. de Jong E, Walther F, Kroes A, et al. Parvovirus B19 infection in pregnancy: new insights and management. Prenat Diagn 2011;31(5):419–25.
56. Human parvovirus. Available at: http://www.cdc.gov/parvovirusb19/pregnancy.html. Accessed October 31, 2014.
57. Bonvicini F, Puccetti C, Salfi N, et al. Gestational and fetal outcomes in B19 maternal infection: a problem of diagnosis. J Clin Microbiol 2011;49:3514–8.

58. Dijkmans A, de Jong E, Dijkmans B, et al. Parvovirus B19 in pregnancy: prenatal diagnosis and management of fetal complications. Curr Opin Obstet Gynecol 2012;24(2):95–101.
59. Lamont R, Sobel J, Vaisbuch E, et al. Parvovirus B19 infection in human pregnancy. BJOG 2011;118(2):175–86.
60. Isumi H, Nunoue T, Nishida A, et al. Fetal brain infection with human parvovirus B19. Pediatr Neurol 1999;21:661–3.
61. Heegaard E, Hasle H, Skibsted L, et al. Congenital anemia caused by parvovirus B19 infection. Pediatr Infect Dis J 2000;19(12):1216–8.
62. Hudson A, Montegudo A, Steele R. Congenital human parvovirus B19 infection with persistent viremia. Clin Pediatr 2014;1–5. http://dx.doi.org/10.1177/0009922814533412.
63. De Jong E, Lindenburg I, van Klink J, et al. Intrauterine transfusion for parvovirus B19 infection: long-term neurodevelopmental outcome. Am J Obstet Gynecol 2012;206(3):204.e1–5.
64. Lassen J, Bager P, Wohlfahrt J, et al. Parvovirus B19 infection in pregnancy and subsequent morbidity and mortality in offspring. Int J Epidemiol 2013;42(4):1070–6.
65. Lindenburg I, van Klink J, Smits-Wintjens V, et al. Long-term neurodevelopmental and cardiovascular outcome after intrauterine transfusions for fetal anaemia: a review. Prenat Diagn 2013;33(9):815–22.

PERINATAL HUMAN IMMUNODEFICIENCY VIRUS INFECTION

66. Nesheim S, Taylor A, Lampe MA, et al. A framework for elimination of perinatal transmission of HIV in the United States. Pediatrics 2012;130(4):738–44.
67. Centers for Disease Control and Prevention. HIV surveillance report 2011, vol. 23. 2013. Available at: http://www.cdc.gov/hiv/topics/surveillance/resources/reports/. Accessed October 7, 2014.
68. World Health Organization. Global update on the health sector response to HIV, 2014. 2014. Available at: http://apps.who.int/iris/bitstream/10665/128494/1/9789241507585_eng.pdf?ua=1. Accessed October 31, 2014.
69. John G, Nduati R, Mbori-Ngacha D, et al. Correlates of mother-to-child human immunodeficiency virus type 1 (HIV-1) transmission: association with maternal plasma HIV-1 RNA load, genital HIV-1 shedding and breast infections. J Infect Dis 2001;183:206–12.
70. Fowler MG, Kourtis AP, Aizire J, et al. Breastfeeding and transmission of HIV-1: epidemiology and global magnitude. Adv Exp Med Biol 2012;743:3–25.
71. Drake AL, Wagner A, Richardson B, et al. Incident HIV during pregnancy and postpartum and risk of mother-to-child HIV transmission: a systematic review and meta-analysis. PLoS Med 2014;11(2):e1001608.
72. Kourtis AP, Bulterys M, Nesheim SR, et al. Understanding the timing of HIV transmission from mother to infant. JAMA 2001;285:709.
73. Landesman SH, Kalish LA, Burns DN, et al. Obstetrical factors and the transmission of HIV. Curr HIV Res 2013;11:10.
74. American Academy of Pediatrics Committee on Pediatric AIDS. HIV testing and prophylaxis to prevent mother-to-child transmission in the United States. Pediatrics 2008;122(5):1127–34.
75. Mofenson LM. Technical report: perinatal human immunodeficiency virus testing and prevention of transmission. Committee on Pediatric Aids. Pediatrics 2000;106(6):E88.

76. US Preventive Services Task Force. Screening for HIV: recommendation statement. Ann Intern Med 2005;143(1):32–7.

77. Branson BM, Handsfield HH, Lampe MA, et al. Revised recommendations for HIV testing of adults, adolescents, and pregnant women in health-care settings. MMWR Recomm Rep 2006;55(RR-14):1–17 [quiz: CE1–4].

78. American College of Obstetrics and Gynecology Committee on Obstetric Practice. ACOG Committee Opinion No. 418: prenatal and perinatal human immunodeficiency virus testing: expanded recommendations. Obstet Gynecol 2008; 112(3):739–42.

79. Panel on Treatment of HIV-Infected Pregnant Women and Prevention of Perinatal Transmission. Recommendations for use of antiretroviral drugs in pregnant HIV-1-infected women for maternal health and interventions to reduce perinatal HIV transmission in the United States. Available at: http://aidsinfo. nih.gov/contentfiles/lvguidelines/perinatalgl.pdf. Accessed October 19, 2014.

80. Panel on Antiretroviral Therapy and Medical Management of HIV-Infected Children. Guidelines for the use of antiretroviral agents in pediatric HIV infection. Available at: http://aidsinfo.nih.gov/contentfiles/lvguidelines/pediatric guidelines.pdf. Accessed October 31, 2014.

81. Violari A, Cotton MF, Gibb DM, et al. Early antiretroviral therapy and mortality among HIV-infected infants. N Engl J Med 2008;359(21):2233–44.

82. Laughton B, Cornell M, Grove D, et al. Early antiretroviral therapy improves neurodevelopmental outcomes in infants. AIDS 2012;26(13):1685–90.

83. Persaud D, Gay H, Ziemniak C, et al. Absence of detectable viremia after treatment cessation in an infant. N Engl J Med 2013;369:1828–35.

84. NIH news press release Thursday July 10, 2014. "Mississippi Baby" now has detectable virus, researchers find. Available at: http://www.niaid.nih.gov/news/ newsreleases/2014/Pages/MississippiBabyHIV.aspx. Accessed October 31, 2014.

85. Panel on Treatment of HIV-Infected Pregnant Women and Prevention of Perinatal Transmission. Recommendations for use of antiretroviral drugs in pregnant HIV-1-infected women for maternal health and interventions to reduce perinatal HIV transmission in the United States. Available at: http://aidsinfo.nih.gov/ contentfiles/lvguidelines/PerinatalGL.pdf. Accessed October 29, 2014. [page 27, Table only section].

HEPATITIS B

86. Chang M. Hepatitis B virus infection. Semin Fetal Neonatal Med 2007;12(3):160–7.

87. Karnsahul W, Schwarz K. Hepatitis B. In: Remington J, Klein J, Wilson C, et al, editors. Infectious diseases of the fetus and newborn infant. 7th edition. Philadelphia: Elsevier Saunders; 2011. p. 803–6.

88. American Academy of Pediatrics. Hepatitis B. In: Pickering LK, editor. Red book: 2012 report of the Committee on Infectious Disease. 29th edition. Elk Grove Village (IL): American Academy of Pediatrics; 2012. p. 369–90.

89. Tran T. Immune tolerant hepatitis B: a clinical dilemma. Gastroenterol Hepatol 2011;7(8):511–6.

90. Bleich L, Swenson E. Prevention of neonatal hepatitis B virus transmission. J Clin Gastroenterol 2014;48(9):765–72.

91. Tran T. Hepatitis B: treatment to prevent perinatal transmission. Clin Obstet Gynecol 2012;55(2):541–9.

92. Milich D, Liang T. Exploring the biological basis of hepatitis B e antigen in hepatitis B virus infection. Hepatology 2003;38:1075–86.

93. Hwang E, Cheung R. Global epidemiology of hepatitis B virus (HBV) infection. N Am J Med Sci 2011;4(1):7–13.
94. Available at: https://www.health.ny.gov/diseases/communicable/hepatitis/hepatitis_b/perinatal/docs/program_manual.pdf. Accessed October 30, 2014.
95. US Preventive Services Task Force. Screening for hepatitis B virus infection in pregnancy: US Preventive Services Task Force reaffirmation recommendation statement. Ann Intern Med 2009;150(12):869–73.
96. Kubo A, Shlager L, Marks AR, et al. Prevention of vertical transmission of hepatitis B: an observational study. Ann Intern Med 2014;160(12):828–35.
97. Lee C, Gong Y, Brok J, et al. Hepatitis B immunisation for newborn infants of hepatitis B surface antigen-positive mothers. Cochrane Database Syst Rev 2006;(2):CD004790. http://dx.doi.org/10.1002/14651858.CD004790.pub2.
98. CDC. A comprehensive immunization strategy to eliminate transmission of hepatitis B virus infection in the United States: recommendations of the Advisory Committee on Immunization Practices (ACIP); Part 1: immunization of infants, children, and adolescents. MMWR Recomm Rep 2005;54:RR-16.
99. Available at: http://www.cdc.gov/vaccines/pubs/pinkbook/hepb.html. Accessed October 31, 2014.

HEPATITIS C

100. Karnsahul W, Schwarz K. Hepatitis C. In: Remington J, Klein J, Wilson C, et al, editors. Infectious diseases of the fetus and newborn infant. 7th edition. Philadelphia: Elsevier Saunders; 2011. p. 806–8.
101. American Academy of Pediatrics. Hepatitis C. In: Pickering LK, editor. Red book: 2012 report of the Committee on Infectious Diseases. 29th edition. Elk Grove Village (IL): American Academy of Pediatrics; 2012. p. 391–5.
102. Jahveri R, Swamy G. Hepatitis C virus in pregnancy and early childhood: current understanding and knowledge deficits. J Pediatric Infect Dis Soc 2014; 3(Suppl 1):S13–8.
103. Wen J, Haber B. Maternal–fetal transmission of hepatitis C infection: what is so special about babies? J Pediatr Gastroenterol Nutr 2014;58(3):278–82.
104. Mast E, Hwang L, Seto D, et al. Risk factors for perinatal transmission of hepatitis C virus (HCV) and the natural history of HCV infection acquired in infancy. J Infect Dis 2005;192:1880.
105. Indolfi G, Azzari C, Resti M. Perinatal transmission of hepatitis C virus. J Pediatr 2013;163(6):1549–52.
106. Bevilacqua E, Fabris A, Floreano P, et al, EPHN Collaborators. Genetic factors in mother-to-child transmission of HCV infection. Virology 2009;390:64–70.
107. Benova L, Mohamoud Y, Calvert C, et al. Vertical transmission of hepatitis C virus: systematic review and meta-analysis. Clin Infect Dis 2014;59(6):765–73.
108. Indolfi G, Resti M. Perinatal transmission of hepatitis C virus infection. J Med Virol 2009;81(5):836–43.
109. Available at: http://www.cdc.gov/hepatitis/HCV/Management.htm#section1. Accessed October 29, 2014.
110. Cottrell E, Chou R, Wasson N, et al. Reducing risk for mother-to-infant transmission of hepatitis C virus: a systematic review for the US Preventive Services Task Force. Ann Intern Med 2013;158(2):109–13.
111. Mack CL, Gonzalez-Peralta RP, Gupta N, et al. NASPGHAN practice guidelines: diagnosis and management of hepatitis C infection in infants, children, and adolescents. J Pediatr Gastroenterol Nutr 2012;54:838–55.

112. Available at: http://www.who.int/hiv/pub/hepatitis/hepatitis-c-guidelines/en/. Accessed October 30, 2014.

ADDITIONAL REFERENCE

113. Parasites–toxoplasmosis (*Toxoplasma* infection). Available at: http://www.cdc.gov/parasites/toxoplasmosis/gen_info/pregnant.html. Accessed October 31, 2014.

The Epidemiology and Diagnosis of Invasive Candidiasis Among Premature Infants

Matthew S. Kelly, MD, MPH[a,b], Daniel K. Benjamin Jr, MD, MPH, PhD[a,b,*],
P. Brian Smith, MD, MPH, MHS[a,b]

KEYWORDS

- Neonatal candidiasis • *Candida* • Premature infants • Risk factors

KEY POINTS

- Invasive candidiasis occurs primarily in extremely premature infants and is associated with substantial morbidity and mortality.
- The incidence of invasive candidiasis is strongly related to gestational age and birth weight, but most cases are preventable.
- The diagnosis of invasive candidiasis relies on clinical suspicion and detection of *Candida* in blood culture or cultures from other normally sterile sites.
- Several methods were recently developed that can shorten the time needed for the identification of yeast from a positive culture, but improved diagnostics are still needed.

BACKGROUND

Invasive candidiasis is a leading infectious cause of morbidity and mortality in extremely premature infants. It affects 4% to 8% of extremely low-birth-weight (ELBW; birth weight <1000 g) infants and is associated with 30% mortality.[1–8] Infants with invasive candidiasis who survive frequently have long-term neurological impairment, including cerebral palsy, blindness, hearing impairment, cognitive deficits, and periventricular leukomalacia.[2,5,9–11]

Conflicts of interest: Dr D.K. Benjamin receives support from the US government for his work in pediatric and neonatal clinical pharmacology (1R01HD057956-05, 1K24HD058735-05, UL1TR001117, and National Institute of Child Health and Human Development contract HHSN275201000003I) and the nonprofit organization Thrasher Research Fund for his work in neonatal candidiasis (www.thrasherresearch.org); he also receives research support from industry for neonatal and pediatric drug development (www.dcri.duke.edu/research/coi.jsp). Dr. P.B. Smith receives consultant fees from Astellas Pharma, GlaxoSmithKline, and Pfizer.
a Department of Pediatrics, Duke University, Box 3499, Durham, NC 27710, USA; b Duke Clinical Research Institute, PO Box 17969, Durham, NC 27705, USA
* Corresponding author.
E-mail address: danny.benjamin@duke.edu

Clin Perinatol 42 (2015) 105–117
http://dx.doi.org/10.1016/j.clp.2014.10.008
0095-5108/15/$ – see front matter © 2015 Elsevier Inc. All rights reserved.

The incidence of neonatal candidiasis rose rapidly in the 1980s and 1990s with the improved survival of ELBW infants and the increased use of central venous catheters.[12] However, this trend has reversed, with the incidence of invasive candidiasis among premature infants declining substantially over the past 15 years.[13–15] In one study that included data from 322 neonatal intensive care units (NICUs), the incidence of invasive candidiasis decreased from 3.6 episodes per 1000 infants in 1997 to 1.4 episodes per 1000 infants in 2010.[15] Fluconazole prophylaxis, reduced use of broad-spectrum antibacterial antibiotics, empirical antifungal therapy, and improved care of central venous catheters have contributed to the declining incidence of invasive candidiasis.[13,15]

PATHOGENESIS

Candida species are yeast that frequently colonize skin, the gastrointestinal (GI) tract, and the female genitourinary tract.[16] Infants admitted to the NICU are colonized by *Candida* rapidly after birth, with the GI and respiratory tracts being the most frequent sites during the first 2 weeks of life.[17–21] Colonization during this age period may be related to the birthing process; infants delivered vaginally have higher rates of colonization than infants born by Caesarean section, and the colonizing *Candida* species are identical to those isolated from the maternal genitourinary tract in most cases.[17,20–22] Colonization of infants greater than 2 weeks of age frequently occurs on the skin and may be related to contact with maternal skin or the hands of health care providers.[20] In particular, health care workers may be the primary source of *Candida parapsilosis* colonization in the NICU environment.[22,23]

Colonization of infants by *Candida* species is not sufficient for the development of invasive candidiasis (**Fig. 1**), although up to 5% to 10% of very low-birth-weight (VLBW; birth weight <1500 g) infants colonized by *Candida* develop invasive disease.[18,20,24,25] Premature infants are predisposed to invasive candidiasis for several reasons. First, the typical barriers to invasion by *Candida* species are not fully developed in premature infants. The epidermis of the infant born at less than 30 weeks gestational age is thin and poorly formed compared with the skin of term infants.[26] Moreover, immaturity of the barrier and immune functions of the GI tract predispose to translocation by *Candida*.[27] Cellular immunity is also impaired; premature infants have fewer neutrophils and T lymphocytes than term infants, and both groups have altered neutrophil chemotaxis and phagocytosis compared with older children and adults.[28–30] Finally, virulence factors of the colonizing yeast isolate also seem to be important in determining the risk of progression to invasive disease. Bliss and colleagues[31] observed enhanced virulence characteristics among more than half of *Candida* isolates from infants with invasive candidiasis.

Once *Candida* species invade across mucosal surfaces or enter the bloodstream, they have a predilection for tissue invasion in the central nervous system, kidneys, liver, spleen, heart, and retina. Within the central nervous system, *Candida* can cause meningoencephalitis, cerebral abscesses, and ventriculitis with obstructive hydrocephalus.[32,33] *Candida* can also infiltrate with or without abscess formation in the liver, spleen, and (most commonly) the kidneys.[32,34] Finally, endocarditis and endogenous endophthalmitis may result from seeding of the heart valves or eyes during fungemia.

RISK FACTORS

Neonatal candidiasis generally occurs after the first 2 weeks of life in the setting of extreme prematurity or among infants of any gestational age with GI processes.[35]

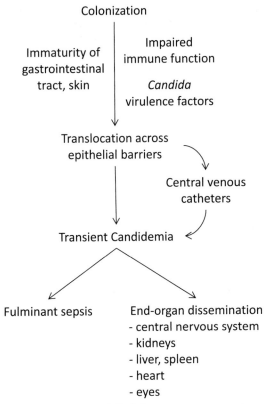

Fig. 1. Pathophysiology of invasive candidiasis in premature neonates.

Over the past decade, investigators identified risk factors for invasive candidiasis in several large cohorts of infants.

Prematurity and Birth Weight

Extreme prematurity is the strongest risk factor for the development of invasive candidiasis.[2,4,15] The incidence of invasive candidiasis is low (0.06%) among infants admitted to the NICU with a birth weight greater than 1500 g.[36] In comparison, invasive candidiasis develops in 2% to 5% of VLBW infants, whereas 4% to 16% of ELBW infants have historically been affected.[2,6,15,37–39] The incidence of invasive candidiasis is inversely related to birth weight even among ELBW infants, with infants born at less than 750 g being at least twice as likely to develop invasive candidiasis as infants with birth weights between 751 and 1000 g.[2,15] Mortality from invasive candidiasis is also inversely related to birth weight, approaching 50% for infants less than 750 g.[10]

Neonatal Intensive Care Unit Site

NICU site is strongly related to the risk of invasive candidiasis.[8] In a cohort of ELBW infants admitted to 12 NICUs, the incidence of invasive candidiasis ranged from 2.4% to 20.4%.[2] Empirical use of third-generation cephalosporins correlated with the center-specific incidence observed in this study.[2] Use of antifungal prophylaxis might also contribute to the differing incidence by center. However, substantial variation in the incidence of invasive candidiasis was still observed among infants receiving placebo in several recent trials of antifungal prophylaxis (**Table 1**).[24,25,40–42]

Broad-Spectrum Antibiotics

The strongest modifiable risk factor is antibiotic exposure and, more importantly, the choice of antibiotics for routine empirical therapy. Antibacterial therapy increases the density of *Candida* colonization by reducing the competitive pressure exerted by commensal bacteria, and receipt of broad-spectrum antibacterial antibiotics (eg, third-generation cephalosporins) is among the most consistently identified risk factors for neonatal candidiasis.[2,4,8,17,23,37,43] Studies suggest that exposure to third-generation cephalosporins is associated with an approximate doubling of the risk of invasive candidiasis among ELBW infants.[2,38] Carbapenems are likely to be increasingly used in NICUs with the emergence of multidrug-resistant gram-negative bacteria.[44] In one study of VLBW infants, receipt of a carbapenem or third-generation cephalosporin in the prior 7 days was associated with invasive candidiasis, although no studies have assessed the risk specifically associated with carbapenem use.[4]

Central Venous Catheters

Central venous catheters are indispensable in the treatment of critically ill premature infants, minimizing the need for venipuncture and facilitating the administration of parenteral nutrition, blood products, and inotropic therapy. However, these devices also play a critical role in the pathogenesis of invasive candidiasis, providing a portal of entry for *Candida* as well as a foreign surface for adhesion and biofilm formation.[1,3,8,43] The portion of central venous catheters that is within the vessel lumen frequently becomes covered by a fibrin sheath.[45] *Candida* species can grow within this fibrin matrix while remaining protected from host immune defenses and antifungal therapy.[46] As a result, central venous catheter removal is often necessary to clear candidemia, whereas delayed catheter removal (>1 day after initiation of antifungal therapy) is associated with an increased risk of death or neurodevelopmental impairment from invasive candidiasis.[38]

Table 1
Variation in the cumulative incidence of definite invasive candidiasis among placebo recipients in recent clinical trials of antifungal prophylaxis among premature infants

Study, Year	Patient Population (Birth Weight, Age)	Patients (N)	Cumulative Incidence of Invasive Candidiasis (%)	Patients, Birth Weight <750 g (n)	Cumulative Incidence of Invasive Candidiasis, Birth Weight <750 g (%)
Kicklighter et al,[24] 2001	<1500 g, 0–28 d	50	0	10	0
Kaufman et al,[25] 2001	<1000 g, 0–42 d	50	20	24	25
Manzoni et al,[41] 2007	1000–1500 g, 0–30 d <1000 g, 0–45 d	106	13	18	17
Parikh et al,[42] 2007	<1500 g, 0–28 d	60	25	0	—
Benjamin et al,[40] 2014	<750 g, 0–42 d	173	7	173	7

Other Risk Factors

Translocation across the GI tract is generally thought to be the most frequent source of invasive candidiasis.[47] Necrotizing enterocolitis, congenital GI anomalies (eg, gastroschisis),[3,32] spontaneous intestinal perforation,[48] and prior abdominal surgery[43,49] are all associated with an increased risk of invasive candidiasis among premature infants. Histamine-2-receptor antagonists (H2 antagonists) encourage overgrowth of *Candida* in the GI tract through suppression of gastric acid production and may facilitate invasion by *Candida* species through inhibition of the neutrophil oxidative burst.[50,51] In a study conducted among infants in 6 NICUs, H2 antagonists more than doubled the risk of invasive candidiasis.[1] Data also suggest that corticosteroid treatment increases the risk of invasive candidiasis among premature infants.[52,53] Corticosteroids alter the number and function of T lymphocytes and result in hyperglycemia, which facilitates growth and inhibits phagocytosis of *Candida* species in vitro.[54,55] In a placebo-controlled trial, dexamethasone increased the risk of sepsis and meningitis among VLBW infants, with *Candida* species accounting for roughly one-quarter of these infections.[53] Finally, in a prospective cohort study of more than 1500 infants, the presence of an endotracheal tube increased the risk of invasive candidiasis by more than 50%.[8] Although the mechanism for this association has not been defined, endotracheal intubation can result in abrasion of the respiratory mucosa, which may enable invasion by *Candida* species.[56]

MICROBIOLOGY

Although there are more than 150 species of *Candida*, most cases of invasive candidiasis among infants are caused by relatively few species. *C albicans* is generally the most commonly isolated species, accounting for 45% to 55% of episodes of invasive candidiasis among infants.[2,3,8,13,57] In most cohorts, *C parapsilosis* is the most frequent nonalbicans *Candida* species (20%–35%), followed by *C tropicalis* (1%–6%).[3,13,39,58] Nonalbicans species may be responsible for a growing proportion of neonatal candidiasis.[13,14,57] *C krusei* and *C glabrata* warrant special consideration given their inherent or potential resistance to fluconazole.[57] However, these species still account for a relatively small proportion (<5%) of neonatal candidiasis; no increase in disease caused by these species was observed in recent cohorts.[8,13,14,39]

C albicans is also the most pathogenic species of *Candida*. In some studies, mortality associated with invasive candidiasis caused by *C albicans* was higher than for disease caused by *C parapsilosis*.[2,12,22,59,60] Moreover, the mortality differences in several of these studies were substantial, as in a cohort whereby the case fatality rates for invasive candidiasis caused by *C albicans* and *C parapsilosis* were 24% and 3%, respectively.[59] However, this mortality difference was not observed in some studies; a recent meta-analysis concluded that invasive candidiasis caused by *C parapsilosis* is associated with a mortality rate of approximately 10% among premature infants.[37,58]

DIAGNOSIS

Delayed initiation of appropriate antifungal therapy is associated with increased mortality from invasive candidiasis.[61,62] However, the identification of infants with candidiasis is challenging, as infants typically have nonspecific symptoms and diagnostic capabilities are currently limited.

Clinical Findings

Infants with invasive candidiasis frequently present with features suggestive of sepsis, including lethargy or apnea, feeding intolerance, cardiorespiratory instability, and hyperbilirubinemia.[46] Hyperthermia, a generally unreliable marker for infection in infants, is present in only half of infants with invasive candidiasis.[35,39] Thrombocytopenia lacks specificity for a diagnosis of invasive candidiasis, and studies reporting the sensitivity of this finding yielded conflicting results.[4,63,64] Glucose intolerance and leukopenia or leukocytosis are also common findings, although the white blood cell count is normal in 40% of infants with fungal sepsis.[39] Finally, C-reactive protein and procalcitonin are often elevated in infants with fungal sepsis, but the specificity of these results is poor.[65,66]

Clinical judgment in determining the risk of invasive candidiasis among ELBW infants was evaluated in one study.[8] At the time that blood cultures were obtained for sepsis, the bedside clinician was asked to estimate the probability of invasive candidiasis. Of the sepsis episodes resulting in a diagnosis of invasive candidiasis, only 25% were deemed to have been *probably* or *highly likely* to be caused by *Candida* by the treating clinician.[8] Moreover, the accuracy of clinical judgment was similar across levels of medical training (resident, fellow, and attending).[8]

Culture-Based Methods

Blood culture remains the gold standard for diagnosis of neonatal candidiasis. However, autopsy studies suggest that the sensitivity of blood culture for invasive candidiasis is less than 50% even when an optimal volume of blood (7.5–10 mL) is obtained for culture.[67,68] Blood culture yield varies based on the number of organs that are involved, ranging from 28% when one vital organ is involved to 78% when at least 4 vital organs are involved.[67] Blood culture sensitivity may be even lower in premature infants because of the small volumes that are typically used to inoculate blood culture bottles in this patient population. Substantial improvements in blood culture technology were made since these original autopsy studies. The precise impact of these advances on the yield of blood cultures for invasive candidiasis is unknown, but blood culture likely remains an insensitive test for invasive candidiasis.[69]

Once growth of *Candida* in blood culture occurs, a lengthy process to identify the species generally ensues. Over the past decade, several techniques became available that can reduce the time needed for identification of yeast species from positive blood cultures. Matrix-assisted laser desorption/ionization–time-of-flight mass spectrometry (MALDI-TOF MS) emerged as a powerful technique for the rapid identification of bacteria and fungi from growth on solid media. MALDI-TOF MS uses mass spectrometry to identify bacterial and fungal species based on the ribosomal protein patterns, often providing results in less than 1 hour.[70] Several studies confirm that the MALDI-TOF MS identifies *Candida* species from solid growth with 90% to 95% accuracy, effectively reducing the time needed for species identification following blood culture positivity.[70–72]

Peptide nucleic acid fluorescent in situ hybridization (PNA-FISH) enables rapid detection of *Candida* directly from liquid media, including positive blood cultures.[73,74] One such test, the PNA-FISH Yeast Traffic Light Assay (AdvanDx, Inc, Woburn, MA), uses species-specific fluorescent probes and is capable of identifying the 5 most commonly isolated species of *Candida* within 90 minutes.[73] When viewed under a fluorescent microscope, green fluorescence is seen in the presence of *C albicans* or *C parapsilosis*, yellow fluorescence with *C tropicalis*, and red fluorescence in the presence of *C glabrata* or *C krusei*.[73,74] For each of the probes, the sensitivity and specificity are more than 90%; this assay generally identifies blood culture isolates more quickly than the MALDI-TOF MS, as it does not require growth on solid media.[73,74]

Polymerase chain reaction (PCR) holds great promise for earlier identification of *Candida* species from positive blood cultures. Several PCR-based assays are commercially available that can identify yeast species from positive blood cultures with sensitivity and specificity greater than 98%.[75–77] Moreover, like the PNA-FISH Yeast Traffic Light Assay, PCR does not require growth on solid media; the total time needed for this technique is generally less than 4 hours.[75] Given its ability to detect small quantities of fungal DNA, PCR is also being evaluated for the direct detection of *Candida* species from whole blood.[78–80] Among the most studied assays for this purpose is the LightCycler SeptiFast (Roche Diagnostics GmbH, Mannheim, Germany), which can detect *Candida* species from whole blood in approximately 60% of patients with culture-confirmed candidemia.[78]

Fungal Antigens

There are several fungal antigens that may be detectable in the blood of patients with invasive candidiasis. These fungal antigens include mannan, a component of the outer cell wall of *Candida* species, and 1-3-β-$_D$-glucan, found in the middle layers of the cell wall.[81] The Platelia *Candida* Antigen Plus assay (Bio-Rad, Marnes-la-Coquette, France) is most frequently used for the detection of mannan antigen in blood. The available data indicate that the specificity of this assay for invasive candidiasis in adults is excellent (>90%), but the sensitivity is poor (30%–60%).[81–84] Few studies have been conducted in infants, although mannan antigen was positive in 11 of 12 infants with proven invasive candidiasis in one small study.[85] Mannan is poorly expressed by *C parapsilosis*, and the sensitivity of mannan antigen for invasive candidiasis caused by this species is likely to be lower.[82,83]

There are several commercially available kits for the detection of 1-3-β-$_D$-glucan from clinical specimens, including the Fungitell assay (Associates of Cape Cod, Inc, Falmouth, MA) and the Fungitec G-test (Seikagaku Corporation, Tokyo, Japan). Reports suggest that 1-3-β-$_D$-glucan may be a useful screening test for invasive fungal infection in certain populations.[86–88] A recent meta-analysis including 19 studies concluded that 1-3-β-$_D$-glucan assays have a sensitivity of 81% and a specificity of 81% for the diagnosis of invasive candidiasis, although most of the included data were from adults.[89] Goudjil and colleagues[87] retrospectively examined serum 1-3-β-$_D$-glucan levels in 61 infants with clinical suspicion of fungal infection. Among 18 infants who were diagnosed with invasive candidiasis, the mean 1-3-β-$_D$-glucan level was 364 pg/mL (range 131–976) compared with 89 pg/mL (range 30–127) among noninfected control infants. However, healthy children and infants have higher 1-3-β-$_D$-glucan levels than adults, suggesting that age-specific cutoffs may be necessary; larger prospective studies are needed before use of 1-3-β-$_D$-glucan assays can be recommended for the diagnosis of neonatal candidiasis.[90,91]

TREATMENT

Indications and neonatal dosing for specific antifungal agents are discussed in detail elsewhere in this issue. However, for the bedside clinician, 2 aspects of invasive candidiasis warrant special consideration: (1) involvement of the kidneys should guide the choice of antifungal therapy and (2) central nervous system involvement should be presumed in the infant with invasive candidiasis. More specifically, liposomal formulations of amphotericin B should not be used for infants with renal candidiasis given the suboptimal penetration of these agents into the renal parenchyma.[92] Central nervous system involvement should be presumed because the incidence of meningoencephalitis exceeds 15% in neonates with invasive candidiasis,[33] cerebrospinal fluid parameters (white blood cells, glucose, protein) and culture unreliably detect disease, and imaging is not sufficiently sensitive to exclude central nervous system involvement.

The optimal duration of antifungal therapy for neonatal candidiasis has not been defined, but guidelines are available from the Infectious Diseases Society of America.[92] Candidemia without evidence of end-organ dissemination should be treated with 3 weeks of antifungal therapy from clearance of blood cultures and resolution of signs of infection. Infants with *Candida* meningoencephalitis should receive antifungal therapy until these conditions are met and cerebrospinal fluid abnormalities have completely resolved. Native valve endocarditis should be treated with 6 weeks or more of antifungal therapy and may require valve replacement. Central venous catheters should be promptly removed or replaced in the setting of bloodstream infection, as this reduces the duration of candidemia, the rate of end-organ dissemination, and mortality.[32,38,59]

SUMMARY

Although improved recognition of risk factors led to a substantial reduction in neonatal candidiasis over the past decade, this infection remains a barrier to achieving further reductions in the morbidity and mortality associated with extreme prematurity. The diagnosis of invasive candidiasis continues to rely on clinical suspicion and the detection of candidemia. Several methods were recently developed that can shorten the duration of time needed for the identification of yeast from positive blood cultures. However, improved diagnostics that can rapidly identify infants with invasive candidiasis and permit initiation of prompt antifungal therapy are still needed.

Best practices

What is the current practice?

- Blood cultures are sent routinely from premature infants with signs of sepsis.
- The decision of whether to start empirical antifungal therapy is determined by the clinician's suspicion for invasive candidiasis based on local epidemiology and infant-specific risk factors.
- Widespread variation exists in the practices of antifungal prophylaxis and empirical antifungal therapy for premature infants with sepsis.

What changes in current practice are likely to improve outcomes?

- Further research to determine what accounts for the variation in the incidence of invasive candidiasis across NICUs
- Improved molecular or fungal antigen-based diagnostics that can rapidly identify *Candida* species from blood or other normally sterile sites
- Determining optimal duration of antifungal therapy for invasive candidiasis among premature infants

Major recommendations

- Minimize exposure to modifiable risk factors for invasive candidiasis (broad-spectrum antibacterials, central venous catheters) in caring for premature infants.
- Consider empirical antifungal therapy for premature infants with signs of sepsis, particularly in the setting of established infant risk factors.
- Infants with invasive candidiasis should be treated presumptively for central nervous system disease.

REFERENCES

1. Saiman L, Ludington E, Pfaller M, et al. Risk factors for candidemia in neonatal intensive care unit patients. The National Epidemiology of Mycosis Survey study group. Pediatr Infect Dis J 2000;19(4):319–24.
2. Cotten CM, McDonald S, Stoll B, et al. The association of third-generation cephalosporin use and invasive candidiasis in extremely low birth-weight infants. Pediatrics 2006;118(2):717–22.
3. Feja KN, Wu F, Roberts K, et al. Risk factors for candidemia in critically ill infants: a matched case-control study. J Pediatr 2005;147(2):156–61.
4. Benjamin DK Jr, DeLong ER, Steinbach WJ, et al. Empirical therapy for neonatal candidemia in very low birth weight infants. Pediatrics 2003;112(3 Pt 1):543–7.
5. Friedman S, Richardson SE, Jacobs SE, et al. Systemic Candida infection in extremely low birth weight infants: short term morbidity and long term neurodevelopmental outcome. Pediatr Infect Dis J 2000;19(6):499–504.
6. Stoll BJ, Hansen N, Fanaroff AA, et al. Late-onset sepsis in very low birth weight neonates: the experience of the NICHD Neonatal Research Network. Pediatrics 2002;110(2 Pt 1):285–91.
7. Benjamin DK, DeLong E, Cotten CM, et al. Mortality following blood culture in premature infants: increased with gram-negative bacteremia and candidemia, but not gram-positive bacteremia. J Perinatol 2004;24(3):175–80.
8. Benjamin DK Jr, Stoll BJ, Gantz MG, et al. Neonatal candidiasis: epidemiology, risk factors, and clinical judgment. Pediatrics 2010;126(4):e865–73.
9. Mittal M, Dhanireddy R, Higgins RD. Candida sepsis and association with retinopathy of prematurity. Pediatrics 1998;101(4 Pt 1):654–7.
10. Adams-Chapman I, Bann CM, Das A, et al. Neurodevelopmental outcome of extremely low birth weight infants with Candida infection. J Pediatr 2013;163(4):961–7.e3.
11. Stoll BJ, Hansen NI, Adams-Chapman I, et al. Neurodevelopmental and growth impairment among extremely low-birth-weight infants with neonatal infection. JAMA 2004;292(19):2357–65.
12. Kossoff EH, Buescher ES, Karlowicz MG. Candidemia in a neonatal intensive care unit: trends during fifteen years and clinical features of 111 cases. Pediatr Infect Dis J 1998;17(6):504–8.
13. Chitnis AS, Magill SS, Edwards JR, et al. Trends in Candida central line-associated bloodstream infections among NICUs, 1999-2009. Pediatrics 2012;130(1):e46–52.
14. Fridkin SK, Kaufman D, Edwards JR, et al. Changing incidence of Candida bloodstream infections among NICU patients in the United States: 1995-2004. Pediatrics 2006;117(5):1680–7.
15. Aliaga S, Clark RH, Laughon M, et al. Changes in the incidence of candidiasis in neonatal intensive care units. Pediatrics 2014;133(2):236–42.
16. Bendel CM. Nosocomial neonatal candidiasis. Pediatr Infect Dis J 2005;24(9):831–2.
17. Saiman L, Ludington E, Dawson JD, et al. Risk factors for Candida species colonization of neonatal intensive care unit patients. Pediatr Infect Dis J 2001;20(12):1119–24.
18. Huang YC, Li CC, Lin TY, et al. Association of fungal colonization and invasive disease in very low birth weight infants. Pediatr Infect Dis J 1998;17(9):819–22.
19. Manzoni P, Farina D, Galletto P, et al. Type and number of sites colonized by fungi and risk of progression to invasive fungal infection in preterm neonates in neonatal intensive care unit. J Perinat Med 2007;35(3):220–6.

20. Baley JE, Kliegman RM, Boxerbaum B, et al. Fungal colonization in the very low birth weight infant. Pediatrics 1986;78(2):225–32.

21. Ali GY, Algohary EH, Rashed KA, et al. Prevalence of Candida colonization in preterm newborns and VLBW in neonatal intensive care unit: role of maternal colonization as a risk factor in transmission of disease. J Matern Fetal Neonatal Med 2012;25(6):789–95.

22. Waggoner-Fountain LA, Walker MW, Hollis RJ, et al. Vertical and horizontal transmission of unique Candida species to premature newborns. Clin Infect Dis 1996; 22(5):803–8.

23. Bendel CM. Colonization and epithelial adhesion in the pathogenesis of neonatal candidiasis. Semin Perinatol 2003;27(5):357–64.

24. Kicklighter SD, Springer SC, Cox T, et al. Fluconazole for prophylaxis against candidal rectal colonization in the very low birth weight infant. Pediatrics 2001;107(2): 293–8.

25. Kaufman D, Boyle R, Hazen KC, et al. Fluconazole prophylaxis against fungal colonization and infection in preterm infants. N Engl J Med 2001;345(23): 1660–6.

26. Evans NJ, Rutter N. Development of the epidermis in the newborn. Biol Neonate 1986;49(2):74–80.

27. Neu J. Gastrointestinal development and meeting the nutritional needs of premature infants. Am J Clin Nutr 2007;85(2):629s–34s.

28. Carr R. Neutrophil production and function in newborn infants. Br J Haematol 2000;110(1):18–28.

29. Correa-Rocha R, Perez A, Lorente R, et al. Preterm neonates show marked leukopenia and lymphopenia that are associated with increased regulatory T-cell values and diminished IL-7. Pediatr Res 2012;71(5):590–7.

30. Bektas S, Goetze B, Speer CP. Decreased adherence, chemotaxis and phagocytic activities of neutrophils from preterm neonates. Acta Paediatr Scand 1990;79(11):1031–8.

31. Bliss JM, Wong AY, Bhak G, et al. Candida virulence properties and adverse clinical outcomes in neonatal candidiasis. J Pediatr 2012;161(3):441–7.e2.

32. Chapman RL, Faix RG. Persistently positive cultures and outcome in invasive neonatal candidiasis. Pediatr Infect Dis J 2000;19(9):822–7.

33. Benjamin DK Jr, Poole C, Steinbach WJ, et al. Neonatal candidemia and end-organ damage: a critical appraisal of the literature using meta-analytic techniques. Pediatrics 2003;112(3 Pt 1):634–40.

34. Bryant K, Maxfield C, Rabalais G. Renal candidiasis in neonates with candiduria. Pediatr Infect Dis J 1999;18(11):959–63.

35. Wang LW, Lin CH, Liu CC, et al. Systemic fungal infection in very low-birth-weight infants. Zhonghua Min Guo Xiao Er Ke Yi Xue Hui Za Zhi 1996;37(4):272–7.

36. Lee JH, Hornik CP, Benjamin DK Jr, et al. Risk factors for invasive candidiasis in infants >1500 g birth weight. Pediatr Infect Dis J 2013;32(3):222–6.

37. Benjamin DK Jr, Ross K, McKinney RE Jr, et al. When to suspect fungal infection in neonates: a clinical comparison of Candida albicans and Candida parapsilosis fungemia with coagulase-negative staphylococcal bacteremia. Pediatrics 2000; 106(4):712–8.

38. Benjamin DK Jr, Stoll BJ, Fanaroff AA, et al. Neonatal candidiasis among extremely low birth weight infants: risk factors, mortality rates, and neurodevelopmental outcomes at 18 to 22 months. Pediatrics 2006;117(1):84–92.

39. Makhoul IR, Kassis I, Smolkin T, et al. Review of 49 neonates with acquired fungal sepsis: further characterization. Pediatrics 2001;107(1):61–6.

40. Benjamin DK Jr, Hudak ML, Duara S, et al. Effect of fluconazole prophylaxis on candidiasis and mortality in premature infants: a randomized clinical trial. JAMA 2014;311(17):1742–9.
41. Manzoni P, Stolfi I, Pugni L, et al. A multicenter, randomized trial of prophylactic fluconazole in preterm neonates. N Engl J Med 2007;356(24):2483–95.
42. Parikh TB, Nanavati RN, Patankar CV, et al. Fluconazole prophylaxis against fungal colonization and invasive fungal infection in very low birth weight infants. Indian Pediatr 2007;44(11):830–7.
43. Yu Y, Du L, Yuan T, et al. Risk factors and clinical analysis for invasive fungal infection in neonatal intensive care unit patients. Am J Perinatol 2013;30(7):589–94.
44. Hornik CP, Herring AH, Benjamin DK Jr, et al. Adverse events associated with meropenem versus imipenem/cilastatin therapy in a large retrospective cohort of hospitalized infants. Pediatr Infect Dis J 2013;32(7):748–53.
45. Suojanen JN, Brophy DP, Nasser I. Thrombus on indwelling central venous catheters: the histopathology of "fibrin sheaths". Cardiovasc Intervent Radiol 2000;23(3):194–7.
46. Benjamin DK Jr, Garges H, Steinbach WJ. Candida bloodstream infection in neonates. Semin Perinatol 2003;27(5):375–83.
47. Cole GT, Halawa AA, Anaissie EJ. The role of the gastrointestinal tract in hematogenous candidiasis: from the laboratory to the bedside. Clin Infect Dis 1996; 22(Suppl 2):S73–88.
48. Coates EW, Karlowicz MG, Croitoru DP, et al. Distinctive distribution of pathogens associated with peritonitis in neonates with focal intestinal perforation compared with necrotizing enterocolitis. Pediatrics 2005;116(2):e241–6.
49. Shetty SS, Harrison LH, Hajjeh RA, et al. Determining risk factors for candidemia among newborn infants from population-based surveillance: Baltimore, Maryland, 1998-2000. Pediatr Infect Dis J 2005;24(7):601–4.
50. Boero M, Pera A, Andriulli A, et al. Candida overgrowth in gastric juice of peptic ulcer subjects on short- and long-term treatment with H2-receptor antagonists. Digestion 1983;28(3):158–63.
51. Ciz M, Lojek A. Modulation of neutrophil oxidative burst via histamine receptors. Br J Pharmacol 2013;170(1):17–22.
52. Botas CM, Kurlat I, Young SM, et al. Disseminated candidal infections and intravenous hydrocortisone in preterm infants. Pediatrics 1995;95(6):883–7.
53. Stoll BJ, Temprosa M, Tyson JE, et al. Dexamethasone therapy increases infection in very low birth weight infants. Pediatrics 1999;104(5):e63.
54. Gunn T, Reece ER, Metrakos K, et al. Depressed T cells following neonatal steroid treatment. Pediatrics 1981;67(1):61–7.
55. Hostetter MK, Lorenz JS, Preus L, et al. The iC3b receptor on Candida albicans: subcellular localization and modulation of receptor expression by glucose. J Infect Dis 1990;161(4):761–8.
56. Bishop MJ. Mechanisms of laryngotracheal injury following prolonged tracheal intubation. Chest 1989;96(1):185–6.
57. Steinbach WJ, Roilides E, Berman D, et al. Results from a prospective, international, epidemiologic study of invasive candidiasis in children and neonates. Pediatr Infect Dis J 2012;31(12):1252–7.
58. Pammi M, Holland L, Butler G, et al. Candida parapsilosis is a significant neonatal pathogen: a systematic review and meta-analysis. Pediatr Infect Dis J 2013; 32(5):e206–16.
59. Karlowicz MG, Hashimoto LN, Kelly RE Jr, et al. Should central venous catheters be removed as soon as candidemia is detected in neonates? Pediatrics 2000; 106(5):E63.

60. Faix RG. Invasive neonatal candidiasis: comparison of albicans and parapsilosis infection. Pediatr Infect Dis J 1992;11(2):88–93.
61. Garey KW, Rege M, Pai MP, et al. Time to initiation of fluconazole therapy impacts mortality in patients with candidemia: a multi-institutional study. Clin Infect Dis 2006;43(1):25–31.
62. Cahan H, Deville JG. Outcomes of neonatal candidiasis: the impact of delayed initiation of antifungal therapy. Int J Pediatr 2011;2011:813871.
63. Guida JD, Kunig AM, Leef KH, et al. Platelet count and sepsis in very low birth weight neonates: is there an organism-specific response? Pediatrics 2003;111(6 Pt 1):1411–5.
64. Manzoni P, Mostert M, Galletto P, et al. Is thrombocytopenia suggestive of organism-specific response in neonatal sepsis? Pediatr Int 2009;51(2):206–10.
65. Montagna MT, Coretti C, Rella A, et al. The role of procalcitonin in neonatal intensive care unit patients with candidemia. Folia Microbiol (Praha) 2013;58(1):27–31.
66. Oguz SS, Sipahi E, Dilmen U. C-reactive protein and interleukin-6 responses for differentiating fungal and bacterial aetiology in late-onset neonatal sepsis. Mycoses 2011;54(3):212–6.
67. Berenguer J, Buck M, Witebsky F, et al. Lysis-centrifugation blood cultures in the detection of tissue-proven invasive candidiasis. Disseminated versus single-organ infection. Diagn Microbiol Infect Dis 1993;17(2):103–9.
68. Thaler M, Pastakia B, Shawker TH, et al. Hepatic candidiasis in cancer patients: the evolving picture of the syndrome. Ann Intern Med 1988;108(1):88–100.
69. Alexander BD. Diagnosis of fungal infection: new technologies for the mycology laboratory. Transpl Infect Dis 2002;4(Suppl 3):32–7.
70. Marklein G, Josten M, Klanke U, et al. Matrix-assisted laser desorption ionization-time of flight mass spectrometry for fast and reliable identification of clinical yeast isolates. J Clin Microbiol 2009;47(9):2912–7.
71. Bader O, Weig M, Taverne-Ghadwal L, et al. Improved clinical laboratory identification of human pathogenic yeasts by matrix-assisted laser desorption ionization time-of-flight mass spectrometry. Clin Microbiol Infect 2011;17(9): 1359–65.
72. Sendid B, Ducoroy P, Francois N, et al. Evaluation of MALDI-TOF mass spectrometry for the identification of medically-important yeasts in the clinical laboratories of Dijon and Lille hospitals. Med Mycol 2013;51(1):25–32.
73. Stone NR, Gorton RL, Barker K, et al. Evaluation of PNA-FISH yeast traffic light for rapid identification of yeast directly from positive blood cultures and assessment of clinical impact. J Clin Microbiol 2013;51(4):1301–2.
74. Calderaro A, Martinelli M, Motta F, et al. Comparison of peptide nucleic acid fluorescence in situ hybridization assays with culture-based matrix-assisted laser desorption/ionization-time of flight mass spectrometry for the identification of bacteria and yeasts from blood cultures and cerebrospinal fluid cultures. Clin Microbiol Infect 2013;20:O468–75.
75. Aittakorpi A, Kuusela P, Koukila-Kahkola P, et al. Accurate and rapid identification of Candida spp. frequently associated with fungemia by using PCR and the microarray-based Prove-it Sepsis assay. J Clin Microbiol 2012;50(11): 3635–40.
76. Balada-Llasat JM, LaRue H, Kamboj K, et al. Detection of yeasts in blood cultures by the Luminex xTAG fungal assay. J Clin Microbiol 2012;50(2):492–4.
77. Paolucci M, Foschi C, Tamburini MV, et al. Comparison between MALDI-TOF MS and FilmArray Blood Culture Identification panel for rapid identification of yeast from positive blood culture. J Microbiol Methods 2014;104:92–3.

78. Chang SS, Hsieh WH, Liu TS, et al. Multiplex PCR system for rapid detection of pathogens in patients with presumed sepsis - a systemic review and meta-analysis. PLoS One 2013;8(5):e62323.
79. Dunyach C, Bertout S, Phelipeau C, et al. Detection and identification of Candida spp. in human serum by LightCycler real-time polymerase chain reaction. Diagn Microbiol Infect Dis 2008;60(3):263–71.
80. Khlif M, Mary C, Sellami H, et al. Evaluation of nested and real-time PCR assays in the diagnosis of candidaemia. Clin Microbiol Infect 2009;15(7):656–61.
81. Poissy J, Sendid B, Damiens S, et al. Presence of Candida cell wall derived polysaccharides in the sera of intensive care unit patients: relation with candidaemia and Candida colonisation. Crit Care 2014;18(3):R135.
82. Held J, Kohlberger I, Rappold E, et al. Comparison of (1->3)-beta-D-glucan, mannan/anti-mannan antibodies, and Cand-Tec Candida antigen as serum biomarkers for candidemia. J Clin Microbiol 2013;51(4):1158–64.
83. Mikulska M, Calandra T, Sanguinetti M, et al. The use of mannan antigen and anti-mannan antibodies in the diagnosis of invasive candidiasis: recommendations from the Third European Conference on Infections in Leukemia. Crit Care 2010; 14(6):R222.
84. Alam FF, Mustafa AS, Khan ZU. Comparative evaluation of (1, 3)-beta-D-glucan, mannan and anti-mannan antibodies, and Candida species-specific snPCR in patients with candidemia. BMC Infect Dis 2007;7:103.
85. Oliveri S, Trovato L, Betta P, et al. Experience with the Platelia Candida ELISA for the diagnosis of invasive candidosis in neonatal patients. Clin Microbiol Infect 2008;14(4):391–3.
86. Mularoni A, Furfaro E, Faraci M, et al. High levels of beta-D-glucan in immunocompromised children with proven invasive fungal disease. Clin Vaccine Immunol 2010;17(5):882–3.
87. Goudjil S, Kongolo G, Dusol L, et al. (1-3)-beta-D-glucan levels in candidiasis infections in the critically ill neonate. J Matern Fetal Neonatal Med 2013;26(1):44–8.
88. Mackay CA, Ballot DE, Perovic O. Serum 1,3-betaD-glucan assay in the diagnosis of invasive fungal disease in neonates. Pediatr Rep 2011;3(2):e14.
89. Onishi A, Sugiyama D, Kogata Y, et al. Diagnostic accuracy of serum 1,3-beta-D-glucan for pneumocystis jiroveci pneumonia, invasive candidiasis, and invasive aspergillosis: systematic review and meta-analysis. J Clin Microbiol 2012;50(1): 7–15.
90. Smith PB, Benjamin DK Jr, Alexander BD, et al. Quantification of 1,3-beta-D-glucan levels in children: preliminary data for diagnostic use of the beta-glucan assay in a pediatric setting. Clin Vaccine Immunol 2007;14(7):924–5.
91. Mokaddas E, Burhamah MH, Khan ZU, et al. Levels of (1->3)-beta-D-glucan, Candida mannan and Candida DNA in serum samples of pediatric cancer patients colonized with Candida species. BMC Infect Dis 2010;10:292.
92. Pappas PG, Kauffman CA, Andes D, et al. Clinical practice guidelines for the management of candidiasis: 2009 update by the Infectious Diseases Society of America. Clin Infect Dis 2009;48(5):503–35.

Staphylococcal Infections in Infants

Updates and Current Challenges

Ana C. Blanchard, MDCM[a], Caroline Quach, MD, MSc, FRCPC[b,c,d],
Julie Autmizguine, MD, MHS, FRCPC[a,e,f,*]

KEYWORDS

- Coagulase-negative staphylococci • *Staphylococcus aureus* • Infants
- Neonatal intensive care unit • Sepsis • Bloodstream infection • Resistance
- Heteroresistance

KEY POINTS

- Staphylococci are a leading cause of late-onset sepsis in infants.
- Coagulase-negative staphylococcal definition needs harmonization.
- Emergence of antibiotic resistance affects choice of empirical antibiotic therapy.

INTRODUCTION

Staphylococci are common pathogens in the neonatal period, especially after 3 days of life, causing up to 90% of late-onset sepsis (LOS) in hospitalized infants.[1,2] *Staphylococcus aureus* (SA) represents around 10% of LOS, whereas the proportion of coagulase-negative staphylococci (CoNS) ranges from 30% to 60%.[1,3,4] Variability in rates of CoNS sepsis is partly explained by inconsistent definitions in the literature and clinical practice. Establishing the diagnosis of a CoNS sepsis is challenging, because of the difficulty in discriminating culture contamination from true infection.

Disclosure Statement: The authors have indicated they have no financial relationships relevant to this article to disclose.
[a] Department of Pediatrics, CHU Sainte Justine, University of Montreal, 3175 Chemin Côte Sainte-Catherine, Montreal, Quebec H3T 1C5, Canada; [b] Division of Infectious Diseases, Department of Medical Microbiology, The Montreal Children's Hospital, McGill University Health Centre, 2300 Tupper Street, Suite C1242, Montreal, Quebec H3H 1P3, Canada; [c] Department of Pediatrics, The Montreal Children's Hospital, McGill University Health Centre, 2300 Tupper Street, Suite C1242, Montreal, Quebec H3H 1P3, Canada; [d] Department of Epidemiology, Biostatistics and Occupational Health, McGill University, 1020 Pine Avenue West, Montreal, Quebec H3A 1A2, Canada; [e] Department of Pharmacology, University of Montreal, 2900 Boulevard Edouard-Montpetit, Montreal, Quebec H3T 1J4, Canada; [f] Research Center CHU Sainte-Justine, 3175 Chemin Côte Sainte Catherine, Montreal, Quebec H3T 1C5, Canada
* Corresponding author.
E-mail address: julie.autmizguine@umontreal.ca

Staphylococcal infections are associated with prolonged hospitalization, mortality, and neurodevelopmental impairment (NDI).[5] Treatment is increasingly complicated by the emergence of antibiotic resistance. The prevalence of methicillin-resistant SA (MRSA) has been reported as less than 1% to 8% among all infants in neonatal intensive care units (NICUs), with wide variations across NICUs,[6,7] and more recently, the emergence of vancomycin resistance in SA and CoNS has challenged treatment even further,[8–10] especially in infants for whom safety and effectiveness of new antistaphylococcal drugs are not well established.

In this article, the changing epidemiology and the challenges of diagnosing and treating neonatal staphylococcal infections in the NICUs are discussed. A better understanding of the current data will help optimize management of infants and identify areas of prevention and future research.

EPIDEMIOLOGY

Humans are the principal reservoir of staphylococci. Staphylococcal acquisition occurs directly via contact of hands or body fluids from colonized individuals.[11] Transmission can also occur via indirect contact of colonized objects including stethoscopes, clothing, and equipment.[11] Staphylococci from the infant's skin may cause infection, typically after disruption of the skin or integrity of the mucosal membranes with catheters and tubes.[11] It has been suggested since the 1960s that health care workers are a major source of staphylococcal infection, but recent data have shown that maternal colonization also increases the risk of newborn staphylococcal colonization, through vertical transmission and breastfeeding.[12,13]

Staphylococcus aureus

Prevalence/incidence and risk factors
SA frequently colonizes infants, with up to 50% colonization rates in the first days of life.[1,14–16] SA is a rare cause of early-onset sepsis (EOS) (<1%) and responsible for 8% to 15% of LOS.[4] Over a period of 10 years, a study[16] showed a slight but significant increase in SA bacteremia (0.91% in 2000–2003 and 1.73% in 2004–2009, $P<.001$) in the NICU.

MRSA is an increasing concern, representing up to 55% of SA infections in NICUs.[16–19] MRSA incidence is increasing as reported by the Centers for Disease Control and Prevention's (CDC) National Nosocomial Infections Surveillance system (0.7–3.1 per 10,000 infants infected from 1995 to 2004).[19] Thirty percent of participating NICUs had no MRSA infections, indicating that differences in geographic location, hospital-specific infection control policy, and compliance to preventive measures may contribute to variation in infection rates.[19]

Infants with MRSA and meticillin-susceptible SA (MSSA) infection were shown to have similar gestational age (GA) and birth weight (BW).[20,21] However, those with MRSA infection tended to be younger at time of diagnosis compared with those with MSSA (median age of 23 vs 32 days, $P = .03$).[20] In addition to postnatal age, MRSA colonization was also shown to increase the risk of MRSA infection (relative risk: 2.64; 95% confidence interval [CI]: 2.34–2.98).[6]

Outcomes
Overall, SA-related mortality ranges from 5% to 18%, but it is as high as 25% in very low BW infants (VLBW; <1500 g BW).[14,16,18,21,22] In a study conducted in 20 US NICUs,[14] MRSA and MSSA infections were associated with similar mortality (26% and 24%, respectively) and morbidity in VLBW infants. In contrast, a study including all infants admitted to 17 Australian NICUs[22] observed a higher

mortality for MRSA than MSSA infection (25% vs 10%, P<.001). However, mortality related to EOS caused by MSSA was higher (39%) than with LOS caused by MSSA (7%).[22] When compared with a group of controls (infants with no positive MRSA cultures), MRSA colonization and infection were both associated with increased morbidity and financial burden but were not independently associated with mortality (colonization: hazard ratio [HR] 0.9; 95% CI 0.5–1.5; infection: HR 1.1; 95% CI 0.7–1.8).[23] NDI has been described in 18% to 37% of infants with previous SA infection.[21]

Coagulase-Negative Staphylococci

Prevalence/incidence and risk factors

CoNS, especially *S. epidermidis*, are ubiquitous on healthy human skin. By 4 days of life, 83% of infants are colonized with CoNS, and rates increase to nearly 100% after 2 weeks.[24] Two percent to 22.5% of EOS are caused by CoNS.[3,25,26] After 3 days of life, up to 10% of VLBW infants develop CoNS sepsis, and 50% of late-onset bloodstream infections (BSI) are caused by CoNS.[1,4,27,28] In blood cultures, most commonly identified CoNS species are *S. epidermidis*, *S. haemolyticus*, *S. warneri*.[29] The increase in CoNS sepsis incidence is believed to be related to improved survival, prolonged hospitalization of premature infants, and increasing need for invasive procedures.[1,30,31]

Infants born prematurely are at increased risk of CoNS sepsis,[32–34] presumably because of the lack of an efficient immune response. However, prematurity is also associated with longer hospital stay, more invasive iatrogenic procedures, including central line (CL), which are risk factors for CoNS sepsis.[32] Of all CL types, umbilical catheters were associated with higher BSI rates (rate ratio 2.4; 95% CI 1.2–4.9).[35] The number of venous CLs in place before the occurrence of sepsis was also identified as a risk factor for CoNS infection (odds ratio 3.5; 95% CI: 1.4–8.3 for each additional CL inserted).[32] The contribution of CL dwell time to the risk of CoNS sepsis is not consistent across studies; a few suggested that longer dwell time was a risk factor.[35,36] In a retrospective study of 21 cases of BSI, the BSI incidence increased by 4% per day in the first 18 days after peripherally inserted central catheter (PICC) insertion (incidence rate ratio (IRR) 1.14; 95% CI: 1.04–1.25) and by 33% per day at 36 to 60 days after PICC insertion (IRR: 1.33; 95% CI: 1.12–1.57).[36] However, other studies did not identify duration of CL as a risk factor.[32,37,38] Therefore, CLs should be removed as soon as possible when they are no longer needed, but elective replacement of CL is not recommended as a preventive strategy.[32,37,39]

Despite numerous epidemiologic studies reporting neonatal CoNS sepsis rates, the burden and trend of CoNS-related disease are difficult to assess, because of inconsistent definitions across studies (**Box 1**). A positive blood culture can reflect catheter or culture contamination rather than true infection, potentially leading to overestimation and high variability in CoNS sepsis rates. Nonetheless, 1 study[34] observed no difference in mortality between infants with definite, probable and possible CoNS infections (see **Box 1**).

Outcomes

Mortality after CoNS sepsis was estimated at 1.6% to 8% lower than sepsis caused by gram-negative rods or *Candida* sp.[18,33,40] CoNS BSI has been associated with increased morbidity, including intraventricular hemorrhage, retinopathy of prematurity, bronchopulmonary dysplasia, and cerebral palsy.[25,41,42] Moreover, CoNS sepsis has been shown to increase the incidence of NDI in VLBW infants.[43] However, these

---

Box 1
Definitions of coagulase-negative *Staphylococcus* sepsis in infants

CDC–National Healthcare Safety Network[46]

2 positive blood cultures drawn on separate occasion within 48 hours

and appropriate treatment

and 1 or more signs/symptoms:

  Fever (>38°C, rectal)

  Hypothermia (<37°C, rectal)

  Apnea or bradycardia

and signs, symptoms, and laboratory results not related to an infection at another site

National Institute of Child Health and Human Development–Neonatal Research Network[4]

Definite

  2 positive blood cultures drawn within 48 hours

  or 1 positive blood culture and increased C-reactive protein levels (>1 mg/L) within 48 hours of blood culture

Possible

  1 positive blood culture

  and treatment with vancomycin, oxacillin, or a semisynthetic antistaphylococcal agent for 5 or more days

Australasian Study Group for Neonatal Infections[33]

1 positive blood culture

and clinical sepsis

and abnormal hematology test (high or low peripheral neutrophil count or abnormal immature/total white cell ratio, or thrombocytopenia <150 × 10^9/L)

Others[3,34]

Definite

  2 positive blood cultures on the same day

Probable

  2 positive blood cultures within 4 days

  or 3 positive blood cultures within 7 days

  or 4 positive blood cultures within 10 days

Possible

  Positive blood cultures that do not meet criteria for definite or probable CoNS infection above

---

results were not confirmed in a more recent study including premature infants.[44] Again, these inconsistent results may reflect differences in definitions of CoNS sepsis in the literature. CoNS infection in VLBW infants was also associated with prolongation of hospital stay (approximately of 7 days longer) and increase in care costs ($6000–$12,000).[5]

CLINICAL MANIFESTATIONS AND DIAGNOSIS

Staphylococcal infection may present as bacteremia, skin and soft tissue infection, bone and joint infection, endocarditis, and meningitis.[18] SA is more likely to present as disseminated disease, whereas CoNS presents mainly as BSI.[18,28,34] Manifestations of staphylococcal infections are nonspecific and frequently indistinguishable from neonatal sepsis caused by other organisms.[27]

Staphylococcus aureus

Diagnosis of SA sepsis relies on a positive culture from a normally sterile body site. Because SA is associated with disseminated disease, bacteremia should prompt investigation to rule out secondary pyogenic foci, especially if more than 1 blood culture is positive.[18] Among neonates with SA bacteremia, 46% were shown to have a second SA focus of infection, including superficial abscess, cellulitis, and osteoarticular infection.[45] Those infants tended to be older (median age 12 vs 5 days; $P = .02$) and had longer duration of illness before presentation (4 vs 2 days; $P = .04$) compared with infants with only SA bacteremia.[45]

Coagulase-Negative Staphylococci

Diagnosis of CoNS sepsis is challenging, because isolation of CoNS from a single blood culture may reflect CL colonization or culture contamination. Some evidence supports the use of 2 positive blood cultures within 48 hours to establish a diagnosis; however, doubling the quantity of blood drawn in precarious infants may affect adherence to recommendations.[46,47] A single positive blood culture is sometimes considered as sufficient in the presence of signs and symptoms of sepsis or laboratory results that indicate infection, such as white blood cell levels greater than $20,000/mm^3$ or less than $5000/mm^3$, platelet levels less than $150,000/mm^3$, or increased C-reactive protein levels at 24 to 48 hours of presentation (>12 mg/L).[48,49]

Conflicting definitions (see **Box 1**) have resulted in inconsistent practice and possible inappropriate use of antibiotics, such as overuse of vancomycin.[2,50] This lack of consensus was shown by a multicenter survey of neonatologists,[51] in which 83% obtained 1 blood culture from infants with suspected sepsis without a CL and 50% of clinicians routinely interpreted a single positive blood culture to indicate sepsis and completed a course of antimicrobial therapy. In cases in which 2 blood cultures were obtained and 1 grew CoNS, nearly half of neonatologists completed a full course of antimicrobial therapy.[51]

RESISTANCE
Methicillin Resistance

Methicillin resistance in SA is mediated through the staphylococcal chromosomal cassette (SCC) *mecA*, which codes for an altered penicillin-binding protein (PBP2a), leading to reduced affinity for β-lactam antibiotics.[52] Two types of MRSA clones infect and colonize infants; community-associated MRSA (CA-MRSA) and hospital-associated MRSA (HA-MRSA). CA-MRSA clones carry a different SCCmec, show less resistance to multiple classes of agents, and more frequently produce the Panton-Valentine leukocidin.[53] Molecular analysis of MRSA isolates showed a shift from HA-MRSA to CA-MRSA from 2001 to 2008 in the NICU.[54,55] Although distinguishing CA-MRSA from HA-MRSA is important to guide therapy and prevention strategies, the impact of this changing epidemiology on clinical outcomes is unknown.

β-Lactams are not typically used as empirical therapy for CoNS, because of frequent methicillin resistance (80%).[56]

Vancomycin Resistance

Reduced susceptibility to vancomycin has emerged as a new therapeutic challenge in both SA and CoNS. Transfer of *vanA* gene from Enterococci to SA is believed to be the underlying mechanism of vancomycin-resistant SA (VRSA).[8] No cases of VRSA have been reported in infants.

In vancomycin-intermediate SA (VISA), decreased susceptibility is believed to be related to thickening of the cell wall, leading to trapping of vancomycin molecules.[57–59] Decreased glycopeptide susceptibility can manifest as heteroresistance, found in SA (hVISA) and CoNS. Heteroresistance indicates that within a single isolate cultured from a clinical specimen, lies a minor subpopulation of staphylococci with a minimum inhibitory concentration (MIC) in the intermediate range, whereas the vancomycin MIC for the whole bacterial population remains susceptible.[47,60] There has been no report of hVISA infection in infants, but cases of infections with heteroresistant CoNS have been described.[9,10] Infants are at increased risk of colonization with heteroresistant CoNS when exposed to vancomycin for greater than 10 days.[61] The clinical significance of glycopeptide heteroresistance in staphylococci has not been well established, but heteroresistant staphylococci may cause prolonged bacteremia (≥7 days) and refractory thrombocytopenia and have been possibly associated with increased mortality in small, retrospective studies.[62,63] Vancomycin heteroresistance may not be initially apparent with standard laboratory susceptibility testing, and suspicion should arise when an infant has persistent bacteremia despite vancomycin therapy and removal of CLs.

TREATMENT

Duration of antibiotic therapy is mainly derived from empirical observations and experts' opinion and depends on the type of infection and clinical response. It ranges from 7 days in uncomplicated BSI to 4 to 6 weeks in osteoarticular infections.[64]

Antistaphylococcal Penicillin

Oxacillin or nafcillin represent first-line therapy for MSSA. Although limited data have been reported on pharmacokinetics (PK), safety, and efficacy in infants, clinicians have extensive experience with dosing recommended in **Table 1**.[64]

Vancomycin

For neonatal MRSA and CoNS infections, vancomycin is the recommended first-line therapy.[65] Multiple studies have described vancomycin PK, resulting in different dosing strategies based on postmenstrual age or serum creatinine levels.[66] Most of those dosing strategies yield similar vancomycin serum trough concentrations, and there is no evidence that 1 regimen is superior.[66] In addition to this lack of consensus on initial dosing recommendations, optimal trough concentrations are unknown in infants. Adult guidelines for invasive MRSA recommend targeting a vancomycin 24-hour area under the curve (AUC)/MIC greater than 400, which was found to be associated with better outcome.[65] For adults, this target is usually achieved with troughs of 15 to 20 mg/L. However, recent data have suggested that lower troughs (7–10 mg/L) are associated with adequate

Table 1					
Dosing of antistaphylococcal agents in infants					
			Dose	Dosing Interval (h)	References
Oxacillin/ nafcillin	**Weight (kg)**	**Postnatal age (d)**			64
	<1.2	0–28	25–50 mg/kg/dose	12	
	1.2–2	0–7	IV or IM	12	
		>7		8	
	>2	0–7		8	
		>7		6	
Vancomycin	**Postnatal age (d)**				66,78
	0–7		Loading dose: 15 mg/kg/dose IV	12–24	
	>7		Maintenance dose: 10 mg/kg/dose IV	6–8	
Clindamycin	**Postmenstrual age (wk)**				69
	≤32		5 mg/kg/dose IV	8	
	>32–40		7 mg/kg/dose IV		
	>40–60		9 mg/kg/dose IV		
Linezolid	**GA (wk)**	**Postnatal age (d)**			71,79
	≤34	0–7	10 mg/kg/dose IV or orally	12	
		>7		8	
	≥35	All		8	

Abbreviations: IM, intramuscularly; IV, intravenously.

AUC_{0-24} exposure in children.[45,67] In infants, the relationship between vancomycin trough and AUC is not well characterized, but a recent PK study[68] showed that troughs of 10 mg/L or greater were predictive of an AUC_{0-24} greater than 400 mg.h/L. For CoNS, no specific target exposure has been established. To improve safe and effective use of vancomycin, further studies are needed to establish optimal vancomycin trough concentrations and more standardized initial dosing regimens.

Clindamycin

Clindamycin is recommended as an alternative to vancomycin in neonatal MRSA infection caused by susceptible isolates.[65] Recently, a large PK study across the pediatric age range, including infants,[69] yielded clindamycin age-based dosing recommendations (see **Table 1**). This dosing regimen was selected to match adult exposure after recommended dosing for treatment of MRSA infection.[65]

Linezolid

Linezolid is the alternative choice against staphylococci with decreased vancomycin susceptibility.[70] A PK study[71] suggested that in infants older than 7 days, dosing of 10 mg/kg every 8 hours would achieve similar systemic exposure as in adults with conventional dosing. Because of lower clearance in the first week of life, it was hypothesized that dosing of 10 mg/kg every 12 hours would be sufficient, but this regimen still needs validation.[71] Safety and efficacy of 10 mg/kg every 8 hours have been reported in infants with gram-positive infections (80%

were staphylococci).[70] Pathogen eradication was similar to vancomycin, whereas adverse events, including abnormal kidney function and oral/skin candidiasis, were less frequent with linezolid (32% vs 12%; $P = .06$).[70] Although the findings were not statistically significant, thrombocytopenia occurred more frequently with linezolid (5% vs 0%; $P = .34$), which is consistent with adult data.[70,72] This reversible toxicity generally occur after 2 weeks of therapy and is especially concerning in infants with platelets already low because of sepsis. In an open-label trial of linezolid versus vancomycin in 63 infants,[73] no significant differences were noted in thrombocytopenia (linezolid, 1.9% vs vancomycin, 0%; $P = .17$) or other drug-related hematologic events. In the 2 trials described earlier, mean linezolid treatment duration was less than 2 weeks. More data are needed on linezolid safety for infants who need treatment longer than 2 weeks, or in those with marked thrombocytopenia caused by sepsis.

Novel Antistaphylococcal Antibiotics

Recent developments in antistaphylococcal antibiotics have led to approval of daptomycin, quinupristin/dalfopristin, telavancin, tigecycline, ceftaroline, and dalbavancin for treatment of MRSA infections in adults. Of those antibiotics, daptomycin is the only drug for which PK and safety data in infants are available,[74] but data remain limited, and routine use of this antibiotic is not recommended. Pediatric trials are ongoing for ceftaroline, telavancin, daptomycin, and dalbavancin; however, none of these studies includes infants.

Empirical Therapy

Empirical therapy for suspected staphylococcal infection (antibiotic therapy while awaiting culture results) is not universally accepted. Although it may improve outcomes in infants who are truly infected, it also increases antibiotic exposure and contributes to the emergence of antibiotic resistance.[75] Appropriate agents for empirical antibiotic therapy depend on clinical characteristics and local susceptibility patterns. Limited data are available on the impact of empirical therapy on neonatal outcomes.

A 10-year review of LOS in a NICU[76] showed that CoNS infections are rarely fulminant and that duration of sepsis did not change when clinicians stopped using empirical vancomycin therapy. Similarly, a large retrospective cohort of infants,[77] from 348 US NICUs, showed that empirical vancomycin for CoNS BSI did not significantly improve survival. In this study, no data were available on NDI outcomes.

For infants with MRSA sepsis, no data have been published on the impact of empirical vancomycin on clinical outcomes. Therefore, empirical use of vancomycin should be considered when MRSA is suspected.

SUMMARY

Staphylococci are a leading cause of sepsis in infants. Invasive staphylococcal disease is increasing in the NICU as a result of increased survival of premature infants and use of invasive procedure. For CoNS infection, the use of consistent definitions is critical in evaluating the epidemiology and risk factors, which allows appropriate preventive strategies. Emerging antibiotic resistance influences the use of empirical antibiotic therapy and creates the need for new antibiotics. Better evidence is needed regarding the safe and rational use of antibiotics in neonatal staphylococcal disease.

Best practices

What is the current practice?

Neonatal Staphylococcal Infections

Best Practice/Guideline/Care Path Objective(s)

- Promptly diagnose staphylococcal infections with cultures from infected body site
- Begin empirical antistaphylococcal antibiotics, based on local surveillance susceptibility patterns
- Decrease mortality and risk of long-term NDI

What changes in current practice are likely to improve outcomes?

- Distinguish true CoNS infection from culture contamination
- Rational use of antibiotics to prevent emerging resistant staphylococci
- Implementation of effective preventive measures, with systematic surveillance of staphylococcal infections and outcomes

Major Recommendations

- Perform cultures from normally sterile body sites in all neonates with symptoms of sepsis (grade 2A). Two distinct positive blood cultures for CoNS are required to confirm CoNS bacteremia diagnosis (grade 2B)
- The need for empirical therapy, while culture results are pending, should be assessed based on clinical presentation. Targeting *S. aureus* should be considered; however specific treatment of CoNS may warrant waiting for confirmation of infection (grade 3C)
- The following antistaphylococcal agents are recommended for first-line treatment of septic neonates with positive cultures:

    Oxacillin or nafcillin for MSSA (grade 2A)

    Vancomycin for MRSA and CoNS (grade 2A)

    Linezolid for staphylococci with decreased susceptibility to vancomycin (grade 2B)

- Failure to sterilize cultures from infected body site should prompt further investigation to rule out secondary pyogenic foci, and removal of central catheter (grade 2A)

Summary statement

Rigorous preventive measures, as well as rapid diagnosis and appropriate treatment, contribute to reduction of morbidity and mortality associated with staphylococcal infections in neonates.

Data from Refs.[18,47,80]

REFERENCES

1. Van den Hoogen A, Gerards LJ, Verboon-Maciolek MA, et al. Long-term trends in the epidemiology of neonatal sepsis and antibiotic susceptibility of causative agents. Neonatology 2010;97(1):22–8.
2. Stoll BJ, Gordon T, Korones SB, et al. Late-onset sepsis in very low birth weight neonates: a report from the National Institute of Child Health and Human Development Neonatal Research Network. J Pediatr 1996;129(1):63–71.
3. Hornik CP, Fort P, Clark RH, et al. Early and late onset sepsis in very-low-birthweight infants from a large group of neonatal intensive care units. Early Hum Dev 2012;88(Suppl 2):S69–74.

4. Stoll BJ, Hansen N, Fanaroff AA, et al. Late-onset sepsis in very low birth weight neonates: the experience of the NICHD Neonatal Research Network. Pediatrics 2002;110(2 Pt 1):285–91.

5. Payne NR, Carpenter JH, Badger GJ, et al. Marginal increase in cost and excess length of stay associated with nosocomial bloodstream infections in surviving very low birth weight infants. Pediatrics 2004;114(2):348–55.

6. Huang YC, Chou YH, Su LH, et al. Methicillin-resistant *Staphylococcus aureus* colonization and its association with infection among infants hospitalized in neonatal intensive care units. Pediatrics 2006;118(2):469–74.

7. McAdams RM, Ellis MW, Trevino S, et al. Spread of methicillin-resistant *Staphylococcus aureus* USA300 in a neonatal intensive care unit. Pediatr Int 2008;50(6): 810–5.

8. de Niederhausern S, Bondi M, Messi P, et al. Vancomycin-resistance transferability from VanA *enterococci* to *Staphylococcus aureus*. Curr Microbiol 2011; 62(5):1363–7.

9. Rasigade JP, Raulin O, Picaud JC, et al. Methicillin-resistant *Staphylococcus capitis* with reduced vancomycin susceptibility causes late-onset sepsis in intensive care neonates. PLoS One 2012;7(2):e31548.

10. Van Der Zwet WC, Debets-Ossenkopp YJ, Reinders E, et al. Nosocomial spread of a *Staphylococcus capitis* strain with heteroresistance to vancomycin in a neonatal intensive care unit. J Clin Microbiol 2002;40(7):2520–5.

11. Fonseca SN, Ehrenkranz RA, Baltimore RS. Epidemiology of antibiotic use in a neonatal intensive care unit. Infect Control Hosp Epidemiol 1994;15(3):156–62.

12. Jimenez-Truque N, Tedeschi S, Saye EJ, et al. Relationship between maternal and neonatal *Staphylococcus aureus* colonization. Pediatrics 2012;129(5):e1252–9.

13. Leshem E, Maayan-Metzger A, Rahav G, et al. Transmission of *Staphylococcus aureus* from mothers to newborns. Pediatr Infect Dis J 2012;31(4):360–3.

14. Shane AL, Hansen NI, Stoll BJ, et al. Methicillin-resistant and susceptible *Staphylococcus aureus* bacteremia and meningitis in preterm infants. Pediatrics 2012; 129(4):e914–22.

15. de Almeida Silva H, Steffen Abdallah VO, Carneiro CL, et al. Infection and colonization by *Staphylococcus aureus* in a high risk nursery of a Brazilian teaching hospital. Braz J Infect Dis 2003;7(6):381–6.

16. Dolapo O, Dhanireddy R, Talati AJ. Trends of *Staphylococcus aureus* bloodstream infections in a neonatal intensive care unit from 2000–2009. BMC Pediatr 2014;14:121.

17. Healy CM, Hulten KG, Palazzi DL, et al. Emergence of new strains of methicillin-resistant *Staphylococcus aureus* in a neonatal intensive care unit. Clin Infect Dis 2004;39(10):1460–6.

18. Healy CM, Palazzi DL, Edwards MS, et al. Features of invasive staphylococcal disease in neonates. Pediatrics 2004;114(4):953–61.

19. Lessa FC, Edwards JR, Fridkin SK, et al. Trends in incidence of late-onset methicillin-resistant *Staphylococcus aureus* infection in neonatal intensive care units: data from the National Nosocomial Infections Surveillance System, 1995–2004. Pediatr Infect Dis J 2009;28(7):577–81.

20. Carey AJ, Duchon J, Della-Latta P, et al. The epidemiology of methicillin-susceptible and methicillin-resistant *Staphylococcus aureus* in a neonatal intensive care unit, 2000–2007. J Perinatol 2010;30(2):135–9.

21. Cohen-Wolkowiez M, Benjamin DK Jr, Fowler VG Jr, et al. Mortality and neurodevelopmental outcome after *Staphylococcus aureus* bacteremia in infants. Pediatr Infect Dis J 2007;26(12):1159–61.

22. Isaacs D, Fraser S, Hogg G, et al. *Staphylococcus aureus* infections in Australasian neonatal nurseries. Arch Dis Child Fetal Neonatal Ed 2004;89(4):F331–5.
23. Song X, Perencevich E, Campos J, et al. Clinical and economic impact of methicillin-resistant *Staphylococcus aureus* colonization or infection on neonates in intensive care units. Infect Control Hosp Epidemiol 2010;31(2):177–82.
24. Goldmanln DA. Bacterial colonization and infection in the neonate. Am J Med 1981;70(2):417–22.
25. Mularoni A, Madrid M, Azpeitia A, et al. The role of coagulase-negative staphylococci in early onset sepsis in a large European cohort of very low birth weight infants. Pediatr Infect Dis J 2014;33(5):e121–5.
26. Stoll BJ, Hansen N, Fanaroff AA, et al. Changes in pathogens causing early-onset sepsis in very-low-birth-weight infants. N Engl J Med 2002;347(4):240–7.
27. Schmidt BK, Kirpalani HM, Corey M, et al. Coagulase-negative staphylococci as true pathogens in newborn infants: a cohort study. Pediatr Infect Dis J 1987;6(11):1026–31.
28. Sohn AH, Garrett DO, Sinkowitz-Cochran RL, et al. Prevalence of nosocomial infections in neonatal intensive care unit patients: results from the first national point-prevalence survey. J Pediatr 2001;139(6):821–7.
29. Raimundo O, Heussler H, Bruhn JB, et al. Molecular epidemiology of coagulase-negative staphylococcal bacteraemia in a newborn intensive care unit. J Hosp Infect 2002;51(1):33–42.
30. Bizzarro MJ, Raskind C, Baltimore RS, et al. Seventy-five years of neonatal sepsis at Yale: 1928–2003. Pediatrics 2005;116(3):595–602.
31. Verstraete E, Boelens J, De Coen K, et al. Healthcare-associated bloodstream infections in a neonatal intensive care unit over a 20-year period (1992–2011): trends in incidence, pathogens, and mortality. Infect Control Hosp Epidemiol 2014;35(5):511–8.
32. Healy CM, Baker CJ, Palazzi DL, et al. Distinguishing true coagulase-negative *Staphylococcus* infections from contaminants in the neonatal intensive care unit. J Perinatol 2013;33(1):52–8.
33. Isaacs D. A ten year, multicentre study of coagulase negative staphylococcal infections in Australasian neonatal units. Arch Dis Child Fetal Neonatal Ed 2003;88(2):F89–93.
34. Jean-Baptiste N, Benjamin DK Jr, Cohen-Wolkowiez M, et al. Coagulase-negative staphylococcal infections in the neonatal intensive care unit. Infect Control Hosp Epidemiol 2011;32(7):679–86.
35. Yumani DF, van den Dungen FA, van Weissenbruch MM. Incidence and risk factors for catheter-associated bloodstream infections in neonatal intensive care. Acta Paediatr 2013;102(7):e293–8.
36. Sengupta A, Lehmann C, Diener-West M, et al. Catheter duration and risk of CLA-BSI in neonates with PICCs. Pediatrics 2010;125(4):648–53.
37. Casado-Flores J, Barja J, Martino R, et al. Complications of central venous catheterization in critically ill children. Pediatr Crit Care Med 2001;2(1):57–62.
38. Greenberg RG, Cochran KM, Smith PB, et al. Effect of dwell time on central line associated bloodstream infection in infants. Presented at The Pediatric Academic Societies Annual Conference. Vancouver, May 4, 2014.
39. de Jonge RC, Polderman KH, Gemke RJ. Central venous catheter use in the pediatric patient: mechanical and infectious complications. Pediatr Crit Care Med 2005;6(3):329–39.
40. Benjamin DK, DeLong E, Cotten CM, et al. Mortality following blood culture in premature infants: increased with Gram-negative bacteremia and candidemia, but not Gram-positive bacteremia. J Perinatol 2004;24(3):175–80.

41. Schlapbach LJ, Aebischer M, Adams M, et al. Impact of sepsis on neurodevelopmental outcome in a Swiss National Cohort of extremely premature infants. Pediatrics 2011;128(2):e348–57.

42. Liljedahl M, Bodin L, Schollin J. Coagulase-negative staphylococcal sepsis as a predictor of bronchopulmonary dysplasia. Acta Paediatr 2004;93(2): 211–5.

43. Stoll BJ, Hansen NI, Adams-Chapman I, et al. Neurodevelopmental and growth impairment among extremely low-birth-weight infants with neonatal infection. JAMA 2004;292(19):2357–65.

44. Hemels MA, Nijman J, Leemans A, et al. Cerebral white matter and neurodevelopment of preterm infants after coagulase-negative staphylococcal sepsis. Pediatr Crit Care Med 2012;13(6):678–84.

45. Ladhani S, Konana OS, Mwarumba S, et al. Bacteraemia due to *Staphylococcus aureus*. Arch Dis Child 2004;89(6):568–71.

46. Horan TC, Andrus M, Dudeck MA. CDC/NHSN surveillance definition of health care-associated infection and criteria for specific types of infections in the acute care setting. Am J Infect Control 2008;36(9):655.

47. Struthers S, Underhill H, Albersheim S, et al. A comparison of two versus one blood culture in the diagnosis and treatment of coagulase-negative *Staphylococcus* in the neonatal intensive care unit. J Perinatol 2002;22(7): 547–9.

48. Ng PC, Cheng SH, Chui KM, et al. Diagnosis of late onset neonatal sepsis with cytokines, adhesion molecule, and C-reactive protein in preterm very low birth-weight infants. Arch Dis Child Fetal Neonatal Ed 1997;77(3):F221–7.

49. St Geme JW 3rd, Bell LM, Baumgart S, et al. Distinguishing sepsis from blood culture contamination in young infants with blood cultures growing coagulase-negative staphylococci. Pediatrics 1990;86(2):157–62.

50. Huang YC, Wang YH, Su LH, et al. Determining the significance of coagulase-negative staphylococci identified in cultures of paired blood specimens from neonates by species identification and strain clonality. Infect Control Hosp Epidemiol 2006;27(1):70–3.

51. Rubin LG, Sanchez PJ, Siegel J, et al. Evaluation and treatment of neonates with suspected late-onset sepsis: a survey of neonatologists' practices. Pediatrics 2002;110(4):e42.

52. Hiramatsu K, Cui L, Kuroda M, et al. The emergence and evolution of methicillin-resistant *Staphylococcus aureus*. Trends Microbiol 2001;9(10):486–93.

53. Methods for dilution antimicrobial susceptibility tests for bacteria that grow aerobically, 7th edition. Approved standard M7-A7. Wayne, PA: Clinical and Laboratory Standards Institute; 2006;26(2).

54. Carey AJ, Della-Latta P, Huard R, et al. Changes in the molecular epidemiological characteristics of methicillin-resistant *Staphylococcus aureus* in a neonatal intensive care unit. Infect Control Hosp Epidemiol 2010;31(6):613–9.

55. Seybold U, Halvosa JS, White N, et al. Emergence of and risk factors for methicillin-resistant *Staphylococcus aureus* of community origin in intensive care nurseries. Pediatrics 2008;122(5):1039–46.

56. Clinical and Laboratory Standards Institute. Performance standards for antimicrobial susceptibility testing: sixteenth informational supplement. M100–S16 methods for dilution antimicrobial susceptibility tests for bacteria that grow aerobically: Approved Standard. Wayne (PA): CLSI; 2006.

57. Hiramatsu K. Vancomycin resistance in staphylococci. Drug Resist Updat 1998; 1(2):135–50.

58. Cui L, Iwamoto A, Lian JQ, et al. Novel mechanism of antibiotic resistance originating in vancomycin-intermediate *Staphylococcus aureus*. Antimicrob Agents Chemother 2006;50(2):428–38.

59. Hiramatsu K. Vancomycin-resistant *Staphylococcus aureus*: a new model of antibiotic resistance. Lancet Infect Dis 2001;1(3):147–55.

60. Dunne WM Jr, Qureshi H, Pervez H, et al. *Staphylococcus epidermidis* with intermediate resistance to vancomycin: elusive phenotype or laboratory artifact? Clin Infect Dis 2001;33(1):135–7.

61. Center KJ, Reboli AC, Hubler R, et al. Decreased vancomycin susceptibility of coagulase-negative staphylococci in a neonatal intensive care unit: evidence of spread of *Staphylococcus warneri*. J Clin Microbiol 2003;41(10):4660–5.

62. Dimitriou G, Fouzas S, Giormezis N, et al. Clinical and microbiological profile of persistent coagulase-negative staphylococcal bacteraemia in neonates. Clin Microbiol Infect 2011;17(11):1684–90.

63. Wong SS, Ho PL, Woo PC, et al. Bacteremia caused by staphylococci with inducible vancomycin heteroresistance. Clin Infect Dis 1999;29(4):760–7.

64. Remington JS, Klein JO. Infectious diseases of the fetus and newborn, 7th edition. Philadelphia: Saunders/Elsevier; 2010.

65. Liu C, Bayer A, Cosgrove SE, et al. Clinical practice guidelines by the Infectious Diseases Society of America for the treatment of methicillin-resistant *Staphylococcus aureus* infections in adults and children. Clin Infect Dis 2011;52(3):e18–55.

66. de Hoog M, Mouton JW, van den Anker JN. Vancomycin: pharmacokinetics and administration regimens in neonates. Clin Pharmacokinet 2004;43(7):417–40.

67. Frymoyer A, Guglielmo BJ, Hersh AL. Desired vancomycin trough serum concentration for treating invasive methicillin-resistant staphylococcal infections. Pediatr Infect Dis J 2013;32(10):1077–9.

68. Frymoyer A, Hersh AL, Gaskari S, et al. What is the goal vancomycin trough for neonates with invasive MRSA? Poster Presentation. Presented at The Pediatric Academic Societies Annual Conference. Vancouver, May 3, 2014.

69. Gonzalez D, Melloni C, Yogev R, et al. Use of opportunistic clinical data and a population pharmacokinetic model to support dosing of clindamycin for premature infants to adolescents. Clin Pharmacol Ther 2014;96:429–37.

70. Deville JG, Adler S, Azimi PH, et al. Linezolid versus vancomycin in the treatment of known or suspected resistant gram-positive infections in neonates. Pediatr Infect Dis J 2003;22(Suppl 9):S158–63.

71. Kearns GL, Jungbluth GL, Abdel-Rahman SM, et al. Impact of ontogeny on linezolid disposition in neonates and infants. Clin Pharmacol Ther 2003;74(5):413–22.

72. Gerson SL, Kaplan SL, Bruss JB, et al. Hematologic effects of linezolid: summary of clinical experience. Antimicrob Agents Chemother 2002;46(8):2723–6.

73. Meissner HC, Townsend T, Wenman W, et al. Hematologic effects of linezolid in young children. Pediatr Infect Dis J 2003;22(Suppl 9):S186–92.

74. Cohen-Wolkowiez M, Watt KM, Hornik CP, et al. Pharmacokinetics and tolerability of single-dose daptomycin in young infants. Pediatr Infect Dis J 2012;31(9):935–7.

75. Ofek-Shlomai N, Benenson S, Ergaz Z, et al. Gastrointestinal colonization with ESBL-producing *Klebsiella* in preterm babies–is vancomycin to blame? Eur J Clin Microbiol Infect Dis 2012;31(4):567–70.

76. Karlowicz MG, Buescher ES, Surka AE. Fulminant late-onset sepsis in a neonatal intensive care unit, 1988–1997, and the impact of avoiding empiric vancomycin therapy. Pediatrics 2000;106(6):1387–90.

77. Ericson JE, Hornik CP, Thaden J, et al. Empirical vancomycin therapy for coagulase-negative staphylococcal sepsis in infants. Neonatology Poster session. Presented at The Pediatric Academic Societies Annual Conference. Vancouver, May 3, 2014.
78. Vancomycin [package insert]. Lake Forest IA-S, LLC. 2009. Available at: http://dailymed.nlm.nih.gov/dailymed/lookup.cfm?setid=622b9406-1c06-4323-8ca2-873cb9112dd4. Accessed November 24, 2014.
79. Linezolid [package insert]. Kalamazoo MPUC. 2002. Available at: http://dailymed.nlm.nih.gov/dailymed/lookup.cfm?setid=6e70e63b-bfd5-478d-a8ee-8ba22c9efabd. Accessed November 24, 2014.
80. Karlowicz MG, Furigay PJ, Croitoru DP, et al. Central venous catheter removal versus in situ treatment in neonates with coagulase-negative staphylococcal bacteremia. Pediatr Infect Dis J 2002;21(1):22–7.

Infectious Causes of Necrotizing Enterocolitis

Sarah A. Coggins, BA[a], James L. Wynn, MD[b], Jörn-Hendrik Weitkamp, MD[b,*]

KEYWORDS

- Necrotizing enterocolitis • Neonate • Bacteria • Virus • Fungi

KEY POINTS

- Necrotizing enterocolitis (NEC) is the most common cause of gastrointestinal morbidity and mortality in premature infants.
- The exact role of microbes in the pathogenesis of NEC is still incompletely understood.
- The presence of specific bacteria, viruses, and fungi has been associated with NEC predominantly in relatively rare outbreak situations.
- Aberrant bacterial colonization seems necessary for NEC development but is unlikely to cause disease by itself.
- Future studies are needed to determine how therapeutic interventions on microbial communities may prevent the development of NEC.

INTRODUCTION

Necrotizing enterocolitis (NEC) is the most common surgical emergency in premature infants, affecting approximately 7% of infants with less than 1500 g birth weights.[1] Universally described risk factors include prematurity, aberrant microbial colonization, and lack of human milk feeding.[2] NEC's clinical presentation is nonspecific and can range from signs limited to the gastrointestinal (GI) tract (eg, feeding intolerance, ileus, abdominal distention, hematochezia) to catastrophic illness with multiorgan failure (eg, lethargy, apnea, metabolic acidosis, shock, disseminated intravascular coagulopathy) and death.[3] Since its first mention in the medical

Disclosures: J.L. Wynn is supported by funding from the National Institutes of Health/National Institute of General Medical Sciences (NIH/NIGMS) GM106143. J.H. Weitkamp has been supported by award number K08HD061607 from the Eunice Kennedy Shriver National Institute of Child Health & Human Development (NIH/NICHD), the Vanderbilt University Medical Center's Digestive Disease Research Center sponsored by NIH grant P30DK058404 and CTSA award No. UL1TR000445 from the National Center for Advancing Translational Sciences (NCATS).

[a] Vanderbilt University School of Medicine, 2215 Garland Avenue, Nashville, TN 37232, USA;
[b] Department of Pediatrics, Monroe Carell Jr. Children's Hospital at Vanderbilt, Vanderbilt University, 2215 B Garland Avenue, 1125 MRB IV/Light Hall, Nashville, TN 37232, USA
* Corresponding author.
E-mail address: hendrik.weitkamp@vanderbilt.edu

Clin Perinatol 42 (2015) 133–154
http://dx.doi.org/10.1016/j.clp.2014.10.012   **perinatology.theclinics.com**

literature more than 150 years ago, NEC has stimulated intensive research in its cause; despite seminal discoveries of epidemiologic and molecular risk factors and pathways, the pathogenesis remains unclear.[4] One reason for the lack in progress is inclusion of diseases closely resembling classic NEC as a complication of preterm birth, such as spontaneous intestinal perforation (SIP), NEC in term infants, cow-milk intolerance, and viral enteritis.[5]

The role of bacteria as significant contributors to NEC has been identified since the first systematic descriptions of this disease.[6,7] Pneumatosis intestinalis and portal venous gas are pathognomonic radiographic signs of NEC[8] and thought to be caused by anaerobic bacteria, specifically clostridia.[9] Gram-negative bacteria have been most frequently associated with NEC, and the epithelial receptor and innate immune sensor Toll-like receptor (TLR) 4 is elevated in the premature intestine and required for the development of experimental NEC.[10,11] NEC can occur in clusters, and seasonal outbreaks of virus-associated NEC cases have been reported.[12–16] Here the authors attempted to summarize the main published data on the role of microbes in NEC.

BACTERIA

Bacteria are clearly involved in the pathogenesis of NEC (**Table 1**); despite the paucity of randomized control trials to determine the optimal antimicrobial regimen in premature infants, treatment with intravenous broad-spectrum antibiotics remains a mainstay of the clinical management.[17,18] However, many open questions remain, including the role of specific bacterial overgrowth as the cause or the consequence of NEC, timing of bacterial colonization during fetal/neonatal development, and type of molecular interactions between different microbes and their host.[19] Despite the abundance of bacteria in the premature intestine early in life[20] and the clinical appearance of gram-negative sepsis, a positive blood culture is uncommon in infants with NEC.[21,22] This finding is surprising given the frequent growth of bacteria in peritoneal fluid.[23] In 80 cases of NEC with intestinal perforation, *Enterobacteriaceae* were present in the peritoneal fluid in 75% of cases, coagulase-negative *Staphylococci*

Table 1		
Infectious causes of NEC		
Bacterial	**Viral**	**Fungal**
Clostridium spp	Astrovirus[15,184,185]	*Candida*
Butyricum[83–89]	Cytomegalovirus[163–165]	spp[194,197–199]
Difficile[76,79,80]	Coronavirus[167,168]	
Perfringens[61–68]	Coxsackievirus B2[176,177]	
Cronobacter (Enterobacter)	Echovirus[180]	
sakazakii[91,101–103,105]	Human immunodeficiency virus	
Enterococcus (VRE)[205]	(maternal exposure)[186–188]	
Escherichia coli[22,114,116–119]	Norovirus[16,147,149,150]	
Klebsiella spp[22,112–116]	Rotavirus[14,133–135]	
Pseudomonas aeruginosa[123–125]	Torovirus[170,171]	
Salmonella[206,207]		
Staphylococcus aureus (MRSA)[208]		
Staphylococcus epidermidis[48,212]		
Ureaplasma urealyticum[25,128,129]		

Abbreviations: MRSA, methicillin-resistant *Staphylococcus aureus*; VRE, vancomycin-resistant enterococci.

(CoNS) in 14%, and anaerobes in 6%.[23] Despite similar age at the time of intestinal perforation and similar mortality, the distribution of predominant organisms cultured from peritoneal fluid differed significantly between patients with NEC and SIP. *Candida* species (44%) and CoNS (50%) dominated samples from 36 patients with SIP.[23] Specific bacteria have been suggested as important contributing factors in NEC,[24,25] and NEC occurs typically after the first week post partum after the intestine has been colonized. In contrast, one study on human NEC samples using laser capture microdissection and subsequent sequencing combined with fluorescent in situ hybridization and bacterial rRNA-targeting oligonucleotide probes did not detect dominating potential pathogenic bacteria and suggested that NEC is a "non-infectious syndrome."[9]

Bacteria shape normal immune development including the development of T regulatory cells (Treg), which are critical for reducing inflammation-mediated injury.[26–29] Another example is recruitment of intestinal intraepithelial lymphocytes (IEL) after microbial colonization of germ-free mice.[30] IEL are reduced in human NEC suggesting that paucity of normal commensals in the newborn gut may alter intestinal immune development.[31] Infectious complications of pregnancy, such as chorioamnionitis, increase the risk for NEC either by direct bacterial colonization or through the anatomic and immunologic changes following the inflammatory challenge of the developing intestine.[25,32–36] Independent epidemiologic association between chorioamnionitis and NEC is difficult to prove, as chorioamnionitis is also the most important risk factor for prematurity and most severe NEC cases occur in extremely premature infants. However, after adjustment for antenatal steroid prophylaxis, gestational age, and surfactant treatment, the presence of intrauterine infection and the fetal inflammatory response syndrome (FIRS) remained independent predictors for NEC in several studies.[32,33] Increased gastric neutrophil counts have been demonstrated in chorioamnionitis-exposed preterm infants, reflecting a proinflammatory state of the gut shortly after birth.[37] Moreover, presence of microbes and inflammatory markers in the gut mirror that of the amniotic fluid when chorioamnionitis is present.[38] Preterm labor and chorioamnionitis are also linked with abnormal intestinal development and fetal proliferation of activated T cells in the immature intestinal mucosa.[35] At the same time, ileum Treg cell proportions are reduced in chorioamnionitis, whereas activated T effector cells are increased.[39,40] Reduced Treg proportions in the small intestinal lamina propria characterize NEC in human disease and in animal models, suggesting the possibility of bacteria-induced fetal immune priming as a risk factor for NEC.[41–43]

Gram-Positive Bacteria

The C-type lectin RegIIIγ and its human counterpart, hepatocarcinoma-intestine-pancreas/pancreatic-associated protein (HIP/PAP), are antimicrobial proteins that bind peptidoglycan, a molecule that is exposed on the surface of gram-positive bacteria. RegIIIγ expression is developmentally regulated and dependent on normal microbial ecology.[44] Although the exact role and developmental regulation of HIP/PAP is unknown in human infants, lower levels, especially in preterm infants, could lead to aberrant intestinal colonization with gram-positive bacteria.

Staphylococcus epidermidis

Colonization of the maternal genital tract with *Staphylococcus* sp has been associated with a significantly increased risk for chorioamnionitis (odds ratio 18.4).[33] The small intestine is colonized with staphylococci shortly after birth and in patients with or without NEC, specifically in infants delivered via cesarean section.[20,45] CoNS were found to preferentially translocate through the intestinal wall after ischemia-reperfusion injury in mice.[46] Importantly, a lack of enteral nutrition and exposure to total parenteral nutrition alone reduce intestinal barrier function.[47] CoNS are frequently cultured from postnatal stool samples and seem to increase the risk for NEC development.[48]

Clostridia species

Clostridia are spore-forming anaerobic motile gram-positive rods. They can be found in soil and the human GI tract and can be considered part of the normal intestinal flora in newborns, especially premature infants exposed to the neonatal intensive care unit (NICU) environment and infants fed formula.[49,50] Therefore, when isolated during disease, it is difficult to establish if they are pathogens or normal flora.[51] However, patients with NEC with positive cultures for Clostridia spp have more extensive pneumatosis intestinalis, a higher incidence of portal venous gas, faster progression to more severe necrosis, and intestinal perforation with higher mortality.[52,53] Clostridium spp were significantly more prevalent among samples from a preterm piglet model of NEC.[54] Clostridia spp have been implicated in NEC for many years because the clinical presentation of diseases caused by these toxin-producing strains often resemble NEC. For example, pseudomembranous colitis as a result of overgrowth of toxin-producing Clostridium difficile in the colon can present with hematochezia and multiorgan failure.[55] Enteritis necroticans, known as pigbel in Papua New Guinea, is a segmental necrotizing infection of the jejunum and ileum caused by Clostridium perfringens, type C.[56,57]

Clostridium perfringens

Clostridium perfringens frequently colonizes the intestine of preterm infants within the first 2 weeks post partum.[58] Clostridium perfringens types A to E form 12 different toxins: major toxins (eg, α-toxin = phospholipase C), collagenase, protease, hyaluronidase, deoxyribonuclease, enterotoxin, and neuraminidase.[59] Clostridium perfringens α-toxin is produced by all 5 types of bacteria (A–E); increases capillary permeability; induces platelet aggregation, hemolysis, and myonecrosis; decreases cardiac contractility; and is lethal.[60] Clostridium perfringens was identified as a causative agent of NEC in 22% of cases in one study.[61] Compared with the control group (n = 32), the onset of disease was earlier in life, portal venous gas was more common (77%), the clinical course was more severe, and the mortality rate was more than twice as high (44%).[61] Another study isolated Clostridium perfringens in patients with fatal outcomes and suggested it has the potential to trigger a fulminant and often lethal course.[62] Clostridium perfringens has been declared as a possible risk factor for NEC as it was recognized by molecular techniques in the first 2 weeks post partum in 3 infants who later developed the disease.[63] In one study, Clostridium perfringens was isolated from intestinal flora in 40% of infants with NEC compared with 13% of controls (P = .03)[64] and has been associated with an NICU outbreak of NEC in another.[65] Clostridium perfringens has also been associated with NEC in several animal models.[66–68]

Clostridium difficile

Clostridium difficile is part of the commensal intestinal flora in humans but has recently attracted the attention of researchers because of its role as the most common cause of severe and refractory health care–associated diarrhea.[69] After intestinal overgrowth following antimicrobial use, toxigenic strains can cause pseudomembranous colitis, ranging from mild diarrhea to fulminant colitis. Clostridium difficile's 2 major toxins, Clostridium difficile toxin A (TcdA) and Clostridium difficile toxin B (TcdB), disrupt host cell function by inactivating small GTPases that regulate the actin cytoskeleton.[70]

Both toxins can manifest disease on their own.[71] During infancy, asymptomatic colonization with toxin-producing *Clostridium difficile* is common and has been associated with changes in the intestinal microbiome composition.[58,72–75] Delivery or exposure to human flora has no effect on colonization, and *Clostridium difficile* originates from the NICU environment rather than maternal transmission.[76,77] The involvement of *Clostridium difficile* in NEC is controversial because toxin-producing *Clostridium difficile* strains are not more frequently recovered in NEC.[78] However, *Clostridium difficile–associated* NEC cases have been described during a *Clostridium difficile* outbreak.[79,80]

Clostridium butyricum

Clostridium butyricum produces butyric acid through fermentation and a specific strain (MIYAIRI 588 strain of *Clostridium butyricum*) is widely used as a probiotic in Asia.[81] It can be isolated from soil, feces of healthy children and adults, as well as soured milk and cheeses. Type E can produce a neurotoxin and has been implicated in cases of botulism.[82] Several reports state isolation of toxin-producing *Clostridium butyricum* from peritoneal fluid, blood, and cerebrospinal fluid of patients with NEC.[83] *Clostridium butyricum* has been suggested as the primary cause of NEC in outbreak situations; but because of a lack of adequate controls, its primary role has been questioned.[84,85] Isolation of *Clostridium butyricum* in blood samples of infants with NEC may have resulted from mucosal breakdown and transmigration of these bacteria into the bloodstream.[86] In a community analysis of bacteria found in tissue specimens from infants with NEC, the presence of *Clostridium butyricum* and *Clostridium parputrificum* highly correlated with histologic pneumatosis intestinalis.[21] *Clostridium butyricum* strains isolated from NEC cases can cause cecal lesions in animals with gas cysts, hemorrhagic ulceration, and necrosis.[87–89] Lactose fermentation and production of butyric acid seem to be a prerequisite, and colonization with bifidobacterium was protective.[67,90] Attachment of *Clostridium butyricum* to the ileal mucosa has been associated with NEC in preterm, cesarean-derived, and formula-fed piglets.[54]

Gram-Negative Bacteria

Cronobacter sakazakii

With a reported incidence of one infection per 10,660 very low birth weight (VLBW, <1500 g) infants,[91] *Cronobacter sakazakii* (formerly *Enterobacter sakazakii*)[92,93] infection is rare. *Cronobacter sakazakii* has been isolated from powdered infant formula worldwide,[94,95] and NICU outbreaks of invasive disease have been reported.[96–100] Meningitis is the most prominent clinical manifestation,[101] but outbreaks of NEC occurred in NICUs with isolation of *Cronobacter sakazakii* from multiple patients' body fluids and cans with powdered infant formula.[102,103] *Cronobacter sakazakii* is commonly found in soil, food items, and other environmental sources.[104] Therefore, inappropriate hygiene practices including storage, temperature control, and hand, nipple, and bottle cleaning after powdered formula reconstitution may contribute to infection. Powdered formula is not a sterile product, and the World Health Organization recommends formula reconstitution with hot water (>70°C) (http://www.who.int/foodsafety/publications/micro/pif2007/en/).

 Cronobacter sakazakii binds to villi in the distal small intestine and can induce NEC from a direct toxic effect to gut epithelium in the rat pup model.[105] *Cronobacter sakazakii*'s best-characterized virulence factor, outer membrane protein A (*ompA*), binds and invades human epithelial cells[103] and brain endothelial cells,[106–108] whereas its enterotoxin functions similarly to lipopolysaccharide (LPS) and modulates the activation of TLR 4.[109] *OmpA* also mediates recruitment of dendritic cells at the expense of neutrophils and macrophages leading to epithelial injury through transforming growth factor-β production and iNOS activation.[110,111]

Klebsiella species

Klebsiella sp have been described in NEC outbreaks with nosocomial origin.[112,113] It is also one of the most common organisms responsible for bacteremia in NEC.[22,114,115] A 1998 outbreak in Johannesburg was significant for isolation of a single clone of an extended-spectrum beta-lactamase–producing Klebsiella in blood cultures of patients with NEC, notable for sudden decompensation leading to shock and severe thrombocytopenia in all cases and for the absence of diarrhea or hematochezia.[112]

Escherichia coli

E coli is a similarly common organism found in normal gut flora; among infants with NEC, it has been isolated in blood in up to one-third of cases.[22,114] Both E coli and Klebsiella were isolated in feces at markedly higher rates in infants with NEC than those without.[116] Several outbreaks of NEC associated with E coli have been described.[117,118] In one report, 15 of 16 infants with suspected or confirmed NEC had either enterotoxigenic E coli or its heat-labile enterotoxin recovered in stool.[118] A report of NEC associated with E coli O157:H7 in a term infant resulted in death secondary to widespread intestinal necrosis.[119]

Pseudomonas

Pseudomonas is well known for its role in nosocomial and immunocompromised infections. It forms biofilms and can colonize hard surfaces and respiratory equipment, with mechanical ventilation as a risk factor for infection. However, Pseudomonas also colonizes the GI tracts of 10% to 42% of newborns[120,121] and 25% to 35% of normal adults.[122] Among VLBW infants, it is primarily responsible for late-onset disease (sepsis, pneumonia, NEC). There are several reports of Pseudomonas-associated NEC. A Taiwanese study reports 45 infants with Pseudomonas in the stool, of whom one had NEC, 4 had colonic perforations, and 2 infants died of sepsis.[123] Other studies noted an increased rate of NEC in infants with Pseudomonas bacteremia compared with nonbacteremic infants (36% vs 7%, respectively) and with it a much higher mortality rate (up to 50%), especially when signs of septic shock were present.[124,125]

Atypical Bacteria

Unique in their lack of a cell wall, Ureaplasma are obligate intracellular mycoplasma that colonize human adult genital tracts. They may be vertically transmitted intrapartum, with nasopharyngeal colonization reported among 22% of NICU patients.[126] Colonization is associated with chorioamnionitis,[127] a known risk factor for NEC. However, the existence of a direct relationship between colonization with Ureaplasma and development of NEC is controversial. One study found a 2-fold increase in incidence of stage 2 or greater NEC associated with elevated interleukin (IL)-6 and IL-1 beta among infants colonized with Ureaplasma (12.3% vs 5.5%).[25] Two other groups disagreed and found no increased incidence of NEC associated with Ureaplasma colonization.[128,129]

VIRUSES
Rotavirus

A double-stranded DNA member of the Reovirus family, rotavirus causes GI disease by invading enterocytes and disrupting their absorptive and digestive activities.[130] Fecal excretion of rotavirus can be found in up to half of infants in the newborn nursery.[131] Although most infants shed the virus asymptomatically, 8% to 30% of infants present with vomiting and diarrhea.[131,132] Rotavirus infection tends to peak in the late winter/early spring, though introduction of a vaccine in young children has interrupted this seasonality.[130] Several outbreaks of NEC have been associated with rotavirus infection with virus isolated from stool or serologic diagnosis and concomitant evidence of infection among a significant portion of NICU staff members.[133,134] Risk factors for the development of serious GI disease included low birth weight and younger age.[133] Notably, rotavirus-associated NEC has been found to cause less severe disease compared with NEC without rotavirus.[14] Anatomic distinctions were also noted: left-sided, more distal colonic pneumatosis intestinalis in rotavirus NEC compared with right-sided, ileal pneumatosis in nonrotavirus NEC.[14,135]

Norovirus

Norovirus (Norwalk virus), a nonenveloped positive-sense single-stranded RNA virus,[136] is the most important cause of foodborne outbreaks of gastroenteritis[137,138] and the second leading cause (after rotavirus) of gastroenteritis in young children.[139] Both individual infections and outbreaks most commonly occur during winter.[98] Seventeen percent of 75 premature infants less than 32 weeks' gestation shed the virus in their stool over the first 4 weeks after admission in a NICU in Sydney.[140] Norovirus prevalence was 1.9%, representing roughly half of all infants in that cohort who shed the virus.[140] Controversy exists regarding the best methods for viral identification, with one report noting several norovirus-positive cases by enzyme-linked immunosorbent assay that were not corroborated by reverse transcription polymerase chain reaction or electron microscopy.[141] The specificity of each aforementioned method is reportedly greater than 90%, and positivity in 2 of the 3 tests confirms norovirus infection.[142] Norovirus has been thought to primarily affect the small intestine based on pathologic findings of villus blunting, crypt hypertrophy, and edema among adults infected with norovirus[143–145] and mononuclear infiltrate and apoptosis in the jejunum and ileum of pediatric small bowel transplant recipients.[146] However, a recent report described 3 premature infants with norovirus infections with radiographic evidence of extensive colonic pneumatosis and pathologic insult (fibrosis and hyperplastic vessels) limited to the colon.[147] Apnea was noted as the primary presentation of norovirus infection in a preterm infant who subsequently developed watery diarrhea and positive stool cultures.[148] Several small outbreaks associated with NEC have been described. The largest involved 8 cases of NEC with a 25% mortality rate and noted that, in comparison with nonoutbreak NEC cases, those associated with norovirus had significantly lower levels of neutrophil band forms.[149] An outbreak of 8 cases of norovirus among premature infants was marked by abdominal distention, apnea, and increased gastric residuals. Vomiting and acute diarrhea were not predominant clinical features (27% and 0%, respectively), but one infant with proven norovirus developed NEC.[150] A case-control study noted an increased prevalence of norovirus in stools of infants with NEC compared with non-NEC controls (40% vs 9%, respectively) and suggested an etiologic role of norovirus in the pathogenesis of NEC.[16]

Cytomegalovirus

Cytomegalovirus (CMV), a double-stranded DNA herpesvirus, is well known to cause serious neonatal disease in its congenital form but has also been implicated in NEC. CMV transmission may occur via transplacental, intrapartum, or postpartum routes.

Rates of perinatal CMV infection in premature infants have been reported to be as high as 15% to 20%.[151,152] Given their immunocompromised status, premature infants are at particular risk for postnatal infection from breast milk (transmission rates 5%–37%)[153–155] or via transfused blood products.[156–159] Among immunocompromised patients, CMV enteritis is common and marked by diarrhea, hematochezia, and toxic megacolon.[160] In infants, however, CMV enteritis is unusual; the virus is a disputed player in the development of NEC. Patients may present with diarrhea or with disease resembling NEC but without distinguishing features, such as intestinal pneumatosis.[161] However, several case reports linking confirmed cases of NEC to CMV infections have been reported, with clinical manifestations including abdominal compartment syndrome,[162] viremia and sepsis,[163] and colonic strictures.[164] In one particularly severe case, fulminant NEC leading to death was associated with stool culture positive for CMV but with a notable reduction in diversity of bacterial flora, prompting speculation that intestinal CMV infection may predispose infants to NEC by altering intestinal immune responses and promoting secondary bacterial infection.[165]

Coronavirus (Torovirus)

Coronaviruses are enveloped viruses with positive-sense RNA genomes that are known to cause respiratory[166] and serious GI disease among infants.[167,168] A coronavirus outbreak was associated with hemorrhagic NEC, and viral particles were visualized both in intestinal and fecal specimens.[168] In another outbreak of NEC, coronavirus was detected in stool in 23 of 32 (72%) infants. Sixty percent of bedside nurses also shed the virus in stool, prompting speculation of nosocomial transmission.[167] As members of the coronavirus family, toroviruses are a known agent of diarrhea in cattle and horses and have been associated with GI disease in children. Torovirus infections are known to occur year-round, with a substantial portion thought to be acquired nosocomially.[169] Its association in neonatal disease was first described in 1982, when "virus-like particles" similar to coronavirus were detected in the stool of 80% of infants in an outbreak of bloody diarrhea, bilious gastric aspirates, and abdominal distention.[170] Transmission was thought to be vertical because all but one mother had flulike or GI symptoms within 2 weeks of delivery, and viral particles were detected in meconium of several infants.[170] One study reported the detection of torovirus in the stools of 48% of its patients with NEC and in 60% of those with stage III disease, although the presence or absence of torovirus did not affect mortality.[171]

Enteroviruses

Enteroviruses are positive-sense, single-stranded RNA viruses encompassing multiple serotypes, including 2 specific viruses that have been associated with NEC: coxsackievirus and echovirus. These infections are seasonal, with most cases occurring during summer and fall.[172–175] Among 27 infants with enterovirus, 3 had NEC marked by fevers, abdominal distention, and bloody diarrhea and one had coxsackievirus B and died following exploratory surgery revealing dusky jejunum.[176] Another fatal case of NEC associated with widespread coxsackievirus B infection demonstrated ischemic ileum with subserosal hemorrhage; the child's parents were both febrile at the time of birth.[177] The clinical presentation of echovirus infection among premature infants ranges from asymptomatic to diarrheal illness[178] to upper and lower respiratory tract infections.[179] An outbreak of echovirus type 22 in a NICU resulted in a diarrheal illness among 12 premature infants, 6 (50%) of whom developed stage I NEC and one had pneumatosis intestinalis, but all survived.

Identification of echovirus was via stool culture in most infants, though a few only had increased serum antibody titers.[180]

Astrovirus

As single-stranded RNA viruses, astroviruses were first described in infants during an outbreak of gastroenteritis in a newborn nursery.[181] Few reports on the pathology of human astrovirus infection are available, but one study in a child following bone marrow transplant revealed villous blunting and inflammatory cell infiltrate in the duodenum and jejunum (not consistent with graft-versus-host disease).[182] Alternatively, intestinal astrovirus infection in a turkey model leads to rearrangement of the actin cytoskeleton on ultrastructural examination and evidence of sodium malabsorption secondary to redistribution of sodium-hydrogen exchangers.[183] There are multiple reports associating astrovirus with NEC.[15,184,185] One report detected astrovirus in the stools of 6% of infants with either gastroenteritis or NEC. Infants with astrovirus more frequently acquired NEC (9 of 14) than those with norovirus (1 of 8) or rotavirus (2 of 12).[184] Compared with uninfected infants, those with astrovirus had increased hematochezia (54% vs 15%) and Bell stage II and III NEC (21% vs 4%).[185]

Human Immunodeficiency Virus

One case-control study suggests that maternal human immunodeficiency virus (HIV) infection places premature infants at higher risk for the development of NEC (at a rate of 8.8% vs 1.2% in children of HIV-positive and HIV-negative mothers, respectively).[186] Additional case reports describe development of NEC in 2 infants born to HIV-positive mothers; one infant also had trisomy 21.[187,188] All HIV-positive mothers received antiretroviral drugs during pregnancy and/or labor, and all infants received antiretrovirals after birth; no infant was HIV positive. The investigators speculate that the reduced production of IL-12 and/or use of zidovudine may have predisposed infants of HIV-positive mothers to NEC.[186]

FUNGI
Candida

Candida is a classically dimorphic organism that produces both yeast and hyphal forms, though certain species differ slightly (Candida glabrata does not form hyphae, and Candida parapsilosis forms pseudohyphae). In VLBW infants, fungal colonization occurs in the first week of life at an estimated rate of 27%, with Candida spp making up most of the organisms.[189] Candida albicans is isolated in more than 60% of cases of candidemia.[190] Among the NICU population, the risk factors for both colonization and invasive disease include the use of central venous lines, intravenous lipids, and histamine H_2 receptor antagonists.[191–193] It is unclear whether intestinal colonization with Candida spp is protective or a risk factor for NEC. In one study, none of 7 infants with NEC had viable fungal organisms detected in stool.[194] Further complicating the picture is the frequent association of Candida with SIP.[195,196] When Candida is linked to NEC, however, the results can be severe[197]; 27% of fatal cases of surgically treated NEC were associated with Candida sepsis, an outcome complicated by late diagnosis occurring either within 48 hours of death or at autopsy.[198] On pathologic examination of 84 patients with NEC, yeast and pseudohyphae were detected in both the intestinal lumen and wall.[199] Antifungal prophylaxis has been shown in a randomized controlled trial[200] to have benefit in reducing both colonization and invasive disease[201,202] but not NEC[201] or overall mortality.[203]

SUMMARY

NEC is a common and devastating problem for premature infants. Bacterial colonization seems to be a necessary but not sufficient contributor to NEC. Although intestinal pathogens may cause NEC-like illness in animal models or occasional clinical outbreaks, they are not detected in most cases of classic NEC.[204] NEC outbreaks have been associated with clusters of viral GI infections, but the clinical presentation may vary and often affect the large intestine. Future studies are needed to determine the impact of host-specific GI tract microbial communities on the development of NEC.

Best practices

What is the current practice?

NEC

The guidelines of the Surgical Infection Society and the Infectious Diseases Society of America recommend fluid resuscitation, bowel decompression, antimicrobial therapy, and surgical intervention (laparotomy or drainage) if needed.[18] Recommended antibiotics for complicated intra-abdominal infections in infants include combinations of ampicillin, gentamicin, and cefotaxime with or without anaerobic coverage with metronidazole, piperacillin-tazobactam, or meropenem.[17,18] In spite of their frequent use, the safety and efficacy of various antimicrobial combination treatment strategies for NEC has not been established in randomized controlled trials. The American Pediatric Surgical Association Outcomes and Clinical Trials Committee advises probiotics to decrease the incidence of NEC, and human milk should be used when possible.[209] They conclude that there is a lack of evidence-based data to support definitive recommendations for the type of surgical treatment or length of antimicrobial therapy.

What changes in current practice are likely to improve outcomes?

Prevention of NEC is the most effective strategy because once the disease becomes clinically evident, a mucosal and systemic inflammatory cascade has already been activated and multiorgan injury is likely. For the same reasons, earlier diagnosis of NEC before clinical onset is an important goal.[210]

Major recommendations

Medical management consists of bowel decompression, discontinuation of enteral feedings and medications, maintaining intravascular volume and electrolyte balance, and initiating broad-spectrum antibiotics based on known sensitivities of prevalent pathogens in the individual NICU. Typical regimens include ampicillin plus gentamicin to cover for common intestinal bacteria. Often the addition of a third antibiotic that provides more targeted anaerobic coverage (eg, clindamycin or metronidazole) is indicated when there is evidence of pneumatosis or bowel perforation. As an alternative, piperacillin-tazobactam may offer the advantage of broad-spectrum antimicrobial coverage including typical anaerobes of the intestinal flora. However, downsides are variable penetration into the cerebrospinal fluid and concerns for the emergence of drug resistance. Second-line therapy for severely ill infants can include meropenem and vancomycin in cases of positive cultures with resistant organisms, possible central nervous system infection, perforated bowel, and/or failed first-line or alternative therapy. Almost all of the drugs mentioned do not have a Food and Drug Administration label for use in this population because safety and efficacy data are lacking. Supportive management may require respiratory and blood pressure support and correcting anemia and thrombocytopenia and/or other coagulation defects. Serial abdominal radiographs are often recommended to monitor for intestinal pneumatosis, portal venous gas, and pneumoperitoneum. Early consultation with a pediatric surgeon is advised. Intestinal perforation or evidence of bowel necrosis is a common indication for operative management. As a preventive measure, a more consistent practice style including the implementation of early breast milk feedings, standardized feeding regimens, and reduction of unnecessary antibiotics is recommended.

Clinical algorithms

The management of patients with NEC (medical and/or surgical) can be guided by Bell staging criteria as reported recently by Sharma and Hudak[211] (**Fig. 1**).

Rating for the strength of the evidence

C (Recommendation based on consensus, usual practice, expert opinion, disease-oriented evidence, and case series for studies of diagnosis, treatment, prevention, or screening)

Summary statement

NEC is a multifactorial disease, but bacteria and other microorganisms have been uniformly implicated somewhere along the pathogenic process. Because no specific microorganism can be considered causative in most cases of NEC, broad-spectrum antimicrobial therapy remains a mainstay in NEC treatment. More research is needed to determine the optimum therapy and to develop effective strategies for NEC prevention.

Data from Refs.[17,18,209–211]

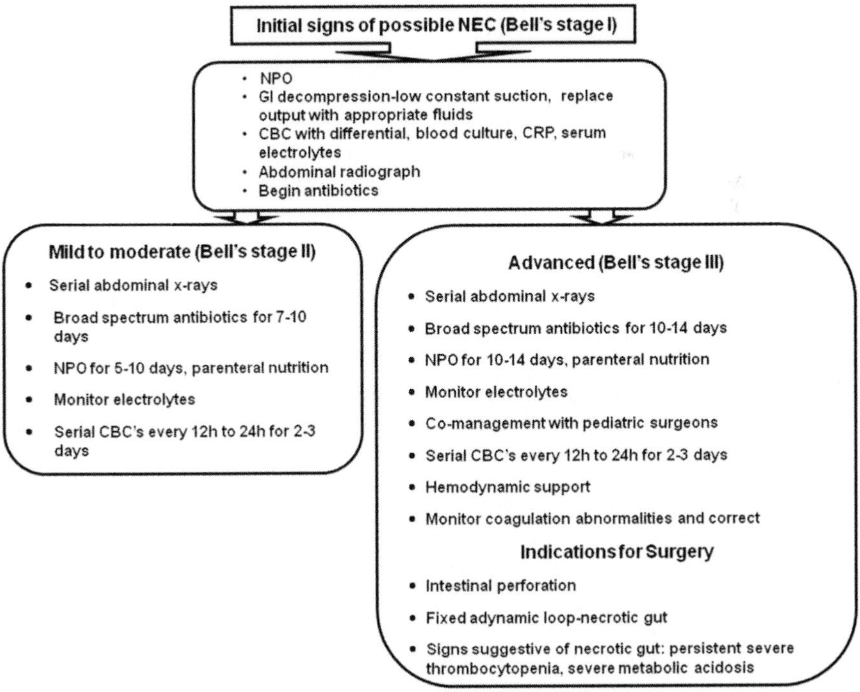

Initial signs of possible NEC (Bell's stage I)

- NPO
- GI decompression-low constant suction, replace output with appropriate fluids
- CBC with differential, blood culture, CRP, serum electrolytes
- Abdominal radiograph
- Begin antibiotics

Mild to moderate (Bell's stage II)

- Serial abdominal x-rays
- Broad spectrum antibiotics for 7-10 days
- NPO for 5-10 days, parenteral nutrition
- Monitor electrolytes
- Serial CBC's every 12h to 24h for 2-3 days

Advanced (Bell's stage III)

- Serial abdominal x-rays
- Broad spectrum antibiotics for 10-14 days
- NPO for 10-14 days, parenteral nutrition
- Monitor electrolytes
- Co-management with pediatric surgeons
- Serial CBC's every 12h to 24h for 2-3 days
- Hemodynamic support
- Monitor coagulation abnormalities and correct

Indications for Surgery

- Intestinal perforation
- Fixed adynamic loop-necrotic gut
- Signs suggestive of necrotic gut: persistent severe thrombocytopenia, severe metabolic acidosis

Fig. 1. Clinical decision algorithms. CBC, complete blood cell count; CRP, C-reactive protein; NPO, nil per os (nothing by mouth). (*Adapted from* Sharma R, Hudak ML. A clinical perspective of necrotizing enterocolitis: past, present, and future. Clin Perinatol 2013;40(1):27–51.)

REFERENCES

1. Lemons JA, Bauer CR, Oh W, et al. Very low birth weight outcomes of the National Institute of Child Health and Human Development Neonatal Research Network, January 1995 through December 1996. NICHD Neonatal Research Network. Pediatrics 2001;107(1):E1.
2. Neu J, Walker WA. Necrotizing enterocolitis. N Engl J Med 2011;364(3):255–64.
3. Kanto WP Jr, Hunter JE, Stoll BJ. Recognition and medical management of necrotizing enterocolitis. Clin Perinatol 1994;21(2):335–46.
4. Obladen M. Necrotizing enterocolitis–150 years of fruitless search for the cause. Neonatology 2009;96(4):203–10.
5. Gordon PV, Swanson JR, Attridge JT, et al. Emerging trends in acquired neonatal intestinal disease: is it time to abandon Bell's criteria? J Perinatol 2007;27(11):661–71.
6. Berdon WE, Grossman H, Baker DH, et al. Necrotizing enterocolitis in the premature infant. Radiology 1964;83:879–87.
7. Willi H. Über eine bösartige Enteritis bei Säuglingen des ersten Trimenons. Ann Pediatr 1944;162:87–112.
8. Buonomo C. The radiology of necrotizing enterocolitis. Radiol Clin North Am 1999;37(6):1187–98, vii.
9. Smith B, Bode S, Petersen BL, et al. Community analysis of bacteria colonizing intestinal tissue of neonates with necrotizing enterocolitis. BMC Microbiol 2011; 11:73.
10. Leaphart CL, Cavallo J, Gribar SC, et al. A critical role for TLR4 in the pathogenesis of necrotizing enterocolitis by modulating intestinal injury and repair. J Immunol 2007;179(7):4808–20.
11. Neal MD, Sodhi CP, Dyer M, et al. A critical role for TLR4 induction of autophagy in the regulation of enterocyte migration and the pathogenesis of necrotizing enterocolitis. J Immunol 2013;190(7):3541–51.
12. Snyder CL, Hall M, Sharma V, et al. Seasonal variation in the incidence of necrotizing enterocolitis. Pediatr Surg Int 2010;26(9):895–8.
13. Meinzen-Derr J, Morrow AL, Hornung RW, et al. Epidemiology of necrotizing enterocolitis temporal clustering in two neonatology practices. J Pediatr 2009; 154(5):656–61.
14. Sharma R, Garrison RD, Tepas JJ 3rd, et al. Rotavirus-associated necrotizing enterocolitis: an insight into a potentially preventable disease? J Pediatr Surg 2004;39(3):453–7.
15. Bagci S, Eis-Hubinger AM, Franz AR, et al. Detection of astrovirus in premature infants with necrotizing enterocolitis. Pediatr Infect Dis J 2008;27(4):347–50.
16. Stuart RL, Tan K, Mahar JE, et al. An outbreak of necrotizing enterocolitis associated with norovirus genotype GII.3. Pediatr Infect Dis J 2010;29(7):644–7.
17. Bell MJ, Ternberg JL, Bower RJ. The microbial flora and antimicrobial therapy of neonatal peritonitis. J Pediatr Surg 1980;15(4):569–73.
18. Solomkin JS, Mazuski JE, Bradley JS, et al. Diagnosis and management of complicated intra-abdominal infection in adults and children: guidelines by the Surgical Infection Society and the Infectious Diseases Society of America. Clin Infect Dis 2010;50(2):133–64.
19. Cilieborg MS, Boye M, Sangild PT. Bacterial colonization and gut development in preterm neonates. Early Hum Dev 2012;88(Suppl 1):S41–9.
20. Romano-Keeler J, Moore DJ, Wang C, et al. Early life establishment of site-specific microbial communities in the gut. Gut Microbes 2014;5(2):192–201.

21. Clark RH, Gordon P, Walker WM, et al. Characteristics of patients who die of necrotizing enterocolitis. J Perinatol 2012;32(3):199–204.
22. Bizzarro MJ, Ehrenkranz RA, Gallagher PG. Concurrent bloodstream infections in infants with necrotizing enterocolitis. J Pediatr 2014;164(1):61–6.
23. Mollitt DL, Tepas JJ 3rd, Talbert JL. The microbiology of neonatal peritonitis. Arch Surg 1988;123(2):176–9.
24. Mollitt DL, Tepas JJ, Talbert JL. The role of coagulase-negative Staphylococcus in neonatal necrotizing enterocolitis. J Pediatr Surg 1988;23(1 Pt 2):60–3.
25. Okogbule-Wonodi AC, Gross GW, Sun CC, et al. Necrotizing enterocolitis is associated with ureaplasma colonization in preterm infants. Pediatr Res 2011; 69(5 Pt 1):442–7.
26. Matsumoto S, Setoyama H, Umesaki Y. Differential induction of major histocompatibility complex molecules on mouse intestine by bacterial colonization. Gastroenterology 1992;103(6):1777–82.
27. Mazmanian SK, Liu CH, Tzianabos AO, et al. An immunomodulatory molecule of symbiotic bacteria directs maturation of the host immune system. Cell 2005; 122(1):107–18.
28. Hooper LV, Littman DR, Macpherson AJ. Interactions between the microbiota and the immune system. Science 2012;336(6086):1268–73.
29. O'Mahony C, Scully P, O'Mahony D, et al. Commensal-induced regulatory T cells mediate protection against pathogen-stimulated NF-kappaB activation. PLoS Pathog 2008;4(8):e1000112.
30. Imaoka A, Matsumoto S, Setoyama H, et al. Proliferative recruitment of intestinal intraepithelial lymphocytes after microbial colonization of germ-free mice. Eur J Immunol 1996;26(4):945–8.
31. Weitkamp JH, Rosen MJ, Zhao Z, et al. Small intestinal intraepithelial TCRgammadelta+ T lymphocytes are present in the premature intestine but selectively reduced in surgical necrotizing enterocolitis. PLoS One 2014;9(6):e99042.
32. Lau J, Magee F, Qiu Z, et al. Chorioamnionitis with a fetal inflammatory response is associated with higher neonatal mortality, morbidity, and resource use than chorioamnionitis displaying a maternal inflammatory response only. Am J Obstet Gynecol 2005;193(3 Pt 1):708–13.
33. Seliga-Siwecka JP, Kornacka MK. Neonatal outcome of preterm infants born to mothers with abnormal genital tract colonisation and chorioamnionitis: a cohort study. Early Hum Dev 2013;89(5):271–5.
34. Been JV, Lievense S, Zimmermann LJ, et al. Chorioamnionitis as a risk factor for necrotizing enterocolitis: a systematic review and meta-analysis. J Pediatr 2013; 162(2):236–42.e2.
35. Wolfs TG, Buurman WA, Zoer B, et al. Endotoxin induced chorioamnionitis prevents intestinal development during gestation in fetal sheep. PLoS One 2009;4(6):e5837.
36. Wolfs TG, Kallapur SG, Knox CL, et al. Antenatal ureaplasma infection impairs development of the fetal ovine gut in an IL-1-dependent manner. Mucosal Immunol 2013;6(3):547–56.
37. Arnon S, Grigg J, Silverman M. Association between pulmonary and gastric inflammatory cells on the first day of life in preterm infants. Pediatr Pulmonol 1993; 16(1):59–61.
38. Miralles R, Hodge R, McParland PC, et al. Relationship between antenatal inflammation and antenatal infection identified by detection of microbial genes by polymerase chain reaction. Pediatr Res 2005;57(4):570–7.
39. Luciano AA, Yu H, Jackson LW, et al. Preterm labor and chorioamnionitis are associated with neonatal T cell activation. PLoS One 2011;6(2):e16698.

40. Wolfs TG, Kallapur SG, Polglase GR, et al. IL-1alpha mediated chorioamnionitis induces depletion of FoxP3+ cells and ileal inflammation in the ovine fetal gut. PLoS One 2011;6(3):e18355.
41. Weitkamp JH, Rudzinski E, Koyama T, et al. Ontogeny of FOXP3(+) regulatory T cells in the postnatal human small intestinal and large intestinal lamina propria. Pediatr Dev Pathol 2009;12(6):443–9.
42. Weitkamp JH, Koyama T, Rock MT, et al. Necrotising enterocolitis is characterised by disrupted immune regulation and diminished mucosal regulatory (FOXP3)/effector (CD4, CD8) T cell ratios. Gut 2013;62(1):73–82.
43. Dingle BM, Liu Y, Fatheree NY, et al. FoxP3(+) regulatory T cells attenuate experimental necrotizing enterocolitis. PLoS One 2013;8(12):e82963.
44. Cash HL, Whitham CV, Behrendt CL, et al. Symbiotic bacteria direct expression of an intestinal bactericidal lectin. Science 2006;313(5790):1126–30.
45. Dominguez-Bello MG, Costello EK, Contreras M, et al. Delivery mode shapes the acquisition and structure of the initial microbiota across multiple body habitats in newborns. Proc Natl Acad Sci U S A 2010;107(26):11971–5.
46. Luo CC, Shih HH, Chiu CH, et al. Translocation of coagulase-negative bacterial staphylococci in rats following intestinal ischemia-reperfusion injury. Biol Neonate 2004;85(3):151–4.
47. Kansagra K, Stoll B, Rognerud C, et al. Total parenteral nutrition adversely affects gut barrier function in neonatal piglets. Am J Physiol Gastrointest Liver Physiol 2003;285(6):G1162–70.
48. Stewart CJ, Marrs EC, Magorrian S, et al. The preterm gut microbiota: changes associated with necrotizing enterocolitis and infection. Acta Paediatr 2012; 101(11):1121–7.
49. Ferraris L, Butel MJ, Campeotto F, et al. Clostridia in premature neonates' gut: incidence, antibiotic susceptibility, and perinatal determinants influencing colonization. PLoS One 2012;7(1):e30594.
50. Stark PL, Lee A. Clostridia isolated from the feces of infants during the first year of life. J Pediatr 1982;100(3):362–5.
51. Alfa MJ, Robson D, Davi M, et al. An outbreak of necrotizing enterocolitis associated with a novel clostridium species in a neonatal intensive care unit. Clin Infect Dis 2002;35(Suppl 1):S101–5.
52. Kosloske AM, Ulrich JA. A bacteriologic basis for the clinical presentations of necrotizing enterocolitis. J Pediatr Surg 1980;15(4):558–64.
53. Kosloske AM, Ulrich JA, Hoffman H. Fulminant necrotising enterocolitis associated with Clostridia. Lancet 1978;2(8098):1014–6.
54. Azcarate-Peril MA, Foster DM, Cadenas MB, et al. Acute necrotizing enterocolitis of preterm piglets is characterized by dysbiosis of ileal mucosa-associated bacteria. Gut Microbes 2011;2(4):234–43.
55. Singer DB, Cashore WJ, Widness JA, et al. Pseudomembranous colitis in a preterm neonate. J Pediatr Gastroenterol Nutr 1986;5(2):318–20.
56. Lallouette P, Bizzini B, Maro B, et al. Studies on the immunostimulating and antitumour activity of a fraction isolated from Corynebacterium granulosum. Dev Biol Stand 1977;38:111–3.
57. Petrillo TM, Beck-Sague CM, Songer JG, et al. Enteritis necroticans (pigbel) in a diabetic child. N Engl J Med 2000;342(17):1250–3.
58. Blakey JL, Lubitz L, Barnes GL, et al. Development of gut colonisation in preterm neonates. J Med Microbiol 1982;15(4):519–29.
59. McDonel JL. Clostridium perfringens toxins (type A, B, C, D, E). Pharmacol Ther 1980;10(3):617–55.

60. Flores-Diaz M, Alape-Giron A. Role of Clostridium perfringens phospholipase C in the pathogenesis of gas gangrene. Toxicon 2003;42(8):979–86.
61. Dittmar E, Beyer P, Fischer D, et al. Necrotizing enterocolitis of the neonate with Clostridium perfringens: diagnosis, clinical course, and role of alpha toxin. Eur J Pediatr 2008;167(8):891–5.
62. Schlapbach LJ, Ahrens O, Klimek P, et al. Clostridium perfringens and necrotizing enterocolitis. J Pediatr 2010;157(1):175.
63. de la Cochetiere MF, Piloquet H, des Robert C, et al. Early intestinal bacterial colonization and necrotizing enterocolitis in premature infants: the putative role of Clostridium. Pediatr Res 2004;56(3):366–70.
64. Blakey JL, Lubitz L, Campbell NT, et al. Enteric colonization in sporadic neonatal necrotizing enterocolitis. J Pediatr Gastroenterol Nutr 1985;4(4):591–5.
65. Kotsanas D, Carson JA, Awad MM, et al. Novel use of tryptose sulfite cycloserine egg yolk agar for isolation of Clostridium perfringens during an outbreak of necrotizing enterocolitis in a neonatal unit. J Clin Microbiol 2010;48(11):4263–5.
66. Miyakawa ME, Saputo J, Leger JS, et al. Necrotizing enterocolitis and death in a goat kid associated with enterotoxin (CPE)-producing Clostridium perfringens type A. Can Vet J 2007;48(12):1266–9.
67. Waligora-Dupriet AJ, Dugay A, Auzeil N, et al. Evidence for clostridial implication in necrotizing enterocolitis through bacterial fermentation in a gnotobiotic quail model. Pediatr Res 2005;58(4):629–35.
68. Cilieborg MS, Boye M, Molbak L, et al. Preterm birth and necrotizing enterocolitis alter gut colonization in pigs. Pediatr Res 2011;69(1):10–6.
69. Dubberke ER, Butler AM, Yokoe DS, et al. Multicenter study of Clostridium difficile infection rates from 2000 to 2006. Infect Control Hosp Epidemiol 2010; 31(10):1030–7.
70. Pruitt RN, Lacy DB. Toward a structural understanding of Clostridium difficile toxins A and B. Front Cell Infect Microbiol 2012;2:28.
71. Kuehne SA, Cartman ST, Heap JT, et al. The role of toxin A and toxin B in Clostridium difficile infection. Nature 2010;467(7316):711–3.
72. Jacquot A, Neveu D, Aujoulat F, et al. Dynamics and clinical evolution of bacterial gut microflora in extremely premature patients. J Pediatr 2011;158(3):390–6.
73. Chang JY, Shin SM, Chun J, et al. Pyrosequencing-based molecular monitoring of the intestinal bacterial colonization in preterm infants. J Pediatr Gastroenterol Nutr 2011;53(5):512–9.
74. Rousseau C, Levenez F, Fouqueray C, et al. Clostridium difficile colonization in early infancy is accompanied by changes in intestinal microbiota composition. J Clin Microbiol 2011;49(3):858–65.
75. Donta ST, Myers MG. Clostridium difficile toxin in asymptomatic neonates. J Pediatr 1982;100(3):431–4.
76. Al-Jumaili IJ, Shibley M, Lishman AH, et al. Incidence and origin of Clostridium difficile in neonates. J Clin Microbiol 1984;19(1):77–8.
77. el-Mohandes AE, Keiser JF, Refat M, et al. Prevalence and toxigenicity of Clostridium difficile isolates in fecal microflora of preterm infants in the intensive care nursery. Biol Neonate 1993;63(4):225–9.
78. Lishman AH, Al Jumaili IJ, Elshibly E, et al. Clostridium difficile isolation in neonates in a special care unit. Lack of correlation with necrotizing enterocolitis. Scand J Gastroenterol 1984;19(3):441–4.
79. Han VK, Sayed H, Chance GW, et al. An outbreak of Clostridium difficile necrotizing enterocolitis: a case for oral vancomycin therapy? Pediatrics 1983;71(6): 935–41.

80. Mathew OP, Bhatia JS, Richardson CJ. An outbreak of Clostridium difficile necrotizing enterocolitis. Pediatrics 1984;73(2):265–6.
81. Seki H, Shiohara M, Matsumura T, et al. Prevention of antibiotic-associated diarrhea in children by Clostridium butyricum MIYAIRI. Pediatr Int 2003;45(1):86–90.
82. McCroskey LM, Hatheway CL, Fenicia L, et al. Characterization of an organism that produces type E botulinal toxin but which resembles Clostridium butyricum from the feces of an infant with type E botulism. J Clin Microbiol 1986;23(1): 201–2.
83. Sturm R, Staneck JL, Stauffer LR, et al. Neonatal necrotizing enterocolitis associated with penicillin-resistant, toxigenic Clostridium butyricum. Pediatrics 1980; 66(6):928–31.
84. Howard FM, Flynn DM, Bradley JM, et al. Outbreak of necrotising enterocolitis caused by Clostridium butyricum. Lancet 1977;2(8048):1099–102.
85. Gothefors L, Blenkharn I. Clostridium butyricum and necrotising enterocolitis. Lancet 1978;1(8054):52–3.
86. Mitchell RG, Etches PC, Day DG. Non-toxigenic clostridia in babies. J Clin Pathol 1981;34(2):217–20.
87. Popoff MR, Ravisse P. Lesions produced by Clostridium butyricum strain CB 1002 in ligated intestinal loops in guinea pigs. J Med Microbiol 1985;19(3): 351–7.
88. Popoff MR, Szylit O, Ravisse P, et al. Experimental cecitis in gnotoxenic chickens monoassociated with Clostridium butyricum strains isolated from patients with neonatal necrotizing enterocolitis. Infect Immun 1985;47(3):697–703.
89. Bousseboua H, Le Coz Y, Dabard J, et al. Experimental cecitis in gnotobiotic quails monoassociated with Clostridium butyricum strains isolated from patients with neonatal necrotizing enterocolitis and from healthy newborns. Infect Immun 1989;57(3):932–6.
90. Butel MJ, Roland N, Hibert A, et al. Clostridial pathogenicity in experimental necrotising enterocolitis in gnotobiotic quails and protective role of bifidobacteria. J Med Microbiol 1998;47(5):391–9.
91. Stoll BJ, Hansen N, Fanaroff AA, et al. Enterobacter sakazakii is a rare cause of neonatal septicemia or meningitis in VLBW infants. J Pediatr 2004;144(6):821–3.
92. Machens HG, Ringe B, Ziemer G, et al. A new procedure for abdominal wound closure after pediatric liver transplantation: the "sandwich" technique. Surgery 1994;115(2):255–6.
93. Kucerova E, Clifton SW, Xia XQ, et al. Genome sequence of Cronobacter sakazakii BAA-894 and comparative genomic hybridization analysis with other Cronobacter species. PLoS One 2010;5(3):e9556.
94. Muytjens HL, Roelofs-Willemse H, Jaspar GH. Quality of powdered substitutes for breast milk with regard to members of the family Enterobacteriaceae. J Clin Microbiol 1988;26(4):743–6.
95. Chap J, Jackson P, Siqueira R, et al. International survey of Cronobacter sakazakii and other *Cronobacter* spp. in follow up formulas and infant foods. Int J Food Microbiol 2009;136(2):185–8.
96. Hoque A, Ahmed T, Shahidullah M, et al. Isolation and molecular identification of *Cronobacter* spp. from powdered infant formula (PIF) in Bangladesh. Int J Food Microbiol 2010;142(3):375–8.
97. Weir E. Powdered infant formula and fatal infection with Enterobacter sakazakii. CMAJ 2002;166(12):1570.
98. Ahmed SM, Lopman BA, Levy K. A systematic review and meta-analysis of the global seasonality of norovirus. PLoS One 2013;8(10):e75922.

99. Bar-Oz B, Preminger A, Peleg O, et al. Enterobacter sakazakii infection in the newborn. Acta Paediatr 2001;90(3):356–8.
100. Clark NC, Hill BC, O'Hara CM, et al. Epidemiologic typing of Enterobacter sakazakii in two neonatal nosocomial outbreaks. Diagn Microbiol Infect Dis 1990; 13(6):467–72.
101. Urmenyi AM, Franklin AW. Neonatal death from pigmented coliform infection. Lancet 1961;1(7172):313–5.
102. van Acker J, de Smet F, Muyldermans G, et al. Outbreak of necrotizing enterocolitis associated with Enterobacter sakazakii in powdered milk formula. J Clin Microbiol 2001;39(1):293–7.
103. Townsend S, Hurrell E, Forsythe S. Virulence studies of Enterobacter sakazakii isolates associated with a neonatal intensive care unit outbreak. BMC Microbiol 2008;8:64.
104. Hunter CJ, Bean JF. Cronobacter: an emerging opportunistic pathogen associated with neonatal meningitis, sepsis and necrotizing enterocolitis. J Perinatol 2013;33(8):581–5.
105. Hunter CJ, Singamsetty VK, Chokshi NK, et al. Enterobacter sakazakii enhances epithelial cell injury by inducing apoptosis in a rat model of necrotizing enterocolitis. J Infect Dis 2008;198(4):586–93.
106. Singamsetty VK, Wang Y, Shimada H, et al. Outer membrane protein A expression in Enterobacter sakazakii is required to induce microtubule condensation in human brain microvascular endothelial cells for invasion. Microb Pathog 2008; 45(3):181–91.
107. Nair MK, Venkitanarayanan K, Silbart LK, et al. Outer membrane protein A (OmpA) of Cronobacter sakazakii binds fibronectin and contributes to invasion of human brain microvascular endothelial cells. Foodborne Pathog Dis 2009; 6(4):495–501.
108. Bensasson M, Perez-Busquier M, Dorfmann H, et al. Special radiographic features of the hand in patients with articular chondrocalcinosis. A controlled study. Ann Radiol (Paris) 1975;18(7):701–10.
109. Pagotto FJ, Nazarowec-White M, Bidawid S, et al. Enterobacter sakazakii: infectivity and enterotoxin production in vitro and in vivo. J Food Prot 2003;66(3): 370–5.
110. Emami CN, Mittal R, Wang L, et al. Recruitment of dendritic cells is responsible for intestinal epithelial damage in the pathogenesis of necrotizing enterocolitis by Cronobacter sakazakii. J Immunol 2011;186(12):7067–79.
111. Emami CN, Mittal R, Wang L, et al. Role of neutrophils and macrophages in the pathogenesis of necrotizing enterocolitis caused by Cronobacter sakazakii. J Surg Res 2012;172(1):18–28.
112. Gregersen N, Van Nierop W, Von Gottberg A, et al. Klebsiella pneumoniae with extended spectrum beta-lactamase activity associated with a necrotizing enterocolitis outbreak. Pediatr Infect Dis J 1999;18(11):963–7.
113. Hill HR, Hunt CE, Matsen JM. Nosocomial colonization with Klebsiella, type 26, in a neonatal intensive-care unit associated with an outbreak of sepsis, meningitis, and necrotizing enterocolitis. J Pediatr 1974;85(3):415–9.
114. Boccia D, Stolfi I, Lana S, et al. Nosocomial necrotising enterocolitis outbreaks: epidemiology and control measures. Eur J Pediatr 2001;160(6):385–91.
115. Stone HH, Kolb LD, Geheber CE. Bacteriologic considerations in perforated necrotizing enterocolitis. South Med J 1979;72(12):1540–4.
116. Bell MJ, Feigin RD, Ternberg JL, et al. Evaluation of gastrointestinal microflora in necrotizing enterocolitis. J Pediatr 1978;92(4):589–92.

117. Speer ME, Taber LH, Yow MD, et al. Fulminant neonatal sepsis and necrotizing enterocolitis associated with a "nonenteropathogenic" strain of *Escherichia coli*. J Pediatr 1976;89(1):91–5.

118. Cushing AH. Necrotizing enterocolitis with *Escherichia coli* heat-labile enterotoxin. Pediatrics 1983;71(4):626–30.

119. Guner YS, Malhotra A, Ford HR, et al. Association of *Escherichia coli* O157:H7 with necrotizing enterocolitis in a full-term infant. Pediatr Surg Int 2009;25(5): 459–63.

120. Borderon E, Thieffry JC, Jamet O, et al. Observations on the intestinal colonization by Pseudomonas aeruginosa in newborn infants. Biol Neonate 1990;57(2):88–97.

121. Jefferies JM, Cooper T, Yam T, et al. Pseudomonas aeruginosa outbreaks in the neonatal intensive care unit–a systematic review of risk factors and environmental sources. J Med Microbiol 2012;61(Pt 8):1052–61.

122. Olson B, Weinstein RA, Nathan C, et al. Epidemiology of endemic Pseudomonas aeruginosa: why infection control efforts have failed. J Infect Dis 1984;150(6): 808–16.

123. Cheng YL, Lee HC, Yeung CY, et al. Clinical significance in previously healthy children of Pseudomonas aeruginosa in the stool. Pediatr Neonatol 2009; 50(1):13–7.

124. Henderson A, Maclaurin J, Scott JM. Pseudomonas in a Glasgow baby unit. Lancet 1969;2(7615):316–7.

125. Leigh L, Stoll BJ, Rahman M, et al. Pseudomonas aeruginosa infection in very low birth weight infants: a case-control study. Pediatr Infect Dis J 1995;14(5): 367–71.

126. Rudd PT, Carrington D. A prospective study of chlamydial, mycoplasmal, and viral infections in a neonatal intensive care unit. Arch Dis Child 1984;59(2): 120–5.

127. Shurin PA, Alpert S, Bernard Rosner BA, et al. Chorioamnionitis and colonization of the newborn infant with genital mycoplasmas. N Engl J Med 1975;293(1):5–8.

128. Ozdemir R, Erdeve O, Yurttutan S, et al. Letter to the editor Re: Okogbule-Wonodi et al. Pediatr Res 69:442–447. Pediatr Res 2011;70(4):423–4 [author reply: 424].

129. Perzigian RW, Adams JT, Weiner GM, et al. Ureaplasma urealyticum and chronic lung disease in very low birth weight infants during the exogenous surfactant era. Pediatr Infect Dis J 1998;17(7):620–5.

130. Cox E, Christenson JC. Rotavirus. Pediatr Rev 2012;33(10):439–45 [quiz: 446–7].

131. Murphy AM, Albrey MB, Crewe EB. Rotavirus infections of neonates. Lancet 1977;2(8049):1149–50.

132. Chrystie IL, Totterdell BM, Banatvala JE. Asymptomatic endemic rotavirus infections in the newborn. Lancet 1978;1(8075):1176–8.

133. Rotbart HA, Nelson WL, Glode MP, et al. Neonatal rotavirus-associated necrotizing enterocolitis: case control study and prospective surveillance during an outbreak. J Pediatr 1988;112(1):87–93.

134. Rotbart HA, Levin MJ, Yolken RH, et al. An outbreak of rotavirus-associated neonatal necrotizing enterocolitis. J Pediatr 1983;103(3):454–9.

135. Keller KM, Schmidt H, Wirth S, et al. Differences in the clinical and radiologic patterns of rotavirus and non-rotavirus necrotizing enterocolitis. Pediatr Infect Dis J 1991;10(10):734–8.

136. Jiang X, Wang M, Wang K, et al. Sequence and genomic organization of Norwalk virus. Virology 1993;195(1):51–61.

137. Scallan E, Hoekstra RM, Angulo FJ, et al. Foodborne illness acquired in the United States–major pathogens. Emerg Infect Dis 2011;17(1):7–15.
138. Widdowson MA, Sulka A, Bulens SN, et al. Norovirus and foodborne disease, United States, 1991–2000. Emerg Infect Dis 2005;11(1):95–102.
139. Patel MM, Widdowson MA, Glass RI, et al. Systematic literature review of role of noroviruses in sporadic gastroenteritis. Emerg Infect Dis 2008;14(8):1224–31.
140. Naing Z, Rayner B, Killikulangara A, et al. Prevalence of viruses in stool of premature neonates at a neonatal intensive care unit. J Paediatr Child Health 2013; 49(3):E221–6.
141. Wiechers C, Bissinger AL, Hamprecht K, et al. Apparently non-specific results found using a norovirus antigen immunoassay for fecal specimens from neonates. J Perinatol 2008;28(1):79–81.
142. Rabenau HF, Sturmer M, Buxbaum S, et al. Laboratory diagnosis of norovirus: which method is the best? Intervirology 2003;46(4):232–8.
143. Agus SG, Dolin R, Wyatt RG, et al. Acute infectious nonbacterial gastroenteritis: intestinal histopathology. Histologic and enzymatic alterations during illness produced by the Norwalk agent in man. Ann Intern Med 1973;79(1):18–25.
144. Schreiber DS, Blacklow NR, Trier JS. The mucosal lesion of the proximal small intestine in acute infectious nonbacterial gastroenteritis. N Engl J Med 1973; 288(25):1318–23.
145. Dolin R, Levy AG, Wyatt RG, et al. Viral gastroenteritis induced by the Hawaii agent. Jejunal histopathology and serologic response. Am J Med 1975;59(6): 761–8.
146. Morotti RA, Kaufman SS, Fishbein TM, et al. Calicivirus infection in pediatric small intestine transplant recipients: pathological considerations. Hum Pathol 2004;35(10):1236–40.
147. Pelizzo G, Nakib G, Goruppi I, et al. Isolated colon ischemia with norovirus infection in preterm babies: a case series. J Med Case Rep 2013;7(1):108.
148. Kamaluddeen M, Lodha A, Akierman A. Non-Rotavirus infection causing apnea in a neonate. Indian J Pediatr 2009;76(10):1051–2.
149. Turcios-Ruiz RM, Axelrod P, St John K, et al. Outbreak of necrotizing enterocolitis caused by norovirus in a neonatal intensive care unit. J Pediatr 2008;153(3):339–44.
150. Armbrust S, Kramer A, Olbertz D, et al. Norovirus infections in preterm infants: wide variety of clinical courses. BMC Res Notes 2009;2:96.
151. Mussi-Pinhata MM, Yamamoto AY, do Carmo Rego MA, et al. Perinatal or early-postnatal cytomegalovirus infection in preterm infants under 34 weeks gestation born to CMV-seropositive mothers within a high-seroprevalence population. J Pediatr 2004;145(5):685–8.
152. de Cates CR, Gray J, Roberton NR, et al. Acquisition of cytomegalovirus infection by premature neonates. J Infect 1994;28(1):25–30.
153. Miron D, Brosilow S, Felszer K, et al. Incidence and clinical manifestations of breast milk-acquired Cytomegalovirus infection in low birth weight infants. J Perinatol 2005;25(5):299–303.
154. Lanzieri TM, Dollard SC, Josephson CD, et al. Breast milk-acquired cytomegalovirus infection and disease in VLBW and premature infants. Pediatrics 2013; 131(6):e1937–45.
155. Hamprecht K, Maschmann J, Vochem M, et al. Epidemiology of transmission of cytomegalovirus from mother to preterm infant by breastfeeding. Lancet 2001; 357(9255):513–8.
156. Adler SP, Chandrika T, Lawrence L, et al. Cytomegalovirus infections in neonates acquired by blood transfusions. Pediatr Infect Dis 1983;2(2):114–8.

157. Yeager AS, Grumet FC, Hafleigh EB, et al. Prevention of transfusion-acquired cytomegalovirus infections in newborn infants. J Pediatr 1981;98(2):281–7.
158. Preiksaitis JK, Brown L, McKenzie M. Transfusion-acquired cytomegalovirus infection in neonates. A prospective study. Transfusion 1988;28(3):205–9.
159. Kim AR, Lee YK, Kim KA, et al. Transfusion-related cytomegalovirus infection among very low birth weight infants in an endemic area. J Korean Med Sci 2006;21(1):5–10.
160. Reyes C, Pereira S, Warden MJ, et al. Cytomegalovirus enteritis in a premature infant. J Pediatr Surg 1997;32(11):1545–7.
161. Cheong JL, Cowan FM, Modi N. Gastrointestinal manifestations of postnatal cytomegalovirus infection in infants admitted to a neonatal intensive care unit over a five year period. Arch Dis Child Fetal Neonatal Ed 2004;89(4):F367–9.
162. Lee SL, Johnsen H, Applebaum H. Cytomegalovirus enterocolitis presenting as abdominal compartment syndrome in a premature neonate. World J Pediatr 2012;8(1):80–2.
163. Tengsupakul S, Birge ND, Bendel CM, et al. Asymptomatic DNAemia heralds CMV-associated NEC: case report, review, and rationale for preemption. Pediatrics 2013;132(5):e1428–34.
164. Gessler P, Bischoff GA, Wiegand D, et al. Cytomegalovirus-associated necrotizing enterocolitis in a preterm twin after breastfeeding. J Perinatol 2004; 24(2):124–6.
165. Tran L, Ferris M, Norori J, et al. Necrotizing enterocolitis and cytomegalovirus infection in a premature infant. Pediatrics 2013;131(1):e318–22.
166. Gagneur A, Sizun J, Vallet S, et al. Coronavirus-related nosocomial viral respiratory infections in a neonatal and paediatric intensive care unit: a prospective study. J Hosp Infect 2002;51(1):59–64.
167. Chany C, Moscovici O, Lebon P, et al. Association of coronavirus infection with neonatal necrotizing enterocolitis. Pediatrics 1982;69(2):209–14.
168. Moscovici O, Chany C, Lebon P, et al. Association of coronavirus infection with hemorrhagic entercolitis in newborn infants. C R Seances Acad Sci D 1980; 290(13):869–72.
169. Jamieson FB, Wang EE, Bain C, et al. Human torovirus: a new nosocomial gastrointestinal pathogen. J Infect Dis 1998;178(5):1263–9.
170. Vaucher YE, Ray CG, Minnich LL, et al. Pleomorphic, enveloped, virus-like particles associated with gastrointestinal illness in neonates. J Infect Dis 1982; 145(1):27–36.
171. Lodha A, de Silva N, Petric M, et al. Human torovirus: a new virus associated with neonatal necrotizing enterocolitis. Acta Paediatr 2005;94(8):1085–8.
172. Pruekprasert P, Stout C, Patamasucon P. Neonatal enterovirus infection. J Assoc Acad Minor Phys 1995;6(4):134–8.
173. Ehrnst A, Eriksson M. Epidemiological features of type 22 echovirus infection. Scand J Infect Dis 1993;25(3):275–81.
174. Moore M, Kaplan MH, McPhee J, et al. Epidemiologic, clinical, and laboratory features of Coxsackie B1-B5 infections in the United States, 1970–79. Public Health Rep 1984;99(5):515–22.
175. Jenista JA, Powell KR, Menegus MA. Epidemiology of neonatal enterovirus infection. J Pediatr 1984;104(5):685–90.
176. Lake AM, Lauer BA, Clark JC, et al. Enterovirus infections in neonates. J Pediatr 1976;89(5):787–91.
177. Johnson FE, Crnic DM, Simmons MA, et al. Association of fatal Coxsackie B2 viral infection and necrotizing enterocolitis. Arch Dis Child 1977;52(10):802–4.

178. Nakao T, Miura R, Sato M. ECHO virus type 22 infection in a premature infant. Tohoku J Exp Med 1970;102(1):61–8.

179. Berkovich S, Pangan J. Recoveries of virus from premature infants during outbreaks of respiratory disease: the relation of ECHO virus type 22 to disease of the upper and lower respiratory tract in the premature infant. Bull N Y Acad Med 1968;44(4):377–87.

180. Birenbaum E, Handsher R, Kuint J, et al. Echovirus type 22 outbreak associated with gastro-intestinal disease in a neonatal intensive care unit. Am J Perinatol 1997;14(8):469–73.

181. Madeley CR, Cosgrove BP. Letter: viruses in infantile gastroenteritis. Lancet 1975;2(7925):124.

182. Sebire NJ, Malone M, Shah N, et al. Pathology of astrovirus associated diarrhoea in a paediatric bone marrow transplant recipient. J Clin Pathol 2004; 57(9):1001–3.

183. Nighot PK, Moeser A, Ali RA, et al. Astrovirus infection induces sodium malabsorption and redistributes sodium hydrogen exchanger expression. Virology 2010;401(2):146–54.

184. Bagci S, Eis-Hubinger AM, Yassin AF, et al. Clinical characteristics of viral intestinal infection in preterm and term neonates. Eur J Clin Microbiol Infect Dis 2010; 29(9):1079–84.

185. Chappe C, Minjolle S, Dabadie A, et al. Astrovirus and digestive disorders in neonatal units. Acta Paediatr 2012;101(5):e208–12.

186. Desfrere L, de Oliveira I, Goffinet F, et al. Increased incidence of necrotizing enterocolitis in premature infants born to HIV-positive mothers. AIDS 2005; 19(14):1487–93.

187. Schmitz T, Weizsaecker K, Feiterna-Sperling C, et al. Exposure to HIV and antiretroviral medication as a potential cause of necrotizing enterocolitis in term neonates. AIDS 2006;20(7):1082–3.

188. van der Meulen EF, Bergman KA, Kamps AW. Necrotising enterocolitis in a term neonate with trisomy 21 exposed to maternal HIV and antiretroviral medication. Eur J Pediatr 2009;168(1):113–4.

189. Baley JE, Kliegman RM, Boxerbaum B, et al. Fungal colonization in the very low birth weight infant. Pediatrics 1986;78(2):225–32.

190. Fridkin SK, Kaufman D, Edwards JR, et al. Changing incidence of Candida bloodstream infections among NICU patients in the United States: 1995–2004. Pediatrics 2006;117(5):1680–7.

191. Saiman L, Ludington E, Dawson JD, et al. Risk factors for Candida species colonization of neonatal intensive care unit patients. Pediatr Infect Dis J 2001;20(12):1119–24.

192. Saiman L, Ludington E, Pfaller M, et al. Risk factors for candidemia in neonatal intensive care unit patients. The National Epidemiology of Mycosis Survey study group. Pediatr Infect Dis J 2000;19(4):319–24.

193. Benjamin DK Jr, Stoll BJ, Gantz MG, et al. Neonatal candidiasis: epidemiology, risk factors, and clinical judgment. Pediatrics 2010;126(4):e865–73.

194. Stewart CJ, Nelson A, Scribbins D, et al. Bacterial and fungal viability in the preterm gut: NEC and sepsis. Arch Dis Child Fetal Neonatal Ed 2013;98(4):F298–303.

195. Coates EW, Karlowicz MG, Croitoru DP, et al. Distinctive distribution of pathogens associated with peritonitis in neonates with focal intestinal perforation compared with necrotizing enterocolitis. Pediatrics 2005;116(2):e241–6.

196. Mintz AC, Applebaum H. Focal gastrointestinal perforations not associated with necrotizing enterocolitis in very low birth weight neonates. J Pediatr Surg 1993; 28(6):857–60.

197. Parra-Herran CE, Pelaez L, Sola JE, et al. Intestinal candidiasis: an uncommon cause of necrotizing enterocolitis (NEC) in neonates. Fetal Pediatr Pathol 2010; 29(3):172–80.
198. Smith SD, Tagge EP, Miller J, et al. The hidden mortality in surgically treated necrotizing enterocolitis: fungal sepsis. J Pediatr Surg 1990;25(10):1030–3.
199. Ballance WA, Dahms BB, Shenker N, et al. Pathology of neonatal necrotizing enterocolitis: a ten-year experience. J Pediatr 1990;117(1 Pt 2):S6–13.
200. Kaufman D, Boyle R, Hazen KC, et al. Fluconazole prophylaxis against fungal colonization and infection in preterm infants. N Engl J Med 2001;345(23): 1660–6.
201. Kaufman DA, Morris A, Gurka MJ, et al. Fluconazole prophylaxis in preterm infants: a multicenter case-controlled analysis of efficacy and safety. Early Hum Dev 2014;90(Suppl 1):S87–90.
202. Healy CM, Campbell JR, Zaccaria E, et al. Fluconazole prophylaxis in extremely low birth weight neonates reduces invasive candidiasis mortality rates without emergence of fluconazole-resistant Candida species. Pediatrics 2008;121(4): 703–10.
203. Benjamin DK Jr, Hudak ML, Duara S, et al. Effect of fluconazole prophylaxis on candidiasis and mortality in premature infants: a randomized clinical trial. JAMA 2014;311(17):1742–9.
204. Ullrich T, Tang YW, Correa H, et al. Absence of gastrointestinal pathogens in ileum tissue resected for necrotizing enterocolitis. Pediatr Infect Dis J 2012; 31(4):413–4.
205. Raskind CH, Dembry LM, Gallagher PG. Vancomycin-resistant enterococcal bacteremia and necrotizing enterocolitis in a preterm neonate. Pediatr Infect Dis J 2005;24(10):943–4.
206. Pumberger W, Novak W. Fatal neonatal Salmonella enteritidis sepsis. J Perinatol 2000;20(1):54–6.
207. Stein H, Beck J, Solomon A, et al. Gastroenteritis with necrotizing enterocolitis in premature babies. Br Med J 1972;2(5814):616–9.
208. Overturf GD, Sherman MP, Scheifele DW, et al. Neonatal necrotizing enterocolitis associated with delta toxin-producing methicillin-resistant Staphylococcus aureus. Pediatr Infect Dis J 1990;9(2):88–91.
209. Downard CD, Renaud E, St Peter SD, et al. American Pediatric Surgical Association Outcomes Clinical Trials Committee. Treatment of necrotizing enterocolitis: an American Pediatric Surgical Association Outcomes and Clinical Trials Committee systematic review. J Pediatr Surg 2012;47(11):2111–22.
210. Weitkamp JH. More than a gut feeling: predicting surgical necrotising enterocolitis. Gut 2014;63(8):1205–6.
211. Sharma R, Hudak ML. A clinical perspective of necrotizing enterocolitis: past, present, and future. Clin Perinatol 2013;40(1):27–51.
212. Ng PC, Lewindon PJ, Siu YK, et al. Bacterial contaminated breast milk and necrotizing enterocolitis in preterm twins. J Hosp Infect 1995;31(2):105–10.

Chorioamnionitis

Implications for the Neonate

Jessica E. Ericson, MD[a], Matthew M. Laughon, MD, MPH[b],*

KEYWORDS

- Neonatal sepsis
- Fetal inflammatory response
- *Mycoplasma*

KEY POINTS

- Chorioamnionitis (CA) is a pathologic diagnosis that is suggested by clinical findings.
- Neonatal sepsis occurs in 1% to 3% of infants exposed to CA.
- Infants exposed to CA require additional monitoring and testing.
- Exposure to CA may lead to a variety of adverse neonatal outcomes, but a causal relationship has been difficult to demonstrate consistently.

Chorioamnionitis (CA) is a perinatal condition characterized by inflammation of the fetal membranes, namely, the chorion and amnion. The incidence of CA increases with decreasing gestational age at birth. Ascending bacterial infection is thought to be the primary mode of acquisition; viruses and fungi are rarely implicated. Although the mechanisms are not entirely clear, CA predisposes infants to premature birth, neonatal sepsis, and other adverse outcomes. In this article, we review the pathophysiology (including definitions), risk factors, management strategies, and neonatal outcomes associated with CA.

DEFINITION

The definition of CA is inconsistent between clinicians and across epidemiologic studies, and this inconsistency has contributed to the conflicting associations

Dr M.M. Laughon receives support from the U.S. government for his work in pediatric and neonatal clinical pharmacology (Government Contract HHSN267200700051C, PI: Benjamin under the Best Pharmaceuticals for Children Act) and from National Institute of Child Health and Human Development (K23HD068497). Dr J.E. Ericson receives support from the National Institute of Child Health and Human Development of the National Institutes of Health under award number 5T32HD060558.
^a Department of Pediatrics, Duke University & Duke Clinical Research Institute, 2400 Pratt Street, Durham, NC 27715, USA; ^b Department of Pediatrics, UNC Hospitals, The University of North Carolina at Chapel Hill, 101 Manning Drive, CB# 7596, 4th Floor, Chapel Hill, NC 275599-7596, USA
* Corresponding author.
E-mail address: matt_laughon@med.unc.edu

between CA and fetal outcomes. The most rigorous definition of CA is inflammation of the chorionic and amniotic layers of the fetal membranes confirmed by pathologic review of the placenta (**Table 1**).[1] The pathologic diagnosis requires the presence of a neutrophilic infiltrate to be present in the placental tissues. Early studies used a threshold of 10 neutrophils per high-power field in at least 10 fields as a definition for histologic CA.[2] More recently, the Extremely Low Gestational Age Newborn (ELGAN) Study group graded the severity of inflammation of each membrane and considers CA to be present when greater than 20 neutrophils are present per 20× field of the chorion or the presence of numerous large or confluent foci of neutrophils or necrosis of the amnion.[1]

Recently, attempts have been made to distinguish between involvement of only the maternal portion of the placenta and inflammation that involves both the maternal and fetal portions because there seem to be differences in neonatal outcomes for infants with more proximal inflammatory changes.[3–6] Inflammation that involves the fetal portion is often referred to as fetal inflammatory response (FIR).[6] CA can be further complicated by involvement of the umbilical cord, a condition called funisitis.[7] Investigators from the ELGAN study group consider funisitis to be present when there is fetal vasculitis with neutrophils noted in the perivascular Wharton jelly.[1] Funisitis is evidence of a vigorous fetal response, and thus is considered a "severe" form of CA. However, even the pathologic diagnosis can vary, depending on how long the placenta was at room temperature before refrigeration, where the placental tissue was sampled, and the skill of the pathologist.

Some investigators define CA as the isolation of bacterial or fungal organisms from the placenta or amniotic fluid, regardless of the presence of inflammation. Histologic CA and the isolation of organisms are highly associated but can occur separately.[2] Organisms can be isolated by culture or polymerase chain reaction (PCR; **Table 2**). Placental cultures may be negative, even in the presence of overt histologic inflammation.[8] One study found that only 4.6% of placental cultures revealed an organism when culture was performed for indications of preterm delivery, prolonged rupture of membranes, suspected infection, or fetal death.[9] This is likely owing to difficulty culturing fastidious or intracellular organisms such as *Mycoplasma* and *Ureaplasma* species, or low colony counts. PCR has been used successfully to increase sensitivity, but fails to detect all pathogens.[10,11] When 150 placentas were cultured and tested via PCR, 141 had no organisms, and 10 had organisms detected by both PCR and culture; PCR alone was positive in 9 cases and culture alone was positive in 6 cases.[12] Fastidious organisms were more likely to be identified by PCR. PCR failed to detect coagulase-negative *Staphylococcus* species, *Bacillus* species, *Peptostreptococcus*

Table 1 Definitions of CA	
Histologic CA	Pathologic diagnosis, inflammatory cells are present in the fetal membranes[19,59]
Clinical CA	Typically maternal fever and at least 2 of uterine tenderness, fetal or maternal tachycardia, maternal leukocytosis, and foul-smelling amniotic fluid.[15,52]
Maternal inflammatory response	Inflammatory changes limited to the subchorion, chorion, and amnion.[5]
Fetal inflammatory response	Umbilical vasculitis, funisitis, elevated inflammatory markers in the cord blood.[5,60]

Abbreviation: CA, chorioamnionitis.

Table 2
Organisms commonly identified in chorioamnionitis

Organism	Prevalence (%)	Reference
Ureaplasma urealyticum	15–62	18,28,61–63
Mycoplasma hominis	7–35	18,61–63
Group B *Streptococcus*	8–11	62,64
Escherichia coli	7–12	62,64
Gardnerella vaginalis	8–25	28,64
Bacteroides sp	8–30	64
Fusobacterium sp	10–67	28,62
Prevotella sp	17	64
Peptostreptococcus sp	16	64

species, and *Gardnerella vaginalis*.[12] Anaerobic and mixed infections are common, which can complicate detection by culture and PCR.[13]

Owing to laboratory limitations, the diagnosis of CA is often made clinically. Fever, uterine tenderness, maternal or fetal tachycardia, maternal leukocytosis, and foul-smelling uterine discharge are commonly considered to represent CA.[14] These findings are nonspecific, however, and have variable relation to histologic CA. Using histologic CA as the reference standard, the sensitivity of maternal fever was only 42%.[15] Maternal tachycardia and fetal tachycardia were 47% and 36% sensitive, respectively.[15] The sensitivity of clinical signs increased to 60% when maternal tachycardia, uterine tenderness, maternal leukocytosis, or malodorous amniotic fluid was present in addition to maternal fever.[16] A study that evaluated placental tissue from 2774 pregnancies found that maternal fever was absent in 92% of histologic CA cases.[17] Conversely, of women with peripartum fever, 59% had findings of CA.[17] The variability and limited sensitivity of findings used to diagnose CA clinically makes comparison of studies and outcomes more difficult.

Inflammatory changes themselves may have a stronger association with adverse outcomes, including preterm birth, than the presence of microorganisms alone.[18] Intra-amniotic interleukin (IL)-6 predicts both preterm birth and neonatal morbidity. Investigators found that mothers presenting in preterm labor with amniotic fluid IL-6 levels greater than 11.3 ng/mL delivered after a median of 1 day; those without elevated IL-6 levels delivered after a median of 25 days.[10] Another cohort of 261 very low birth weight (VLBW; <1500 g birth weight) infants found a C-reactive protein elevated to greater than 10 mg/L was significantly more common in the 99 infants exposed to CA (25% vs 11%; $P = .005$).[19] For 799 infants born at less than 27 weeks gestation, infants exposed to CA were more likely to have an elevated C-reactive protein level (odds ratio [OR], 5.3; 95% CI, 3.0–9.6), as well as elevation of other cytokines.[3] Inflammatory markers may add objective information to the clinical criteria used in diagnosis when pathologic information is unavailable.

PATHOPHYSIOLOGY

The introduction of organisms into the fetal membranes and the placenta is thought to occur via 4 anatomic pathways. The first, and most common, mechanism is ascending infection through the maternal genital tract. Vaginal and enteric flora are often implicated with this route of infection.[20] Second, iatrogenic inoculation can occur after invasive procedures such as amniocentesis.[21] Third, hematogenous spread can occur with migration of organisms from the maternal bloodstream across the placenta.[22]

Listeria monocytogenes in particular has been described to cause infiltration of the placenta after maternal infection.[23] Fourth, and least common, peritoneal infections can enter the intrauterine space via the fallopian tubes. Mothers with chronic kidney or liver disease are most at risk for infection by this mechanism.[24]

Ascending infection can ultimately result in disease of the fetal membranes. Preterm and prolonged rupture of membranes has been associated with increased risk of CA.[4] This may be because removal of the anatomic barrier provided by intact membranes allows for easier migration of organisms from the maternal genital tract into the fetal tissues. Conversely, the membranes may rupture owing to the apparent tendency of infection to weaken the membranes, predisposing them to rupture.[25] Separating which of these is the primary cause of CA is often challenging.

NEONATAL OUTCOMES
Preterm Birth

Preterm birth is the most consistently demonstrated consequence of CA.[26] An early prospective observational study of 2774 mother–infant pairs found that as many as 25% of preterm births are attributable to CA.[17] This was later confirmed in a case-control study demonstrating that premature infants have significantly increased odds of both bacterial isolation and histologic findings of CA.[2] A recent prospective study of 871 pregnancies found that, of those with histologic CA, premature delivery occurred nearly twice as often as those without CA.[27] When *Ureaplasma urealyticum* was detected after preterm premature rupture of membranes of 154 pregnancies, the median gestational age at delivery was 4 weeks less than when it was not detected.[11] Of 50 women who presented in preterm labor with intact membranes, elevated intra-amniotic levels of the proinflammatory cytokines IL-6, IL-1, prostaglandin E2, and tumor necrosis factor-α were associated with progression to preterm birth.[28]

Neonatal Sepsis

Infants born after CA are at increased risk for neonatal infection. Organisms infecting the chorionic membranes are in close proximity to the fetus and can cause fetal infection as a natural consequence of this proximity. The organisms that most often cause early onset neonatal sepsis are those that are also frequent causes of CA: *Escherichia coli* and group B *Streptococcus*.[29] Exposure to CA seems to confer a risk of early onset sepsis of 1% to 3%,[17] which is 10 times greater than the overall risk of early onset sepsis.

Premature infants are particularly susceptible to sepsis after CA. A case control study found that VLBW infants exposed to CA had significantly increased odds of early onset sepsis (OR, 4.7; 95% CI, 1.4–15.9; P = .015).[30] For infants less than 32 weeks gestational age, 145 infants exposed to histologic CA developed clinical criteria consistent with sepsis syndrome significantly more often than 136 infants without CA (39% vs 24%; P = .007).[31]

Term infants are also at risk for neonatal infection after CA. Of 5144 term infants exposed to CA, 1.3% developed culture-proven neonatal sepsis (OR, 2.9; 95% CI, 2.1–4.1).[32] An analysis of 3094 births found that a clinical diagnosis of CA was independently associated with increased odds of early onset neonatal sepsis even with adjustment for initial severity of illness and baseline characteristics (OR, 5.54; 95% CI, 2.87–10.69; P<.001).[33]

Funisitis seems to confer a higher risk of sepsis. When 315 preterm births were considered, 12% of infants with funisitis had a positive blood culture within 72 hours of delivery compared with 1% of infants without funisitis (OR, 7.2; 95% CI, 1.8–29.0).[34] A prospective, observational study of 231 infants found that early-onset sepsis occurred in 18% of infants with funisitis compared with 4% of infants without funisitis (P = .002).[7]

Brain Disease

CA is associated with an increased incidence of early neurologic insults, including severe intraventricular hemorrhage (IVH) and periventricular leukomalacia (PVL), which are established causes of neurodevelopmental impairment in premature infants. A multicenter study of Canadian Neonatal Network hospitals found that CA increased the odds of severe IVH even after adjusting for severity of illness (OR, 1.62; 95% CI, 1.17–2.24).[33] The presence of mononuclear inflammatory cells in the fetal membranes has been found to be associated with increased severe IVH, even after controlling for gestational age (OR, 8.9; 95% CI, 2.1–37.9).[35] A study of 1367 VLBW infants found that exposure to clinical CA increased the odds of both IVH (OR, 2.8; 95% CI, 1.6–4.8) and PVL (OR, 3.4; 95% CI, 1.6–7.3).[36] Recently, inflammatory changes that were classified as FIR were found to increase the odds of grades II to IV IVH (OR, 4.1; 95% CI, 1.3–13.2).[5] However, for the 53 pregnancies where inflammation was isolated to only the maternal placental tissues, there was no increase in IVH compared with the 112 with no placental inflammatory changes (OR, 0.9; 95% CI, 0.2–3.7).[5]

Even when a perinatal diagnosis of IVH or PVL is not documented, CA seems to be associated with an increased risk of cerebral palsy. A case control study of 424 infants with birth weights of greater than 2500 g found that both clinical CA and histologic evidence of placental infection were associated with significantly increased odds of spastic cerebral palsy.[37] Similarly, developmental testing of 33 infants at 18 months of age who had been exposed to clinical CA was significantly worse in cognitive, language, and motor domains than 146 control infants, even though the incidence of PVL and grade III or IV IVH were similar between the 2 groups.[38] The relationship between CA and neurodevelopmental impairment may partially be owing to the intermediate of neonatal sepsis, which has a well-described role in neurodevelopmental impairment.[39–41] However, exposure to inflammatory cytokines likely exerts direct damaging effects on the developing brain.[42–45]

The relationship between CA and poor neurodevelopmental outcome has not been demonstrated in all studies. For 39 infants born at less than 32 weeks gestation who were exposed to CA and then compared with 33 control infants, there was no difference between groups in mental and psychomotor developmental indices.[31] Similarly, a case control study found no difference in performance on the Bayley Scales of Infant Development between the 71 infants exposed and the 259 infants not exposed to CA at 7 months corrected age.[30]

Lung Disease

The relationship of CA and neonatal pulmonary morbidity is conflicting. Various studies have evaluated the risk of respiratory distress syndrome (RDS) and bronchopulmonary dysplasia (BPD) after exposure to CA.

RESPIRATORY DISTRESS SYNDROME

CA has been associated with a lower incidence of RDS in some studies. A lesser incidence of RDS in infants exposed to CA may occur because exposure to prenatal inflammation seems to accelerate lung development and stimulate surfactant production. This rationale is supported by a study that found that RDS was significantly less common in infants exposed to CA than their unexposed counterparts (relative risk [RR], 0.56; 95% CI, 0.34–0.90).[46] A more recent multivariable analysis of 301 premature infants similarly found that CA decreased the odds of severe RDS.[47] Infiltration of the fetal membranes by polymorphonuclear cells was associated with a lower incidence of RDS in infants less than 32 weeks gestational age (OR, 0.4; 95% CI,

0.3–0.7).[35] Another study of 216 infants considered inflammation of the maternal aspect of the placenta alone versus inflammation on the maternal and fetal aspects as 2 distinct pathologies.[5] They found that FIR conferred a protective effect with a reduced odds of RDS compared with placentas with no inflammation or with inflammatory changes only of the maternal placental tissues (OR, 0.08; 95% CI, 0.01–0.62).[5]

However, several studies have found an increase in RDS associated with CA. One study of 95 infants with mean gestational age of 34 weeks found 0 cases of RDS among infants without histologic CA; 23% of infants exposed to CA developed RDS.[48] RDS was also observed more frequently in infants exposed to clinical CA than those who were not in a study of 1367 VLBW infants (OR, 2.9; 95% CI, 1.5–5.5).[36] A multicenter analysis of 3094 infants found that RDS was more common after CA on univariable analysis; however, when gestational age and birth weight were included in a multivariable model, the relationship was no longer significant.[33] A study of 1340 infants less than 27 weeks gestation also found no association between histologic CA or the detection of organisms and respiratory status during the first 2 weeks of life.[49]

BRONCHOPULMONARY DYSPLASIA

The relationship between BPD and CA is also conflicting. The rationale for an increased risk of BPD after CA is that intrauterine exposure to inflammation may cause subsequent lung development to be abnormal leading to BPD.[50] In 1996, the first publication supporting an increased incidence of BPD after CA found an RR of 2.18 (95% CI, 1.07–4.43) for BPD in infants with birth weights of less than 2000 g who were exposed to CA.[46] A meta-analysis including studies from 1994 through 2009 found that histologic, but not clinical, CA was associated with an increased odds of BPD (OR, 2.19; 95% CI, 1.76–2.72).[51]

Data that are not supportive of an association between CA and BPD include a histologic evaluation of 446 placentas that failed to find a difference in BPD incidence for those with and without inflammatory cell infiltration.[35] Evaluation of 529 infants born at less than 29 weeks gestation found that histologic CA with FIR was associated with a decreased incidence of BPD (RR, 0.88; 95% CI, 0.81–0.95).[4]

MANAGEMENT OF CHORIOAMNIONITIS
Prenatal Antibiotics

Randomized, controlled trials support the use of antibiotics in women who present with preterm premature rupture of membranes. Six hundred fourteen women with rupture of membranes between 24 and 32 weeks gestation were randomized to treatment with amoxicillin (or ampicillin IV) or placebo.[52] More women treated with antibiotics were still pregnant at 2 (P = .03), 7 (P = .001), 14 (P = .001), and 21 (P = .008) days later than those given placebo.[52] Infants born to mothers treated with antibiotics had less RDS (RR, 0.83; 95% CI, 0.69–0.99), necrotizing enterocolitis (RR, 0.40; 95% CI, 0.17–0.95), and BPD (RR, 0.64; 95% CI, 0.45–0.92) than those given placebo.[52] A recent Cochrane review found that use of antibiotics after preterm premature rupture of membranes decreased the risk of delivery within 7 days of rupture (RR, 0.79; 95% CI, 0.71–0.89), decreased the incidence of neonatal infection (RR, 0.67; 95% CI, 0.52–0.85), and reduced the incidence of CA (RR, 0.66; 95% CI, 0.46–0.96).[53]

For rupture of membranes occurring after 36 weeks gestation, a recent randomized trial found no reduction in the incidence of early onset sepsis, the need for mechanical ventilation or fetal death for 820 infants exposed to prenatal antibiotics compared with 820 infants exposed to placebo (RR, 1.42; 95% CI, 0.85–2.37).[54]

Postnatal Antibiotics

Owing to the elevated risk of early onset neonatal sepsis in infants exposed to CA, the Committee on the Fetus and Newborn of the American Academy of Pediatrics has recommended that infants exposed to CA have laboratory studies performed and be started on empirical broad-spectrum antibiotics.[55,56] If studies are normal, cultures are negative and the infant is doing well, antibiotics should be stopped at 48 hours.[55] Similarly, the US Centers for Disease Control and Prevention has recommended that infants exposed to CA be started on empirical antibiotics and undergo laboratory evaluation including blood cultures.[57] Neither the American Academy of Pediatrics nor the US Centers for Disease Control and Prevention make a recommendation regarding duration of therapy. If the infant is clinically well and cultures are negative, but the complete blood count or C-reactive protein is suggestive of infection, the role of additional or prolonged antibiotic treatment is unclear.

Antenatal Steroids

The benefits of antenatal steroid administration for preterm delivery are well described. For infants exposed to CA, antenatal steroids also improve outcomes. Exposure to antenatal steroids significantly decreased the incidence of both severe IVH and mortality for 53 infants with histologic CA.[47] A Japanese Neonatal Research Network study of 7896 infants less than 34 weeks gestational age with histologic CA similarly found that RDS (OR, 0.72; $P<.001$), IVH (OR, 0.68; $P<.001$), and mortality (OR, 0.50; $P<.001$) occurred significantly less often in infants whose mothers received antenatal corticosteroid therapy.[58]

SUMMARY

CA is a common problem, especially among preterm deliveries. Diagnosis is most accurately made from pathologic specimens. For preterm premature rupture of membranes, antibiotics should be used to reduce the risk of preterm birth and its subsequent complications. Antibiotic administration to infants born after CA is recommended. Future studies should explore improved diagnostic and treatment modalities.

Best practices

What is the current practice?

- Various strategies are used to define chorioamnionitis (CA).

- Most infants exposed to CA are evaluated for signs and symptoms of infection.

Major Recommendations

- Screen infants exposed to CA with complete blood count and blood culture.

- Evaluate the placentas of infants born prematurely or after prolonged rupture of membranes for evidence of CA.

- Mothers with preterm premature rupture of membranes should receive antibiotic therapy.

Summary Statement

CA predisposes infants to premature birth, neonatal sepsis, and IVH; the role of CA in RDS, BPD, and neurodevelopmental impairment is unclear. Antibiotics for preterm premature rupture of membranes reduces the incidence of CA. Antibiotics are recommended for infants exposed to CA while laboratory studies are being performed.

REFERENCES

1. Hecht JL, Allred EN, Kliman HJ, et al. Histological characteristics of singleton placentas delivered before the 28th week of gestation. Pathology 2008;40(4):372–6.
2. Hillier SL, Martius J, Krohn M, et al. A case-control study of chorioamnionic infection and histologic chorioamnionitis in prematurity. N Engl J Med 1988;319(15): 972–8.
3. Hecht JL, Fichorova RN, Tang VF, et al. Relationship between neonatal blood protein concentrations and placenta histologic characteristics in extremely low GA newborns. Pediatr Res 2011;69(1):68–73.
4. Plakkal N, Soraisham AS, Trevenen C, et al. Histological chorioamnionitis and bronchopulmonary dysplasia: a retrospective cohort study. J Perinatol 2013; 33(6):441–5.
5. Liu Z, Tang Z, Li J, et al. Effects of placental inflammation on neonatal outcome in preterm infants. Pediatr Neonatol 2014;55(1):35–40.
6. Redline RW. Inflammatory response in acute chorioamnionitis. Semin Fetal Neonatal Med 2012;17(1):20–5.
7. Tsiartas P, Kacerovsky M, Musilova I, et al. The association between histological chorioamnionitis, funisitis and neonatal outcome in women with preterm prelabor rupture of membranes. J Matern Fetal Neonatal Med 2013;26(13):1332–6.
8. Queiros da Mota V, Prodhom G, Yan P, et al. Correlation between placental bacterial culture results and histological chorioamnionitis: a prospective study on 376 placentas. J Clin Pathol 2013;66(3):243–8.
9. Bhola K, Al-Kindi H, Fadia M, et al. Placental cultures in the era of peripartum antibiotic use. Aust N Z J Obstet Gynaecol 2008;48(2):179–84.
10. Combs CA, Gravett M, Garite TJ, et al. Amniotic fluid infection, inflammation, and colonization in preterm labor with intact membranes. Am J Obstet Gynecol 2014; 210(2):125.e1–15.
11. Yoon BH, Romero R, Kim M, et al. Clinical implications of detection of *Ureaplasma urealyticum* in the amniotic cavity with the polymerase chain reaction. Am J Obstet Gynecol 2000;183(5):1130–7.
12. DiGiulio DB, Romero R, Amogan HP, et al. Microbial prevalence, diversity and abundance in amniotic fluid during preterm labor: a molecular and culture-based investigation. PLoS One 2008;3(8):e3056.
13. Pankuch GA, Appelbaum PC, Lorenz RP, et al. Placental microbiology and histology and the pathogenesis of chorioamnionitis. Obstet Gynecol 1984;64(6):802–6.
14. Greenberg MB, Anderson BL, Schulkin J, et al. A first look at chorioamnionitis management practice variation among US obstetricians. Infect Dis Obstet Gynecol 2012;2012:628362.
15. Curtin WM, Katzman PJ, Florescue H, et al. Accuracy of signs of clinical chorioamnionitis in the term parturient. J Perinatol 2013;33(6):422–8.
16. Tokumasu H, Hinotsu S, Kita F, et al. Predictive value of clinical chorioamnionitis in extremely premature infants. Pediatr Int 2013;55(1):35–8.
17. Guzick DS, Winn K. The association of chorioamnionitis with preterm delivery. Obstet Gynecol 1985;65(1):11–6.
18. Marconi C, de Andrade Ramos BR, Peracoli JC, et al. Amniotic fluid interleukin-1 beta and interleukin-6, but not interleukin-8 correlate with microbial invasion of the amniotic cavity in preterm labor. Am J Reprod Immunol 2011;65(6):549–56.
19. Lee SY, Leung CW. Histological chorioamnionitis - implication for bacterial colonization, laboratory markers of infection, and early onset sepsis in very-low-birth-weight neonates. J Matern Fetal Neonatal Med 2012;25(4):364–8.

20. Sherman DJ, Tovbin J, Lazarovich T, et al. Chorioamnionitis caused by gram-negative bacteria as an etiologic factor in preterm birth. Eur J Clin Microbiol Infect Dis 1997;16(6):417–23.

21. Rode ME, Morgan MA, Ruchelli E, et al. Candida chorioamnionitis after serial therapeutic amniocenteses: a possible association. J Perinatol 2000;20(5):335–7.

22. Craig S, Permezel M, Doyle L, et al. Perinatal infection with *Listeria monocytogenes*. Aust N Z J Obstet Gynaecol 1996;36(3):286–90.

23. Becroft DM, Farmer K, Seddon RJ, et al. Epidemic listeriosis in the newborn. Br Med J 1971;3(5777):747–51.

24. Tison A, Lozowy C, Benjamin A, et al. Successful pregnancy complicated by peritonitis in a 35- year old CAPD patient. Perit Dial Int 1996;16(Suppl 1):S489–91.

25. Lannon SM, Vanderhoeven JP, Eschenbach DA, et al. Synergy and interactions among biological pathways leading to preterm premature rupture of membranes. Reprod Sci 2014;21:1215–27.

26. Erdemir G, Kultursay N, Calkavur S, et al. Histological chorioamnionitis: effects on premature delivery and neonatal prognosis. Pediatr Neonatol 2013;54(4):267–74.

27. Bastek JA, Weber AL, McShea MA, et al. Prenatal inflammation is associated with adverse neonatal outcomes. Am J Obstet Gynecol 2014;210(5):450.e1–10.

28. Hillier SL, Witkin SS, Krohn MA, et al. The relationship of amniotic fluid cytokines and preterm delivery, amniotic fluid infection, histologic chorioamnionitis, and chorioamnion infection. Obstet Gynecol 1993;81(6):941–8.

29. Hornik CP, Fort P, Clark RH, et al. Early and late onset sepsis in very-low-birth-weight infants from a large group of neonatal intensive care units. Early Hum Dev 2012;88(Suppl 2):S69–74.

30. Dexter SC, Malee MP, Pinar H, et al. Influence of chorioamnionitis on developmental outcome in very low birth weight infants. Obstet Gynecol 1999;94(2):267–73.

31. Arayici S, Kadioglu Simsek G, Oncel MY, et al. The effect of histological chorioamnionitis on the short-term outcome of preterm infants </= 32 weeks: a single-center study. J Matern Fetal Neonatal Med 2014;27(11):1129–33.

32. Alexander JM, McIntire DM, Leveno KJ. Chorioamnionitis and the prognosis for term infants. Obstet Gynecol 1999;94(2):274–8.

33. Soraisham AS, Singhal N, McMillan DD, et al. A multicenter study on the clinical outcome of chorioamnionitis in preterm infants. Am J Obstet Gynecol 2009; 200(4):372.e1–6.

34. Yoon BH, Romero R, Park JS, et al. The relationship among inflammatory lesions of the umbilical cord (funisitis), umbilical cord plasma interleukin 6 concentration, amniotic fluid infection, and neonatal sepsis. Am J Obstet Gynecol 2000;183(5): 1124–9.

35. Andrews WW, Goldenberg RL, Faye-Petersen O, et al. The Alabama Preterm Birth study: polymorphonuclear and mononuclear cell placental infiltrations, other markers of inflammation, and outcomes in 23- to 32-week preterm newborn infants. Am J Obstet Gynecol 2006;195(3):803–8.

36. Alexander JM, Gilstrap LC, Cox SM, et al. Clinical chorioamnionitis and the prognosis for very low birth weight infants. Obstet Gynecol 1998;91(5 Pt 1):725–9.

37. Grether JK, Nelson KB. Maternal infection and cerebral palsy in infants of normal birth weight. JAMA 1997;278(3):207–11.

38. Nasef N, Shabaan AE, Schurr P, et al. Effect of clinical and histological chorioamnionitis on the outcome of preterm infants. Am J Perinatol 2013;30(1):59–68.

39. Alshaikh B, Yusuf K, Sauve R. Neurodevelopmental outcomes of very low birth weight infants with neonatal sepsis: systematic review and meta-analysis. J Perinatol 2013;33(7):558–64.

40. Adams-Chapman I, Bann CM, Das A, et al. Neurodevelopmental outcome of extremely low birth weight infants with Candida infection. J Pediatr 2013;163(4): 961–7.e3.

41. Stoll BJ, Hansen NI, Adams-Chapman I, et al. Neurodevelopmental and growth impairment among extremely low-birth-weight infants with neonatal infection. JAMA 2004;292(19):2357–65.

42. Yoon BH, Romero R, Yang SH, et al. Interleukin-6 concentrations in umbilical cord plasma are elevated in neonates with white matter lesions associated with periventricular leukomalacia. Am J Obstet Gynecol 1996;174(5):1433–40.

43. Yoon BH, Jun JK, Romero R, et al. Amniotic fluid inflammatory cytokines (interleukin-6, interleukin-1beta, and tumor necrosis factor-alpha), neonatal brain white matter lesions, and cerebral palsy. Am J Obstet Gynecol 1997;177(1):19–26.

44. Leviton A, Fichorova RN, O'Shea TM, et al. Two-hit model of brain damage in the very preterm newborn: small for gestational age and postnatal systemic inflammation. Pediatr Res 2013;73(3):362–70.

45. O'Shea TM, Shah B, Allred EN, et al. Inflammation-initiating illnesses, inflammation-related proteins, and cognitive impairment in extremely preterm infants. Brain Behav Immun 2013;29:104–12.

46. Watterberg KL, Demers LM, Scott SM, et al. Chorioamnionitis and early lung inflammation in infants in whom bronchopulmonary dysplasia develops. Pediatrics 1996;97(2):210–5.

47. Been JV, Rours IG, Kornelisse RF, et al. Histologic chorioamnionitis, fetal involvement, and antenatal steroids: effects on neonatal outcome in preterm infants. Am J Obstet Gynecol 2009;201(6):587.e1–8.

48. Jones MH, Corso AL, Tepper RS, et al. Chorioamnionitis and subsequent lung function in preterm infants. PLoS One 2013;8(12):e81193.

49. Laughon M, Allred EN, Bose C, et al. Patterns of respiratory disease during the first 2 postnatal weeks in extremely premature infants. Pediatrics 2009;123(4): 1124–31.

50. Kramer BW, Kallapur S, Newnham J, et al. Prenatal inflammation and lung development. Semin Fetal Neonatal Med 2009;14(1):2–7.

51. Hartling L, Liang Y, Lacaze-Masmonteil T. Chorioamnionitis as a risk factor for bronchopulmonary dysplasia: a systematic review and meta-analysis. Arch Dis Child Fetal Neonatal Ed 2012;97(1):F8–17.

52. Mercer BM, Miodovnik M, Thurnau GR, et al. Antibiotic therapy for reduction of infant morbidity after preterm premature rupture of the membranes. A randomized controlled trial. National Institute of Child Health and Human Development Maternal-Fetal Medicine Units Network. JAMA 1997;278(12):989–95.

53. Kenyon S, Boulvain M, Neilson JP. Antibiotics for preterm rupture of membranes. Cochrane Database Syst Rev 2013;(12):CD001058.

54. Nabhan AF, Elhelaly A, Elkadi M. Antibiotic prophylaxis in prelabor spontaneous rupture of fetal membranes at or beyond 36 weeks of pregnancy. Int J Gynaecol Obstet 2014;124(1):59–62.

55. Polin RA, Committee on Fetus and Newborn. Management of neonates with suspected or proven early-onset bacterial sepsis. Pediatrics 2012;129(5): 1006–15.

56. Committee on Infectious Diseases, Committee on Fetus and Newborn, Baker CJ, et al. Policy statement-recommendations for the prevention of perinatal group B streptococcal (GBS) disease. Pediatrics 2011;128(3):611–6.

57. Verani JR, McGee L, Schrag SJ, Division of Bacterial Diseases, National Center for Immunization and Respiratory Diseases, Centers for Disease Control and

Prevention (CDC). Prevention of perinatal group B streptococcal disease–revised guidelines from CDC, 2010. MMWR Recomm Rep 2010;59(RR-10):1–36.

58. Miyazaki K, Furuhashi M, Ishikawa K, et al, Neonatal Research Network Japan. The effects of antenatal corticosteroids therapy on very preterm infants after chorioamnionitis. Arch Gynecol Obstet 2014;289(6):1185–90.

59. Torricelli M, Voltolini C, Toti P, et al. Histologic chorioamnionitis: different histologic features at different gestational ages. J Matern Fetal Neonatal Med 2014;27(9): 910–3.

60. Gotsch F, Romero R, Kusanovic JP, et al. The fetal inflammatory response syndrome. Clin Obstet Gynecol 2007;50(3):652–83.

61. Kwak DW, Hwang HS, Kwon JY, et al. Co-infection with vaginal *Ureaplasma urealyticum* and Mycoplasma hominis increases adverse pregnancy outcomes in patients with preterm labor or preterm premature rupture of membranes. J Matern Fetal Neonatal Med 2014;27(4):333–7.

62. Mendz GL, Kaakoush NO, Quinlivan JA. Bacterial aetiological agents of intra-amniotic infections and preterm birth in pregnant women. Front Cell Infect Microbiol 2013;3:58.

63. Goldenberg RL, Andrews WW, Goepfert AR, et al. The Alabama Preterm Birth Study: umbilical cord blood *Ureaplasma urealyticum* and Mycoplasma hominis cultures in very preterm newborn infants. Am J Obstet Gynecol 2008;198(1): 43.e1–5.

64. Onderdonk AB, Delaney ML, DuBois AM, et al, Extremely Low Gestational Age Newborns Study Investigators. Detection of bacteria in placental tissues obtained from extremely low gestational age neonates. Am J Obstet Gynecol 2008;198(1): 110.e1–7.

New Antibiotic Dosing in Infants

Leslie C. Pineda, MD[a], Kevin M. Watt, MD[b],*

KEYWORDS

- Neonates • Infants • Antibiotics • Dosing • Pharmacokinetics • Prematurity

KEY POINTS

- Infection is common and devastating in premature infants, and antibiotics are the most commonly used medications in the neonatal intensive care unit.
- Antibiotic dosing regimens in premature infants are often extrapolated from data in adults and older children and may be incorrect because they do not account for developmental changes in infant physiology.
- Pharmacokinetic (PK) studies in infants are scarce because of low study consent rates; limited blood volume available to conduct PK studies; difficulty in obtaining blood from infants; limited use of sensitive, low-volume drug concentration assays; and a lack of expertise in pediatric modeling and simulation.
- New studies using innovative techniques and requiring smaller sample volumes are providing PK data in premature infants.
- PK data in infants provide appropriate dosing regimens for commonly used antibiotics including ampicillin, clindamycin, meropenem, metronidazole, and piperacillin/tazobactam.

INTRODUCTION

Blood culture–proven infection affects approximately 20% of very-low-birth-weight (VLBW; <1500 g birth weight) infants and causes death in up to 18% of infected infants; those with sepsis are three times more likely to die than those without sepsis (35% vs 11%).[1,2] Survivors often suffer from significant morbidities, including periventricular leukomalacia and neurodevelopmental impairment.[3] VLBW infants with sepsis are also exposed to longer periods of mechanical ventilation and are significantly more likely to develop bronchopulmonary dysplasia; they are also more likely to have longer hospital stays, resulting in higher costs of care.[1]

Conflicts of Interest and Source of Funding: L.C. Pineda and K.M. Watt have no relevant conflicts to disclose.
[a] Department of Pediatrics, Duke University Medical Center, Duke University, Box 2739, 2424 Erwin Road, Hock Plaza Suite 504, Durham, NC 27710, USA; [b] Department of Pediatrics, Duke Clinical Research Institute, Duke University Medical Center, Duke University, Box 3046, 2300 Erwin Road, Durham, NC 27710, USA
* Corresponding author.
E-mail address: kevin.watt@duke.edu

Because infection is such a common and significant complication in this population, most infants admitted to the neonatal intensive care unit (NICU) are exposed to antibiotics, with ampicillin and gentamicin being the most commonly prescribed medications in the NICU.[4] Despite the widespread use of antibiotics in premature (<37 weeks gestation) infants, dosing regimens are often extrapolated from data in adults or older children, increasing the risk of drug toxicity and lack of clinical efficacy. Furthermore, these dosing regimens may be incorrect because they do not account for infants' developmental changes in renal function, metabolic capacity, body composition and surface area, gastrointestinal absorption, and immunocompetence.[5]

MECHANISMS FOR THE STUDY OF DRUGS IN CHILDREN

In 2002 and 2003, the Food and Drug Administration (FDA) implemented the Best Pharmaceuticals for Children Act (BPCA), which provides incentives for pediatric drug studies, and the Pediatric Research Equity Act, which requires pediatric studies of safety and effectiveness for drugs that may be of meaningful therapeutic benefit to children. The FDA reauthorized the BPCA and Pediatric Research Equity Act under the FDA Amendments Act in 2007 and made them permanent in 2012 under the FDA Administration Safety and Innovation Act.

Despite these legislative initiatives, infants, especially those born prematurely, continue to be therapeutic orphans because of the inherent difficulties of conducting clinical trials in this unique and vulnerable population. Pharmacokinetic (PK) studies in premature infants have been scarce because of low study consent rates; limited blood volume available to conduct PK studies; difficulty in obtaining blood from infants; limited use of sensitive, low-volume drug concentration assays; and a lack of expertise in pediatric modeling and simulation. However, newer techniques are emerging with minimal-risk study designs, including ultra-low-volume assays, PK modeling and simulation, and opportunistic drug protocols.[6] These new techniques provide more efficient ways to conduct PK studies in infants with smaller blood volumes and less frequent blood sampling.

However, implementation of these techniques has been slow and most drugs used in infants lack FDA labeling. Thus, clinicians often prescribe these drugs "off-label" to infants without evidence-based dosing regimens from clinical trials. In response to this, the Eunice Kennedy Shriver National Institute of Child Health and Human Development sponsored the Pediatric Trials Network (PTN) to conduct pediatric clinical trials to generate or revise pediatric drug labeling in infants and children. With new data emerging from trials conducted by the PTN and other groups, safer, more accurate, antibiotic dosing regimens are becoming available for premature infants.

AMPICILLIN

Ampicillin is a β-lactam antibiotic and is the most commonly prescribed drug in hospitalized infants.[4] In the Eunice Kennedy Shriver National Institute of Child Health and Human Development Neonatal Research Network, 96% of extremely low-birth-weight (<1000 g birth weight) infants received empiric treatment with a combination of two antibiotics, with ampicillin and gentamicin being the most common combination.[7] Despite the frequency of use, the FDA label has no specific dosing of ampicillin for infants.

The PK of ampicillin in infants was recently evaluated by the PTN in the National Institutes of Health (NIH)–sponsored Pharmacokinetics of Understudied Drugs Administered to Children per Standard of Care Study (POPS Trial, clinicaltrials.gov

NCT01431326).[8] The POPS trial enrolls children who are on a drug of interest (eg, ampicillin, clindamycin) as part of standard of care and collects low-volume PK and dried blood spot samples. The ampicillin study included nine centers and 73 infants with postnatal age (PNA) less than 29 days and median gestational age (GA) 36 weeks. Investigators found that postmenstrual age (PMA) and serum creatinine were strongly correlated with clearance (CL). Elimination half-life was inversely proportional to PNA; moreover, ampicillin CL increased by 27% after the first week of life, and increased by 56% from the younger cohort (GA ≤34 weeks) to the older (GA >34 weeks) cohort. These results are consistent with the developmental maturation of renal function in infants and the predominantly renal elimination of ampicillin.

Using the final PK model developed from the POPS Trial, Monte Carlo simulations were used to evaluate the efficacy of multiple dosing regimens, including standard regimens from Neofax[9] and The Harriet Lane Handbook (**Table 1**),[10] and the simplified regimen stratified by GA and PNA suggested by the POPS trial (**Table 2**). The pharmacodynamic target for β-lactams most associated with efficacy is time above minimum inhibitory concentration (T>MIC). The investigators chose MICs of 2 and 8 μg/mL, representing MICs for two pathogens that can cause severe and fatal infections in infants, Listeria monocytogenes and Escherichia coli. The higher doses used in the POPS trial achieved the surrogate target of greater than or equal to 8 μg/mL in greater than 97% of virtual subjects versus 90% of virtual subjects using traditional dosing regimens. The investigators proposed using the simplified dosing regimen suggested from the POPS trial stratified by GA and PNA, because this regimen provides fewer dosing groups, accounts for maturation of renal function, and incorporates less frequent dosing while still achieving the therapeutic target in more than 90% of subjects (see **Table 2**).[8] This study did not account for cerebrospinal fluid penetration of ampicillin, which was reported to be from 11% to 65% in one study of infants with meningitis.[11] Infants with meningitis will likely need higher ampicillin doses for optimal cerebrospinal fluid penetration. The safety and efficacy of the proposed dosing regimen based on GA and PNA is currently being evaluated in a large, multicenter randomized trial comparing antibiotic regimens in infants with complicated intra-abdominal infection (SCAMP Trial, clinicaltrials.gov # NCT01994993).

CLINDAMYCIN

Clindamycin is a lincosamide antibiotic often used to treat anaerobic infections, pneumonia, osteomyelitis, and skin and skin structure infections. Despite its widespread

Table 1
Comparison of antibiotic dosing recommendations extrapolated from adults and older children versus dosing recommendations based on infant PK data

Antibiotic	Previous Recommendation	New Recommendation
Ampicillin	25–100 mg/kg q 4–12 h	50–75 mg/kg q 8–12 h
Clindamycin	5–7.5 mg/kg q 6–12 h	5–9 mg/kg q 8 h
Meropenem	20 mg/kg q 8–12 h	20–30 mg/kg q 8–12 h
Metronidazole	Loading 0–15 mg/kg Maintenance 7.5–15 mg/kg q 6–48 h	Loading 15 mg/kg Maintenance 7.5 mg/kg q 6–12 h
Piperacillin/ tazobactam	75–100 mg/kg q 6–12 h	80–100 mg/kg q 4–8 h

Data from Refs.[8–10,12,18,27,31]

Table 2
Recommended dosing regimen for ampicillin

GA (wk)	PNA (d)	Maintenance Dose (mg/kg)	Dosing Interval (h)
≤34	≤7	50	12
	≥8 and ≤28	75	12
>34	≤28	50	8

Abbreviations: GA, gestational age at birth; PNA, postnatal age.
Data from Tremoulet A, Le J, Poindexter B, et al. Characterization of the population pharmaco-kinetics of ampicillin in neonates using an opportunistic study design. Antimicrob Agents Chemother 2014;58:3013–20.

use, the FDA label does not adequately address dosing in premature infants and infants less than 1 month of age. However, PK data for clindamycin are also emerging using opportunistic study designs.

In the POPS trial, PK samples were collected from 125 children at 24 centers, including 20 infants born at less than or equal to 32 weeks GA receiving intravenous (IV) clindamycin as standard of care. Investigators used ultra-low-volume samples to create a PK model. Investigators found that clindamycin CL increases with increasing body weight and PMA and reaches 50% of adult CL at approximately 44 weeks PMA.[12]

Using the final PK model and Monte Carlo simulations, investigators evaluated multiple pediatric dosing regimens with the goal to match median adult clindamycin exposure following IV administration of 600 mg every 8 hours, the dose recommended in adults for community-acquired methicillin-resistant *Staphylococcus aureus* infections. A virtual adult patient (70 kg weight) administered clindamycin, 600 mg IV every 8 hours, had a median (2.5th, 97.5th percentiles) area under the concentration versus time curve from 0 to 8 hours at steady state (AUC_{0-8ss}) of 42.9 (14.2, 132) µg*h/mL. PMA-based dosing in simulated infants less than 5 months PNA resulted in median AUC_{0-8ss} comparable with the virtual adult estimate (administered every 8 hours): 42.9 µg*h/mL (5 mg/kg; PMA ≤32 weeks); 42.1 µg*h/mL (7 mg/kg; PMA >32–40 weeks); 42.7 µg*h/mL (9 mg/kg; PMA >40–60 weeks). Thus, for infants less than 5 months PNA, investigators recommended a PMA-based dosing regimen (**Table 3**).[12]

The safety and efficacy of the proposed PMA-based dosing regimen is currently being evaluated in the SCAMP Trial (clinicaltrials.gov # NCT01994993). Safety data in infants are scarce, although one retrospective case-control study described an increased risk of necrotizing enterocolitis (NEC) with increased duration of cumulative antibiotic exposure in infants without culture-proven sepsis; there was a

Table 3
Recommended dosing regimen for clindamycin

PMA (wk)	Maintenance Dose (mg/kg)	Dosing Interval (h)
≤32	5	8
>32 and ≤40	7	8
>40 and ≤60	9	8

Abbreviation: PMA, postmenstrual age.
Data from Gonzalez D, Melloni C, Yogev R, et al. Use of opportunistic clinical data and a population pharmacokinetic model to support dosing of clindamycin for premature infants to adolescents. Clin Pharmacol Ther 2014;96(4):429–37.

significantly higher proportion of clindamycin use in the cases diagnosed with NEC compared with matched control subjects without NEC (unadjusted odds ratio, 4.16 [1.29–13.44]).[13]

MEROPENEM

Meropenem is a broad-spectrum carbapenem antibiotic often used in infants with complicated intra-abdominal infections that cause significant morbidity and mortality. NEC is the most common life-threatening emergency of the neonatal gastrointestinal tract and occurs in up to 11% of VLBW infants.[14,15] Reported NEC mortality is 42%; those who survive are at risk for severe growth delay and poor neurodevelopmental outcomes.[16,17] Thus, infants with suspected or confirmed NEC or intra-abdominal infections are often empirically treated with broad-spectrum or combination antibiotic therapy.[18]

Meropenem PK in infants with suspected or confirmed intra-abdominal infection or NEC was evaluated as part of the NIH-sponsored 24-center, prospective, PK study using ultra-low-volume assays under the BPCA mechanism. Based on data from 188 infants with a median GA at birth of 28 weeks, investigators created a PK model showing that meropenem CL was strongly associated with serum creatinine and PMA and was 30% to 40% lower than the average reported CL in adults.[18] This is consistent with meropenem's method of elimination (renal) and the maturation of neonatal renal function because glomerular filtration rate does not reach 90% of the adult glomerular filtration rate until 1 year PNA.[19]

The dosing strategy used in the study was stratified by GA and PNA (**Table 4**) and was based on previous meropenem PK studies in older infants that evaluated regimens to maintain plasma meropenem concentrations above the MIC for different pathogens, including *Pseudomonas aeruginosa*.[18,20] Investigators defined the therapeutic target as T>MIC of 4 µg/mL for 50% of the dose interval and greater than 2 µg/mL for 75% of the dose interval because the MIC breakpoint of meropenem for *P aeruginosa* is less than or equal to 4 µg/mL and more than 80% of isolates are susceptible at MIC of 2 µg/mL. Using the dosing strategy in **Table 4**, more than 90% of infants in the study achieved this therapeutic target. Because trough meropenem concentrations exceeded this therapeutic target (2 µg/mL) in greater than 80% of infants enrolled in this trial, meropenem doses as outlined in this trial should be sufficient for a clinical and microbiologic cure across GA and PNA for infants less than 91 days of age. Using this dosing strategy in critically ill infants with suspected or proven intra-abdominal infection, meropenem was well tolerated with no adverse events probably or definitely related to meropenem.[21]

Table 4			
Recommended dosing regimen for meropenem			
GA (wk)	PNA (d)	Maintenance Dose (mg/kg)	Dosing Interval (h)
< 32	< 14	20	12
	≥ 14	20	8
≥ 32	< 14	20	8
	≥ 14	30	8

Abbreviations: GA, gestational age at birth; PNA, postnatal age.

Data from Smith PB, Cohen-Wolkowiez M, Castro LM, et al. Population pharmacokinetics of meropenem in plasma and cerebrospinal fluid of infants with suspected or complicated intra-abdominal infections. Pediatr Infect Dis J 2011;30:844–9.

METRONIDAZOLE

Metronidazole is a nitroimidazole antibiotic that is FDA-labeled for anaerobic infections, but not specifically labeled for infants. Despite this, it is often used in premature infants for the treatment of NEC, anaerobic bacteremia, and central nervous system infections. Limited PK data of metronidazole in this population have led to various dosing recommendations.[22–24]

Several recent studies evaluated the PK of metronidazole in infants using a variety of innovative techniques including sparse sampling, ultra-low-volume assays, and scavenge and dried blood spot sampling.[25–27] In an NIH-sponsored open-label, multicenter (N = 5), opportunistic study of 32 infants less than or equal to 32 weeks GA and less than 120 days of age receiving IV metronidazole as part of their routine medical care, investigators measured metronidazole concentrations using a combination of ultra-low-volume (0.3 mL) timed plasma samples and scavenged samples. Investigators showed that metronidazole CL increased proportionally with weight and disproportionally with PMA, which accounts for its predominantly hepatic metabolism.[26] The investigators further evaluated the change in metabolism in a second, three-center study. By calculating a parent-metabolite ratio they found that weight-normalized CL increased with increasing metabolic ratio, and older infants had the highest metabolic ratios.[27]

Given these findings, the recommended dosing regimen for metronidazole is based on PMA (**Table 5**). The surrogate efficacy target was defined as a steady state trough concentration greater than or equal to 8 mg/L. This trough was based on the MIC of 8 mg/L as the susceptibility breakpoint for anaerobic organisms. Simulations using the final PK model evaluated dosing available in *Neofax* and *The Harriet Lane Handbook* versus the proposed PMA-based dosing regimen. Less than 70% of subjects achieved the target when using traditional dosing recommendations, whereas 90% of subjects achieved the target when the PMA-based dosing regimen was used in simulated data sets.[26]

Data are lacking on the safety and efficacy of metronidazole in premature infants. The safety and efficacy of the proposed PMA-based dosing regimen for metronidazole is currently being evaluated by the PTN in the SCAMP Trial (clinicaltrials.gov # NCT01994993).

PIPERACILLIN/TAZOBACTAM

Piperacillin is a semisynthetic derivative of ampicillin with enhanced activity against resistant gram-negative bacteria; piperacillin/tazobactam combines a β-lactam antibiotic with a β-lactamase inhibitor and is primarily renally excreted.[28] Piperacillin/tazobactam is FDA-labeled in patients 2 months and older for appendicitis and

Table 5
Recommended dosing regimen for metronidazole

PMA (wk)	Loading Dose (mg/kg)	Maintenance Dose (mg/kg)	Dosing Interval (h)
<34	15	7.5	12
34–40	15	7.5	8
>40	15	7.5	6

Abbreviation: PMA, postmenstrual age.

Data from Cohen-Wolkowiez M, Ouellet D, Smith PB, et al. Population pharmacokinetics of metronidazole evaluated using scavenged samples from preterm infants. Antimicrob Agents Chemother 2012;56:1828–37.

peritonitis, but it is often used in younger infants to treat systemic and intra-abdominal infections.[29]

Piperacillin/tazobactam PK studies in infants have recently been reported using a combination of timed plasma samples, scavenged blood samples, and dried blood spot sampling.[30,31] In an NIH-sponsored open-label PK and safety study using ultra-low-volume samples and involving four centers and 32 infants less than 61 days of age with a mean GA of 30 weeks treated for suspected systemic infection, piperacillin/tazobactam CL was strongly associated with body weight, PMA, PNA, and serum creatinine. Piperacillin/tazobactam CL increased by 100% after the first 2 weeks of life.[31]

The surrogate target end point for piperacillin/tazobactam efficacy was defined as concentration above the MIC for 75% of the dosing interval in greater than 90% of simulated infants. MICs of 16 and 32 mg/L were chosen because they represented the MICs of common pathogens in premature infants, such as *Enterobacteriaceae* (16 mg/L) and *P aeruginosa* (32 mg/L). Using data generated from the previously mentioned study, a population PK model was developed that evaluated the impact of multiple clinically relevant covariates (eg, PMA, GA, PNA, creatinine). A PMA-based PK model was used as the final model for piperacillin CL and was used to perform Monte Carlo simulations to identify the optimal dose for the infant population (**Table 6**). Simulations showed that the PMA-based dosing regimen achieved the surrogate pharmacodynamic target (piperacillin concentrations 32 mg/L for 75% of dosing interval) in greater than 90% of simulated infants. In addition, this dosing regimen achieved comparable exposures with those seen in adult patients receiving piperacillin/tazobactam for intra-abdominal infections.

The performance of dosing regimens currently recommended in pediatric dosing guidelines (*Neofax* and *The Harriet Lane Handbook*) versus PMA-based dosing was also evaluated. The simulation results indicate that the *Neofax* and *The Harriet Lane Handbook* regimens achieved high target attainment rates (>90% patients with concentrations at 75% at steady state [$C75_{ss}$] greater than the MIC) for MICs less than or equal to 8 mg/L. As the MIC increased beyond 8 mg/L, overall target attainment rates of *Neofax* and *The Harriet Lane Handbook* regimens dropped to 75% and 37%, and 78% and 28% for MICs of 16 and 32 mg/L, respectively.

Because prolonged infusions of piperacillin/tazobactam have higher efficacy in adults,[32-34] a PMA-based dosing regimen using prolonged infusion (2–4 hours) was also evaluated. The PMA-based dosing regimen with prolonged infusion was able to achieve greater than 90% target attainment rates for MIC less than or equal to 32 mg/L overall and for each study group; however, no clear advantage was observed over the short (30 minute) infusion. The SCAMP Trial is currently also evaluating the

Table 6		
Recommended dosing regimen for piperacillin/tazobactam		
PMA (wk)	**Maintenance Dose (mg/kg)**	**Dosing Interval (h)**
≤30	100	8
30–35	80	6
35–49	80	4

Abbreviation: PMA, postmenstrual age.

Data from Cohen-Wolkowiez M, Watt KM, Zhou C, et al. Developmental pharmacokinetics of piperacillin and tazobactam using plasma and dried blood spots from infants. Antimicrob Agents Chemother 2014;58:2856–65.

safety and efficacy of the proposed PMA-based dosing regimen (clinicaltrials.gov # NCT01994993).

SUMMARY

Antibiotics are the most commonly used medications in the NICU.[4] To maximize therapeutic benefit and minimize drug toxicity, it is important to determine appropriate dosing regimens for this population. PK studies in premature infants have been scarce, but studies are now more feasible with the emergence of ultra-low-volume assays, PK modeling and simulation, and opportunistic study designs. More appropriate dosing regimens based on PK data are now available for antibiotics commonly used in the NICU, including ampicillin, clindamycin, meropenem, metronidazole, and piperacillin/tazobactam. The discrepancies between previous dosing recommendations and newer dosing regimens based on infant PK studies highlight the need to conduct PK studies specifically for premature infants.

Best practices box

What is the current practice?

Antibiotics are the most commonly used medications in the NICU. Antibiotic dosing regimens in premature infants are often extrapolated from data in adults and older children and may be incorrect because they do not account for developmental changes in infant physiology.

What changes in current practice are likely to improve outcomes?

New studies using innovative techniques and requiring smaller sample volumes are providing PK data in premature infants. PK data in infants provide appropriate dosing regimens for commonly used antibiotics including ampicillin, clindamycin, meropenem, metronidazole, and piperacillin/tazobactam.

Major recommendations

To maximize therapeutic benefit and minimize drug toxicity, it is important to determine appropriate dosing regimens based on infant PK studies. These studies should take advantage of opportunistic study designs, advances in modeling and simulation, alternative sample matrices, and ultra-low-volume assays.

REFERENCES

1. Stoll BJ, Hansen N, Fanaroff AA, et al. Late-onset sepsis in very low birth weight neonates: the experience of the NICHD Neonatal Research Network. Pediatrics 2002;110:285–91.
2. Stoll BJ, Hansen NI, Higgins RD, et al. Very low birth weight preterm infants with early onset neonatal sepsis: the predominance of gram-negative infections continues in the National Institute of Child Health and Human Development Neonatal Research Network, 2002-2003. Pediatr Infect Dis J 2005;24:635–9.
3. Silveira RC, Procianoy RS, Dill JC, et al. Periventricular leukomalacia in very low birth weight preterm neonates with high risk for neonatal sepsis. J Pediatr (Rio J) 2008;84:211–6.
4. Clark RH, Bloom BT, Spitzer AR, et al. Reported medication use in the neonatal intensive care unit: data from a large national data set. Pediatrics 2006;117: 1979–87.
5. Kearns GL, Abdel-Rahman SM, Alander SW, et al. Developmental pharmacology–drug disposition, action, and therapy in infants and children. N Engl J Med 2003;349:1157–67.

6. Autmizguine J, Benjamin DK, Smith PB, et al. Pharmacokinetic studies in infants using minimal-risk study designs. Curr Clin Pharmacol 2014;9:350–8.

7. Cotten CM, Taylor S, Stoll B, et al. Prolonged duration of initial empirical antibiotic treatment is associated with increased rates of necrotizing enterocolitis and death for extremely low birth weight infants. Pediatrics 2009;123:58–66.

8. Tremoulet A, Le J, Poindexter B, et al. Characterization of the population pharmacokinetics of ampicillin in neonates using an opportunistic study design. Antimicrob Agents Chemother 2014;58:3013–20.

9. Thomson Reuters Clinical Editorial Staff. Neofax 2011. Montvale (NJ): Thomson Reuters; 2011.

10. Tschudy MM, Arcara KM, Johns Hopkins Hospital, Children's Medical and Surgical Center. The Harriet Lane handbook: a manual for pediatric house officers. 19th edition. Philadelphia: Elsevier/Mosby; 2012.

11. Kaplan JM, McCracken GH Jr, Horton LJ, et al. Pharmacologic studies in neonates given large dosages of ampicillin. J Pediatr 1974;84:571–7.

12. Gonzalez D, Melloni C, Yogev R, et al. Use of opportunistic clinical data and a population pharmacokinetic model to support dosing of clindamycin for premature infants to adolescents. Clin Pharmacol Ther 2014;96(4):429–37.

13. Alexander VN, Northrup V, Bizzarro MJ. Antibiotic exposure in the newborn intensive care unit and the risk of necrotizing enterocolitis. J Pediatr 2011;159:392–7.

14. Horbar JD, Carpenter JH, Badger GJ, et al. Mortality and neonatal morbidity among infants 501 to 1500 grams from 2000 to 2009. Pediatrics 2012;129:1019–26.

15. Stoll BJ, Hansen NI, Bell EF, et al. Neonatal outcomes of extremely preterm infants from the NICHD Neonatal Research Network. Pediatrics 2010;126:443–56.

16. Fitzgibbons SC, Ching Y, Yu D, et al. Mortality of necrotizing enterocolitis expressed by birth weight categories. J Pediatr Surg 2009;44:1072–5 [discussion: 1075–6].

17. Hintz SR, Kendrick DE, Stoll BJ, et al. Neurodevelopmental and growth outcomes of extremely low birth weight infants after necrotizing enterocolitis. Pediatrics 2005;115:696–703.

18. Smith PB, Cohen-Wolkowiez M, Castro LM, et al. Population pharmacokinetics of meropenem in plasma and cerebrospinal fluid of infants with suspected or complicated intra-abdominal infections. Pediatr Infect Dis J 2011;30:844–9.

19. Rhodin MM, Anderson BJ, Peters AM, et al. Human renal function maturation: a quantitative description using weight and postmenstrual age. Pediatr Nephrol 2009;24:67–76.

20. Blumer JL, Reed MD, Kearns GL, et al. Sequential, single-dose pharmacokinetic evaluation of meropenem in hospitalized infants and children. Antimicrob Agents Chemother 1995;39:1721–5.

21. Cohen-Wolkowiez M, Poindexter B, Bidegain M, et al. Safety and effectiveness of meropenem in infants with suspected or complicated intra-abdominal infections. Clin Infect Dis 2012;55:1495–502.

22. Hall P, Kaye CM, McIntosh N, et al. Intravenous metronidazole in the newborn. Arch Dis Child 1983;58:529–31.

23. Jager-Roman E, Doyle PE, Baird-Lambert J, et al. Pharmacokinetics and tissue distribution of metronidazole in the new born infant. J Pediatr 1982;100:651–4.

24. Upadhyaya P, Bhatnagar V, Basu N. Pharmacokinetics of intravenous metronidazole in neonates. J Pediatr Surg 1988;23:263–5.

25. Suyagh M, Collier PS, Millership JS, et al. Metronidazole population pharmacokinetics in preterm neonates using dried blood-spot sampling. Pediatrics 2011;127:e367–74.

26. Cohen-Wolkowiez M, Ouellet D, Smith PB, et al. Population pharmacokinetics of metronidazole evaluated using scavenged samples from preterm infants. Antimicrob Agents Chemother 2012;56:1828–37.

27. Cohen-Wolkowiez M, Sampson M, Bloom BT, et al. Determining population and developmental pharmacokinetics of metronidazole using plasma and dried blood spot samples from premature infants. Pediatr Infect Dis J 2013;32:956–61.

28. Sorgel F, Kinzig M. The chemistry, pharmacokinetics and tissue distribution of piperacillin/tazobactam. J Antimicrob Chemother 1993;31(Suppl A):39–60.

29. Berger A, Kretzer V, Apfalter P, et al. Safety evaluation of piperacillin/tazobactam in very low birth weight infants. J Chemother 2004;16:166–71.

30. Cohen-Wolkowiez M, Benjamin DK Jr, Ross A, et al. Population pharmacokinetics of piperacillin using scavenged samples from preterm infants. Ther Drug Monit 2012;34:312–9.

31. Cohen-Wolkowiez M, Watt KM, Zhou C, et al. Developmental pharmacokinetics of piperacillin and tazobactam using plasma and dried blood spots from infants. Antimicrob Agents Chemother 2014;58:2856–65.

32. Felton TW, Hope WW, Lomaestro BM, et al. Population pharmacokinetics of extended-infusion piperacillin-tazobactam in hospitalized patients with nosocomial infections. Antimicrob Agents Chemother 2012;56:4087–94.

33. Roberts JA, Kirkpatrick CM, Roberts MS, et al. First-dose and steady-state population pharmacokinetics and pharmacodynamics of piperacillin by continuous or intermittent dosing in critically ill patients with sepsis. Int J Antimicrob Agents 2010;35:156–63.

34. Shea KM, Cheatham SC, Smith DW, et al. Comparative pharmacodynamics of intermittent and prolonged infusions of piperacillin/tazobactam using Monte Carlo simulations and steady-state pharmacokinetic data from hospitalized patients. Ann Pharmacother 2009;43:1747–54.

New Antifungal and Antiviral Dosing

Kelly C. Wade, MD, PhD, MSCE[a],*, Heather M. Monk, PharmD[b]

KEYWORDS

- Neonate • Fluconazole • Amphotericin • Echinocandin • Acyclovir • Ganciclovir

KEY POINTS

- Neonatal antifungal dosing needs to consider treatment of hematogenous candida meningoencephalitis.
- Amphotericin B deoxycholate is recommended for empiric therapy for invasive candidiasis.
- Suppressive therapy with acyclovir for herpes simplex virus and ganciclovir/valganciclovir for cytomegalovirus may provide long-term neurodevelopmental benefits.
- Bone marrow suppression is the most prominent dose-limiting toxicity associated with antiviral therapy.

INTRODUCTION

Neonatal fungal and viral infections are associated with mortality and neurologic impairment among survivors. Advances in pharmacokinetics (PK) and pharmacodynamics (PD) of antimicrobial medications have led to improved dosing guidance designed to optimize outcomes.[1,2] The goals of antimicrobial therapy are simple: eradicate the pathogen, minimize toxicity, and prevent emergence of resistant organisms. Clinicians and pharmacists try to determine what drug dose and interval will lead to the plasma concentrations that have been associated with efficacy. The PK of a drug explains the dose-concentration relationship. The PD of a drug explains the relationship between the concentration of the drug in the body and the therapeutic or toxic response (**Table 1**).

PK/PD relationships allow clinicians to target specific drug concentrations and dosing intervals that have been associated with therapeutic efficacy (see **Table 1**).

Disclosures: None.
[a] Division of Neonatology, Department of Pediatrics, Perelman School of Medicine, Children's Hospital of Philadelphia Newborn Care at Pennsylvania Hospital, 800 Spruce Street, Philadelphia, PA 19107, USA; [b] Department of Pharmacy, Children's Hospital of Philadelphia, 3401 Civic Center Boulevard, Philadelphia, PA 19107, USA
* Corresponding author.
E-mail address: kelly.wade@uphs.upenn.edu

Clin Perinatol 42 (2015) 177–194
http://dx.doi.org/10.1016/j.clp.2014.10.010   **perinatology.theclinics.com**

Table 1
PK/PD relationships for optimal antimicrobial treatment

PD Metric	Definition	Drug Class	PK/PD Target and Dosing Strategy
Concentration dependent with long postantimicrobial effect	Antimicrobial killing is proportional to the maximal concentration achieved relative to the MIC of the causative organism. Antimicrobial properties persist even when concentrations decrease to less than MIC	Amphotericin Echinocandin	C_{max}/MIC Use a high dose to achieve high drug concentrations (C_{max}) with longer dosing interval
Time dependent and concentration independent	Antimicrobial killing is proportional to the amount of time the drug concentration is maintained at more than the MIC of the causative organism. Peak concentration is not related to efficacy	β-Lactams, cephalosporins	% dosing interval time [drug] is >MIC Enhance duration of exposure by using short dosing interval to maintain drug concentration at more than MIC of organism
Time dependent with long postantimicrobial effect	Bacterial killing is proportional to the amount of total drug exposure (AUC) relative to MIC of the causative organism. Antimicrobial properties persist even when concentrations decrease to less than MIC	Fluconazole	AUC/MIC Enhance efficacy by optimizing both drug dose and shorter dosing intervals

Abbreviations: AUC, area less than the concentration curve; C_{max}, peak concentration; MIC, minimum inhibitory concentration.
Data from Refs.[1,2,23,90]

PD characteristics are typically consistent among drugs of the same class and across different species for the same infecting organism.[2] However, unique neonatal PK differences in volume of distribution, protein binding, metabolism, and clearance alter drug exposures. Neonates also have greater likelihood of central nervous system (CNS) involvement. Neonatal dosing needs to consider these differences in order to optimize drug exposures that meet the PD indices associated with efficacy. At this point, PD indices are mostly extrapolated from adults and in vivo and in vitro models. Neonatal PD studies are needed. This article discusses the basic PK/PD properties and dosing of the most common antifungal and antiviral medications used in neonates.

TREATMENT OF INVASIVE FUNGAL INFECTIONS INCLUDING HEMATOGENOUS CANDIDA MENINGOENCEPHALITIS

Invasive fungal infections are serious infections in newborns that primarily affect extremely premature infants. Term infants with central line access and those on extracorporeal membrane oxygenation (ECMO) are also at risk. Most fungal infections in neonates are *Candida albicans* and *Candida parapsilosis*. Other *Candida* species known for high levels of antifungal drug resistance, such as *Candida glabrata* and *Candida krusei*, are less common and noncandida fungal infections (eg, those caused by *Aspergillus*) are rare. Mortality is estimated to be 20% to 30% with significant long-term neurologic impairment in many survivors. Neonates are at high risk for CNS infections known as hematogenous candida meningoencephalitis (HCME).

Treatment failure, defined as death or prolonged candidemia, is common.[3] Early initiation of empiric antifungal therapy is associated with improved survival.[4,5] Doses high enough to treat disseminated disease, including HCME, are needed to promote survival and minimize long-term deficits.

POLYENES: AMPHOTERICIN B DEOXYCHOLATE, LIPOSOMAL AMPHOTERICIN, AND AMPHOTERICIN B LIPID COMPLEX
Antimicrobial Activity

Amphotericin B (AmB) is a potent fungicidal medication that uses its polyene structure to bind the ergosterol in the fungal cell to weaken the cell membrane, and leads to cell death through leakage of essential nutrients and disturbed ion flux.[6] It is active against nearly all fungal species that affect neonates, including most *Candida* spp as well as *Aspergillus*.

Clinical Pharmacology

AmB is only available intravenously (**Table 2**). Solubilization has required either formulation with bile salt AmB deoxycholate (AmB-d) or incorporation into various lipid structures (liposomal AmB [L-AmB] or AmB lipid complex [ABLC]).[6] It is primarily protein bound (>90%). AmB is distributed throughout the body along with lipoproteins and is quickly transferred into solid organs through the reticuloendothelial system.[7] AmB is not metabolized to any relevant degree and is excreted at low concentrations in the urine and feces at a rate proportional to the unbound fraction. AmB formulations penetrate the CNS despite low cerebrospinal fluid (CSF) concentrations and are fungicidal in animal models of HCME.[8,9] Neonates can have CSF concentrations as high as 40% to 90% of serum concentrations.[10] Small case series of premature infants have shown AmB-d and L-AmB to be effective at treating CNS disease.[11–15]

Table 2
Most commonly used antifungal drugs

Drug	Advantages	Disadvantages	Clinical Pharmacology	PK in Preterm Infants	PD Dosing Target	Dose
Amphotericin B deoxycholate	Fungicidal Kills nearly all *Candida* spp	Toxicity, particularly in older patients Long drug infusion time	IV only 90% protein bound Long terminal half-life	Limited and highly variable	$C_{max}/MIC>2-10$	1 mg/kg/d
Fluconazole	IV and PO formulation Minimal side effects High concentrations in tissue, CNS, and urine	Some *Candida* spp are resistant Fungistatic Poor option if infant receiving fluconazole prophylaxis	IV and PO 10% protein bound Renal elimination Active drug concentrated in urine	Yes	AUC 400 $AUC/MIC>50$	12 mg/kg/d Consider loading dose 25 mg/kg Dose adjust for renal insufficiency after 4 d if creatinine remains >1 mg/dL
Liposomal formulations L-AmB ABLC	Fungicidal Kills nearly all *Candida* spp	Toxicity, although less than AmB-d Long drug infusion time	IV only 90% protein bound Long terminal half-life	Limited Only ABLC	C_{max}/MIC	5 mg/kg/d L-AmB range 3-7 mg/kg/d
Micafungin	Fungicidal Kills nearly all *Candida* spp May have properties against biofilms Limited side effects	Liver tumors in rats at high dose	IV only 90% protein bound Hepatic metabolism (not P450)	Yes	$C_{max}/MIC>1-2$ $AUC>166$ mg*h/L for HCME	10 mg/kg/d

See text for detailed references and recent reviews.[1,2,20,23,24,90]
Abbreviations: ABLC, amphotericin lipid complex; IV, intravenous; L-AmB, liposomal amphotericin B; PO, peroral.

Amphotericin B Pharmacokinetics

PK information regarding all formulations of AmB in neonates and young infants is sparse. Three small AmB-d PK studies have included preterm infants and all report extreme interpatient variability.[10,16,17] Some subjects showed drug elimination between doses, whereas others accumulated the drug with minimal elimination. Increasing serum creatinine level was associated with minimal elimination. Only infants receiving 0.8 to 1 mg/kg had detectable serum concentrations after the first dose.[10] Young infants achieved lower concentrations compared with adults because of a higher weight-corrected drug clearance.[16,17] In young infants, an AmB-d dosage of 1 mg/kg/d typically provides serum concentrations of greater than 0.5 μg/mL.[16,17] Even large overdoses in neonates have resulted in minimal toxicity, possibly because of increased weight-normalized clearance.[18]

There is only 1 neonatal PK study for liposomal formulations. The PK of ABLC (2-5 mg/kg/d) were studied in 28 neonates (median gestational age (GA) of 27 weeks, weight of 1kg) who had reported exposure similar to adults; after a 5 mg/kg dose, their mean AmB plasma concentration was 0.45 ug/mL and urinary concentration was 0.35 ug/mL. There was no apparent accumulation with multiple doses and the elimination rate was similar to AmB-d.[19] Weight-normalized drug clearance was nearly 2-fold higher than in children and did not vary with GA. L-AmB PK has not been described in neonates. L-AmB is preferred by some clinicians because it achieves higher CNS concentrations than other liposomal formulations and has evidence for neonatal efficacy.[9] Liposomal formulations may have decreased renal parenchymal penetration and are not optimal for treatment of renal candidiasis.[20]

Safety

AmB-d is associated with significant infusion-related toxicity with fever, chills, and rigors along with nephrotoxicity in older children and adults.[6,21] Lipid formulations have less associated toxicity.[6,13] Neonates experience less AmB-d toxicity, therefore lipid formulations are rarely indicated. Nephrotoxicity and hypokalemia are the most common reported neonatal toxicities; however, it is difficult to distinguish drug-related nephrotoxicity from disease-related effects.[21,22] Renal function and electrolyte monitoring are warranted.

Pharmacodynamics and Recommended Dosing to Achieve Pharmacokinetics/Pharmacodynamics Targets

AmB PD properties follow a concentration-dependent killing pattern with a prolonged postantifungal effect (see **Tables 1** and **2**).[2,9,23] Tissue concentrations increase with total dose. The PK/PD of AmB support infrequent dosing to optimize peak concentrations (C_{max}). A C_{max}/minimum inhibitory concentration (MIC) ratio of 2 to 4 is associated with fungicidal efficacy in murine and in vitro systems of candidiasis.[23] There are no PD efficacy data for neonates.

Inadequate neonatal PK information and large interpatient variability make singular dosing guidance difficult. Treatment failure or toxicity may reflect inadequate dosing. Higher dosages for premature neonates are recommended given the high incidence of CNS disease (HCME). AmB-d dosed at 1 mg/kg/d is recommended as first-line therapy for empiric coverage of HCME in neonates.[20,24] The recommended dosage of lipid formulations of L-AmB and ABLC is typically 3 to 5 mg/kg/d (range, 2.5–7 mg/kg).[20,24] Liposomal formulations are reserved for infants who have not tolerated AmB-d and do not have urinary tract involvement. High-dose L-AmB (5–7 mg/kg/d) achieved cure in greater than 90% of neonates with invasive candidiasis and was well tolerated.[12,25] In small nonrandomized studies, there was no difference in survival, fungal eradication, or side effects between infants receiving AmB-d, L-AmB, or ABLC.[13,26]

TRIAZOLES: FLUCONAZOLE AND VORICONAZOLE
Antimicrobial Activity

The azole antifungals are named for their chemical structure, which contains an azole ring.[27,28] Triazole antifungals are typically fungistatic and lead to weakness of the fungal cell membrane by inhibiting a fungal cytochrome P450–dependent enzyme (lanosterol 14-alpha demethylase), which is responsible for the conversion of lanosterol to ergosterol. Triazoles interact with the cytochrome P450 system, leading to important drug interactions. Fluconazole is effective against *C albicans* and *C parapsilosis* but not *C glabrata*, C *krusei*, or *Aspergillus*. Voriconazole is a second-generation triazole with an expanded spectrum of activity, including *Aspergillus*.

FLUCONAZOLE
Clinical Pharmacology

Fluconazole is one of the most commonly used drugs for invasive candidiasis in neonates (see **Table 2**).[27,28] It is available in both intravenous (IV) and enteral liquid formulations with excellent bioavailability. Its low side effect profile and low protein binding allow infants to achieve high concentrations in solid organs including the CNS. Fluconazole is eliminated through the kidney as active drug and is concentrated in urine. Fluconazole is excellent for urinary tract infections.

Fluconazole Pharmacokinetics

The PK of fluconazole in neonates and young infants has been described in 76 infants, 23 to 40 weeks' GA, and up to 90 days old.[29–32] Neonates have a larger volume distribution, likely because of the increased total body water. Clearance increases with postnatal age (PNA) and postmenstrual age (PMA). Fluconazole can be administered daily given its long half-life (30 hours), although steady state is not typically achieved for 4 to 5 days.[33] A loading dose of 25 mg/kg is needed to rapidly achieve the therapeutic target.[34]

Safety

Fluconazole is well tolerated, with an excellent safety profile. In adults, there was no dose-limiting toxicity at high doses up to 1600 mg/d.[35,36] In children, increased liver enzyme levels, bilirubin levels, or hepatomegaly were reported in less than 5% of patients, although abnormalities may have been related to concomitant medication or serious illness.[37] In neonates, no serious events have been associated with fluconazole prophylaxis. Modest increases in liver enzyme levels are inconsistently shown, although these are not clinically significant, and return to baseline after completing therapy.[38–42]

Pharmacodynamics and Recommended Dosing to Achieve Pharmacokinetics/Pharmacodynamics Targets

Fluconazole PD are well characterized and consistent within the azole class (see **Tables 1** and **2**).[2] Fluconazole is concentration independent, time dependent, and has prolonged postantifungal effect. Efficacy is optimized by total drug exposure (area under the concentration time curve [AUC]) above the MIC of the organism (AUC/MIC>25–50) for invasive disease.[43,44] The MIC susceptibility break point for most *Candida* species is 8, therefore drug dosing must achieve a minimum AUC of 400 mg*h/L. The adult Infectious Diseases Society of America guideline targets this AUC by recommending an 800-mg ($\approx$ 12 mg/kg) loading dose followed by 400 mg/d ($\approx$ 6 mg/kg). Higher doses (800 mg/d) have been used to treat CNS disease and patients with severe critical illness and immunosuppression.[20]

Extremely premature infants are immunocompromised and likely to have HCME, and thus may benefit from high fluconazole exposures. The recommended neonatal dosage (12 mg/kg/d) ensures that at least 90% of 23-week to 29-week GA infants and 80% of 30-week to 40-week GA infants achieve the therapeutic PD target (AUC>400 mg*h/L).[20,24,33] In the 23-week to 29-week GA infants, the median fluconazole exposure of AUC 800 mg*h/L is consistent with high-dose (800 mg/d) therapy in adults.[33] Steady state is not usually achieved until day 5, so a loading dose should be considered, particularly in infants with proven candidiasis. One study showed that a loading dose of 25 mg/kg could achieve an AUC of 400 mg*h/L.[34]

Fluconazole provides excellent treatment of invasive candidiasis among susceptible *Candida* species given the excellent safety profile; wide distribution into tissue, including the CNS and urinary tract; and availability of an enteral formulation.[20,24,45] In the only randomized controlled trial comparing fluconazole with AmB (n = 24 neonates), fluconazole had a lower case fatality rate of 33% compared with 45% for AmB.[46]

Fluconazole Prophylaxis

Several randomized controlled trials show that fluconazole prophylaxis decreases the incidence of invasive candidiasis in premature infants.[38,41,42] However, in infants of less than 750 g birth weight, fluconazole prophylaxis did not decrease the composite outcome of death or candidiasis or improve neurodevelopmental outcomes.[38] The fluconazole dose for prophylaxis for infants of 23 to 29 weeks' GA is 3 or 6 mg/kg/dose twice weekly.[33,38,41] This dosing maintains fluconazole concentrations greater than 2 or 4 µg/mL respectively for half of the dosing interval.[33] There are concerns that fluconazole prophylaxis may increase the incidence of fluconazole resistance.

Prophylaxis for Infants on Extracorporeal Membrane Oxygenation

Candida infections are an important cause of death in infants on ECMO. Fluconazole PK among 10 infants on ECMO receiving a 25-mg/kg weekly dose provided adequate exposure for prophylaxis and showed higher volume of distribution and similar clearance compared with term infants.[47] Oxygenator extraction was minimal.

VORICONAZOLE

Voriconazole has oral and IV formulations and is typically reserved for rare cases of aspergillosis or resistant *Candida*.[48] Voriconazole is highly protein bound and has important drug interactions caused by hepatic cytochrome p450 isoenzyme 2C19 (CYP2C19) metabolism. Voriconazole exposure in young children is highly variable.[49] Overall, children require higher doses because of higher drug clearance and lower bioavailability. Important side effects include visual disturbances, increased hepatic transaminase levels, and skin reactions, particularly when trough concentrations are greater than or equal to 5 to 6 µg/mL. The pediatric dose (ages 2–11 years) is 7 mg/kg IV twice daily to achieve a trough greater than or equal to 1 µg/mL.[50] In neonatal case series, the most common dose is 4 mg/kg twice a day, although dosing has ranged from 8 to 24 mg/kg/d.[48,51–53] Therapeutic drug monitoring is indicated for neonates. Because of the lack of PK data in neonates and potential side effects, voriconazole should not be routinely used in this population.

ECHINOCANDINS: MICAFUNGIN, CASPOFUNGIN, ANIDULAFUNGIN
Antimicrobial Activity

Echinocandins are cyclic hexapeptides that interfere with cell wall biosynthesis by noncompetitive inhibition of 1,3-beta-D-glucan synthase, a fungus-specific enzyme.[54,55] 1,3-Beta-D-glucan is necessary for cell wall stability. Echinocandins are effective against most *Candida* and *Aspergillus* species.

Clinical Pharmacology

Echinocandins are only available in IV form; are highly protein bound; are widely disseminated into tissues; and achieve high tissue concentrations in the liver, spleen, and lung (see **Table 2**).[55] Clearance is primarily through non–cytochrome P450 hepatic metabolism and fecal elimination. Higher serum exposures are necessary to achieve adequate CNS penetration, although CSF concentrations remain low.[56] Echinocandins are also active against the biofilms that complicate central line–associated infections. Advantages include minimal drug interactions and side effects. They do not typically require dose adjustment in patients with renal disease.

Micafungin Pharmacokinetics

Micafungin is the best studied echinocandin in neonates and infants across a wide dosage range of 0.75 to 15 mg/kg/d.[57–61] Premature infants have faster clearance than older infants, possibly because of age-dependent differences in protein binding.[57–61] In a PK study of 12 preterm infants (mean GA, 28 weeks), 15 mg/kg/d achieved similar exposure to adults receiving 5 mg/kg/d. In a multidose PK study, 7 mg/kg/d in infants of more than 1000 g (mean GA, 30 weeks) and 10 mg/kg/d in infants less than 1000 g (mean GA, 25 weeks) achieved the target AUC of 166 mg*h/L associated with efficacy in an animal model of HCME.[56] A population PK model determined that 10 mg/kg/d achieved this target AUC in 83% of young infants.[58]

Caspofungin Pharmacokinetics

Neonatal PK data for caspofungin are limited. Infants 1 to 11 weeks of age with GAs of 24 to 41 weeks who received caspofungin 25 mg/m^2 daily[62] had plasma concentrations similar to adults and children receiving a higher dose (50 mg/m^2/d) for esophageal or oropharyngeal candidiasis.[62] Higher serum trough concentrations suggested lower clearance in neonates.

Anidulafungin Pharmacokinetics

Anidulafungin has recently been studied in neonates. In general, children have SHORTER half-lives (20 hours) than adults (26 hours). In one small study, 8 neonates who received a loading dose of 3 mg/kg followed by 1.5 mg/kg/d for 5 days had similar exposure to adults receiving 100 mg/d.[63] Two neonates on ECMO had lower exposure, suggesting that a 2-fold to 3-fold higher dose may be necessary on ECMO.[63]

Safety

Echinocandins are well tolerated, with rare adverse effects related to gastrointestinal symptoms, increased liver enzyme levels, hypokalemia, or hypersensitivity reactions. All echinocandin drugs include a warning of possible hepatic dysfunction. There is 1 case report of severe hepatitis in a premature infant with invasive candidiasis that resolved with discontinuation of micafungin.[64] In Europe, there is a black box warning regarding increased incidence of hepatic tumors in rats receiving prolonged excessive micafungin exposure.[24] Similar studies have not been performed for other echinocandins. Hypercalcemia and hyperphosphatemia were reported in 1 neonate receiving high-dose caspofungin.[65]

Pharmacodynamics and Recommended Dosing to Achieve Pharmacokinetics/Pharmacodynamics Targets

Echinocandins have concentration-dependent fungicidal effect with prolonged antifungal effect (see **Tables 1** and **2**). In animal models, fungicidal efficacy correlated with both peak/MIC and AUC/MIC targets.[2,66,67] The PD of micafungin in a rabbit model of HCME showed that a micafungin AUC of 166 mg*h/L was associated with maximal decline in fungal burden and efficacy.[56]

National guidelines recommend micafungin or caspofungin for use in neonates with invasive fungal infections not responsive to AmB or fluconazole or who have drug intolerance.[20,24] The micafungin neonatal dosage for invasive candidiasis is 10 mg/kg/d.[24,57,60] Dosages of 10 mg/kg/d provide systemic exposures that target CNS penetration and the AUC-associated efficacy in HCME models. The caspofungin neonatal dosage of 25 mg/m²/d achieves similar exposure to adult treatment of oropharyngeal infections but may not be adequate for HCME.[24] Micafungin has been shown to be noninferior to L-AmB with an improved safety profile in children and adults. In children, treatment success was similar on either therapy, but fewer patients discontinued micafungin.[68] Given the sparse amount of PK and safety data in neonates, anidulafungin is not recommended for use in young infants.

ANTIVIRAL MEDICATIONS

The PK and PD information available for acyclovir and ganciclovir and their associated oral prodrugs, valacyclovir and valganciclovir, is discussed here.

ACYCLOVIR AND VALACYCLOVIR
Antiviral Activity

Acyclovir has inhibitory activity against herpes simplex virus (HSV)-1, HSV-2, and varicella-zoster virus.[69,70] The inhibitory activity of acyclovir is highly selective because of its affinity for the viral enzyme thymidine kinase, which phosphorylates acyclovir. In vitro, acyclovir stops replication of HSV DNA via competitive inhibition and inactivation of viral DNA polymerase.

Clinical Pharmacology

IV acyclovir is the mainstay of HSV treatment in neonates. Concentrations achieved in the CSF are approximately 50% of plasma values.[71] Acyclovir is eliminated as active drug through renal excretion. Valacyclovir is the L-valyl ester of acyclovir, which is rapidly converted to acyclovir after oral administration and retains the same antiviral properties, safety, and resistance patterns as acyclovir.[71,72] Valacyclovir is not routinely used in neonates because of lack of PK data.

Pharmacokinetics of Acyclovir and Valacyclovir

Neonatal acyclovir PK, given intravenously, have been described over a range of 5 to 15 mg/kg/dose.[73,74] Plasma acyclovir concentrations increase in a dose-dependent manner. The 3-hour to 4-hour half-life was slightly longer than in adults. Infants receiving 15 mg/kg/dose 3 times a day (45 mg/kg/d) had similar peak concentrations, half-life, and clearance.[75] Clearance increased with age, consistent with renal maturation.

IV acyclovir PK has recently been described in preterm and term infants.[76] Infants received either 500 mg/m^2 every 8 hours, or dosing based on GA and PNA: 10 mg/kg every 12 hours (23–29 weeks' GA, 0–13 days old), 20 mg/kg every 12 hours (23–29 weeks' GA, 14–44 days old), or 20 mg/kg every 8 hours (30–34 weeks' GA, 0–44 days old). Clearance increased with advancing GA, PNA, and improved renal function. PMA was the most significant covariate for clearance. Clearance increased and half-life decreased 3-fold between the youngest and oldest PMA groups. Oral acyclovir has limited bioavailability (12%) in infants.[71]

The PK of valacyclovir in young infants is limited. In infants less than 1 year old, oral valacyclovir was rapidly absorbed and converted to acyclovir.[72] Older infants had the lowest exposures and highest clearance. The youngest infants had higher mean acyclovir exposures. Bioavailability was estimated to be ≈50%, except in infants 3 to 5 months of age, in whom the bioavailability was 22%.

Safety

Bone marrow suppression and nephrotoxicity are the most common side effects associated with acyclovir/valacyclovir therapy. In neonates treated with high-dose IV acyclovir (60 mg/kg/d), 21% developed neutropenia (absolute neutrophil count [ANC] ≤ 1000/mm^3).[75] There were no reported adverse events secondary to neutropenia. Among infants receiving oral acyclovir suppressive therapy, 46% developed neutropenia.[77] Most infants continued taking acyclovir without interruption and had spontaneous recovery. A recent study of acyclovir oral suppressive therapy revealed no difference in neutropenia compared with placebo; however, this study was likely underpowered.[78] Neutrophil counts should be monitored while on high-dose IV acyclovir therapy and suppressive therapy, with consideration of decreasing the dose or administering granulocyte colony-stimulating factor if neutropenia (ANC<500/mm^3) persists.[75]

Acyclovir also has potential for nephrotoxicity. Precipitation of acyclovir crystals in renal tubules can occur if the maximum solubility of free acyclovir is exceeded or if the drug is administered by bolus injection, and renal tubular damage can produce acute renal failure. Concomitant use of other nephrotoxic drugs, preexisting renal disease, and dehydration make further renal impairment more likely. In a clinical trial of high-dose (60 mg/kg/d) acyclovir, 6% of subjects developed renal insufficiency, and it is unclear whether disease or acyclovir toxicity contributed to this.[75] Renal function should be closely monitored, with consideration for dose adjustment in patients with significant, persistent renal impairment.

Acyclovir-associated neurotoxicity has been described in adults with high serum concentrations (>50–70 mg/L).[79] The relationship between acyclovir concentration and neurotoxicity was likely related to concomitant CNS insults and/or renal failure. When evaluating dosing regimens, it is reasonable to maintain C_{max} less than 50 to 70 mg/L.

Dosing to Achieve Pharmacokinetics/Pharmacodynamics Targets

IV acyclovir at 60 mg/kg/d (20 mg/kg/dose every 8 hours) reduces mortality in neonates with disseminated HSV.[75] In neonates, PD targets are unknown. The following surrogate PD safety and efficacy targets have been proposed: limit C_{max} to less than 50 to 70 mg/L to avoid potential neurotoxicity and maintain acyclovir plasma concentrations at 50% of the dosing interval ($C50_{ss}$) greater than 3 mg/L in order to achieve CSF concentrations of greater than 1 mg/L, thus exceeding the acyclovir half maximal inhibitory concentration (IC50) of neonatal HSV isolates.[80] The following

PMA-based dosing guidelines account for improved clearance with maturation and target proposed surrogate PD targets: infants less than 30 weeks' PMA, 20 mg/kg/dose every 12 hours; infants 30 to less than 36 weeks' PMA, 20 mg/kg/dose every 8 hours; infants 36 to 41 weeks' PMA, 20 mg/kg/dose every 6 hours. In simulated exposures, nearly all infants achieved the $C50_{ss}$ goal of greater than or equal to 3 mg/L and less than 1% had C_{max} greater than 50 mg/L.[76] This proposed dosing guidance needs prospective validation and safety analysis.

The recommended dose of oral acyclovir suppressive therapy of 300 mg/m²/dose 3 times a day for 6 months reduced cutaneous recurrences and improved neurodevelopmental outcomes in a randomized trial.[78] The incidence of neutropenia was similar in infants exposed to placebo and to acyclovir. Higher doses ($\approx$1200–1600 mg/m²/dose twice a day) administered for 2 years also showed improved neurodevelopmental outcomes in an observational study.[81]

GANCICLOVIR AND VALGANCICLOVIR
Clinical Pharmacology

IV ganciclovir is recommended for symptomatic congenital cytomegalovirus (CMV) infections.[71,82] In adults, CSF concentrations are 24% to 70% of plasma concentrations after IV administration. Plasma protein binding is negligible. Active drug is eliminated by glomerular filtration and active tubular secretion in the kidneys. Oral valganciclovir has good bioavailability and is rapidly converted to ganciclovir.[83,84]

Antimicrobial Activity

Ganciclovir inhibits replication of herpes viruses, including CMV and HSV.[71,82] Ganciclovir is phosphorylated preferentially in CMV-infected cells by a CMV-encoded protein kinase and cellular kinases. Ganciclovir triphosphate inhibits viral DNA synthesis by competitive inhibition of viral DNA polymerases, incorporation into viral DNA, and eventual termination of viral DNA elongation. Valganciclovir is converted to ganciclovir and provides the same activity.

Pharmacokinetics

The PK of ganciclovir has been evaluated in neonates.[83,85–87] Mean half-life, volume distribution, and clearance are similar to those reported in adults. Clearance is most affected by creatinine clearance and renal maturation. Oral valganciclovir 16 mg/kg every 12 hours in neonates provides similar exposure to IV ganciclovir 6 mg/kg every 12 hour.[83] Valganciclovir maintains a more consistent AUC over the first 6 weeks of life, likely because, as clearance improves, the bioavailability also increases.[84]

Safety

The most common toxicity associated with ganciclovir and valganciclovir is myelosuppression. Both drug labels contain black box warnings for neutropenia, anemia, and thrombocytopenia in humans as well as potential carcinogenic effects, teratogenic effects, and inhibition of spermatogenesis based on animal studies. Dose adjustment or interruption of therapy may be necessary if hematologic effects occur. The medications are not typically administered if ANC is less than 500/mm³ or platelet count is less than 25,000/mm³. Neutropenia and thrombocytopenia are also known consequences of CMV.

Neutropenia and thrombocytopenia are common in infants with CMV receiving ganciclovir.[82,85] Neutropenia was more common in infants receiving a lower dose (8 vs 12 mg/kg/d).[85] Thrombocytopenia (platelet count $\leq$50,000/mm³) occurred in 38% of infants. Neutropenia and thrombocytopenia were transient and highly variable, therefore ganciclovir was typically continued in the absence of persistent declines. Many infants also experienced increased liver enzyme levels; however, these may have been caused by CMV. In a controlled trial, 63% of ganciclovir recipients (compared with 21% receiving placebo) experienced grade 3 or 4 neutropenia.[88] Among infants with neutropenia, approximately half required dose adjustments, whereas 13% had the drug discontinued. Oral valganciclovir therapy resulted in grade 3 or 4 neutropenia in 38% of patients.[84] Compared with placebo, there was no difference in the development of renal impairment, increased liver enzyme levels, increased bilirubin levels, or thrombocytopenia after 6 months of ganciclovir therapy.[88] Dosing adjustments are routinely made for renal impairment in older populations.

Dosing to Achieve Pharmacokinetics/Pharmacodynamics Targets

Ganciclovir and valganciclovir show time-dependent killing with a proposed target AUC over the 12-hour interval of 27 mg*h/L.[84] IV ganciclovir 6 mg/kg/dose every 12 hours and valganciclovir 16 mg/kg/dose every 12 hours achieve this target in neonates. Ganciclovir and valganciclovir significantly reduce CMV viral load, but CMV rebounds when off therapy.[84,85] Many infants had improvement in retinitis, hearing, and neurodevelopment. Among infants with congenital CMV involving the CNS, IV ganciclovir 6 mg/kg/dose every 12 hours for 6 weeks was associated with less hearing deterioration at 6 months and fewer developmental delays.[88,89] Valganciclovir 16 mg/kg/dose every 12 hours more consistently maintains the AUC target over 6 weeks of therapy given improved bioavailability over time.[84]

SUMMARY: ANTIFUNGAL AND ANTIVIRAL DOSING

National guidelines for the management of candida infections in neonates advocate the use of AmB-d and fluconazole for the treatment of most candida infections caused by C albicans and C parapsilosis.[20,24] Acyclovir and ganciclovir promote improved outcomes for neonates with HSV and CMV respectively. Prolonged viral suppression is associated with improved outcomes. Bone marrow suppression is common with antiviral medications.

Best practices

What is the current practice?

Dosing antifungal and antiviral mediations

  Best practice/guideline/care path objectives

  • Begin antifungal or antiviral therapy without delay

  • Use doses of medication to cover CNS disease associated with fungal and viral infections

  • Reduce mortality and prevent long-term neurodevelopmental impairment

What changes in current practice are likely to improve outcomes?

• Update drug dosing guidance in formularies to reflect recent PK studies

• Provide suppressive therapy for infants with HSV or CMV infections

Major recommendations

• Use antifungal dosing adequate to treat hematogenous meningoencephalitis

  ○ AmB-d 1 mg/kg/d

  ○ Fluconazole 12 mg/kg/d; consider loading dose of 25 mg/kg

  ○ Micafungin 10 mg/kg/d

- Treat infants with HSV with acyclovir
  - Treatment dose: 20 mg/kg/dose every 8 hours; consider dose alteration in very premature infants
  - Suppressive dose: 300 mg/m^2/dose 3 times a day for 6 months
  - Treat infants with congenital CMV and nervous system involvement with IV ganciclovir 6 mg/kg/dose every 12 hours or valganciclovir 16 mg/kg/dose every 12 hours by mouth for 6 weeks
  - Suppressive therapy is under investigation
- Monitor for bone marrow suppression on antiviral therapy
  - At least 1 to 2 times per week and as clinically indicated while on high-dose therapy
  - Suppressive therapy: week 2, week 4, and monthly thereafter
- All infants with a history of serious fungal or viral infections should have neurodevelopmental follow-up

Summary statement

A high-index of suspicion and prompt initiation of antifungal or antiviral therapies are needed to reduce mortality and morbidity.

Data from Refs.[20,24,75,78]

REFERENCES

1. Autmizguine J, Guptill JT, Cohen-Wolkowiez M, et al. Pharmacokinetics and pharmacodynamics of antifungals in children: clinical implications. Drugs 2014;74(8):891–909.
2. Andes D. Pharmacokinetics and pharmacodynamics of antifungals. Infect Dis Clin North Am 2006;20(3):679–97.
3. Benjamin DK, Stoll BJ, Fanaroff AA, et al. Neonatal candidiasis among extremely low birth weight infants: risk factors, mortality rates, and neurodevelopmental outcomes at 18 to 22 months. Pediatrics 2006;117(1):84–92.
4. Morrell M, Fraser VJ, Kollef MH. Delaying the empiric treatment of *Candida* bloodstream infection until positive blood culture results are obtained: a potential risk factor for hospital mortality. Antimicrob Agents Chemother 2005;49(9):3640–5.
5. Greenberg RG, Benjamin DK, Gantz MG, et al. Empiric antifungal therapy and outcomes in extremely low birth weight infants with invasive candidiasis. J Pediatr 2012;161(2):264–9.e2.
6. Hamill RJ. Amphotericin B formulations: a comparative review of efficacy and toxicity. Drugs 2013;73(9):919–34.
7. Atkinson AJ, Bennett JE. Amphotericin B pharmacokinetics in humans. Antimicrob Agents Chemother 1978;13(2):271–6.
8. Nau R, Sörgel F, Eiffert H. Penetration of drugs through the blood-cerebrospinal fluid/blood-brain barrier for treatment of central nervous system infections. Clin Microbiol Rev 2010;23(4):858–83.
9. Groll AH, Giri N, Petraitis V, et al. Comparative efficacy and distribution of lipid formulations of amphotericin B in experimental *Candida albicans* infection of the central nervous system. J Infect Dis 2000;182(1):274–82.
10. Baley JE, Meyers C, Kliegman RM, et al. Pharmacokinetics, outcome of treatment, and toxic effects of amphotericin B and 5-fluorocytosine in neonates. J Pediatr 1990;116(5):791–7.

11. Scarcella A, Pasquariello MB, Giugliano B, et al. Liposomal amphotericin B treatment for neonatal fungal infections. Pediatr Infect Dis J 1998;17(2):146–8.

12. Juster-Reicher A, Flidel-Rimon O, Amitay M, et al. High-dose liposomal amphotericin B in the therapy of systemic candidiasis in neonates. Eur J Clin Microbiol Infect Dis 2003;22(10):603–7.

13. Linder N, Klinger G, Shalit I, et al. Treatment of candidaemia in premature infants: comparison of three amphotericin B preparations. J Antimicrob Chemother 2003; 52(4):663–7.

14. Fernandez M, Moylett EH, Noyola DE, et al. Candidal meningitis in neonates: a 10-year review. Clin Infect Dis 2000;31(2):458–63.

15. Jeon GW, Koo SH, Lee JH, et al. A comparison of AmBisome to amphotericin B for treatment of systemic candidiasis in very low birth weight infants. Yonsei Med J 2007;48(4):619–26.

16. Starke JR, Mason EO, Kramer WG, et al. Pharmacokinetics of amphotericin B in infants and children. J Infect Dis 1987;155(4):766–74.

17. Koren G, Lau A, Klein J, et al. Pharmacokinetics and adverse effects of amphotericin B in infants and children. J Pediatr 1988;113(3):559–63.

18. Koren G, Lau A, Kenyon CF, et al. Clinical course and pharmacokinetics following a massive overdose of amphotericin B in a neonate. J Toxicol Clin Toxicol 1990; 28(3):371–8.

19. Wurthwein G, Groll AH, Hempel G, et al. Population pharmacokinetics of amphotericin B lipid complex in neonates. Antimicrob Agents Chemother 2005;49(12):5092–8.

20. Pappas PG, Kauffman CA, Andes D, et al. Clinical practice guidelines for the management of candidiasis: 2009 update by the Infectious Diseases Society of America. Clin Infect Dis 2009;48(5):503–35.

21. Le J, Adler-Shohet FC, Nguyen C, et al. Nephrotoxicity associated with amphotericin B deoxycholate in neonates. Pediatr Infect Dis J 2009;28(12):1061–3.

22. Holler B, Omar SA, Farid MD, et al. Effects of fluid and electrolyte management on amphotericin B-induced nephrotoxicity among extremely low birth weight infants. Pediatrics 2004;113(6):e608–16.

23. Andes D. In vivo pharmacodynamics of antifungal drugs in treatment of candidiasis. Antimicrob Agents Chemother 2003;47(4):1179–86.

24. Hope WW, Castagnola E, Groll AH, et al. ESCMID* guideline for the diagnosis and management of *Candida* diseases 2012: prevention and management of invasive infections in neonates and children caused by *Candida* spp. Clin Microbiol Infect 2012;18(Suppl 7):38–52.

25. Juster-Reicher A, Leibovitz E, Linder N, et al. Liposomal amphotericin B (AmBisome) in the treatment of neonatal candidiasis in very low birth weight infants. Infection 2000;28(4):223–6.

26. Cetin H, Yalaz M, Akisu M, et al. The efficacy of two different lipid-based amphotericin B in neonatal *Candida* septicemia. Pediatr Int 2005;47(6):676–80.

27. Lass-Flörl C. Triazole antifungal agents in invasive fungal infections: a comparative review. Drugs 2011;71(18):2405–19.

28. Watt K, Manzoni P, Cohen-Wolkowiez M, et al. Triazole use in the nursery: fluconazole, voriconazole, posaconazole, and ravuconazole. Curr Drug Metab 2013; 14(2):193–202.

29. Saxén H, Hoppu K, Pohjavuori M. Pharmacokinetics of fluconazole in very low birth weight infants during the first two weeks of life. Clin Pharmacol Ther 1993; 54(3):269–77.

30. Wade KC, Wu D, Kaufman DA, et al. Population pharmacokinetics of fluconazole in young infants. Antimicrob Agents Chemother 2008;52(11):4043–9.

31. Wenzl TG, Schefels J, Hörnchen H, et al. Pharmacokinetics of oral fluconazole in premature infants. Eur J Pediatr 1998;157(8):661–2.
32. Nahata MC, Tallian KB, Force RW. Pharmacokinetics of fluconazole in young infants. Eur J Drug Metab Pharmacokinet 1999;24(2):155–7.
33. Wade KC, Benjamin DK, Kaufman DA, et al. Fluconazole dosing for the prevention or treatment of invasive candidiasis in young infants. Pediatr Infect Dis J 2009;28(8):717–23.
34. Piper L, Smith PB, Hornik CP, et al. Fluconazole loading dose pharmacokinetics and safety in infants. Pediatr Infect Dis J 2011;30(5):375–8.
35. Rex JH, Pappas PG, Karchmer AW, et al. A randomized and blinded multicenter trial of high-dose fluconazole plus placebo versus fluconazole plus amphotericin B as therapy for candidemia and its consequences in nonneutropenic subjects. Clin Infect Dis 2003;36(10):1221–8.
36. Voss A, de Pauw BE. High-dose fluconazole therapy in patients with severe fungal infections. Eur J Clin Microbiol Infect Dis 1999;18(3):165–74.
37. Novelli V, Holzel H. Safety and tolerability of fluconazole in children. Antimicrob Agents Chemother 1999;43(8):1955–60.
38. Benjamin DK, Hudak ML, Duara S, et al. Effect of fluconazole prophylaxis on candidiasis and mortality in premature infants: a randomized clinical trial. JAMA 2014;311(17):1742–9.
39. Ericson JE, Benjamin DK. Fluconazole prophylaxis for prevention of invasive candidiasis in infants. Curr Opin Pediatr 2014;26(2):151–6.
40. Kaufman DA, Morris A, Gurka MJ, et al. Fluconazole prophylaxis in preterm infants: a multicenter case-controlled analysis of efficacy and safety. Early Hum Dev 2014;90(Suppl 1):S87–90.
41. Manzoni P, Stolfi I, Pugni L, et al. A multicenter, randomized trial of prophylactic fluconazole in preterm neonates. N Engl J Med 2007;356(24):2483–95.
42. Kaufman D, Boyle R, Hazen KC, et al. Fluconazole prophylaxis against fungal colonization and infection in preterm infants. N Engl J Med 2001;345(23):1660–6.
43. Clancy CJ, Staley B, Nguyen MH. In vitro susceptibility of breakthrough Candida bloodstream isolates correlates with daily and cumulative doses of fluconazole. Antimicrob Agents Chemother 2006;50(10):3496–8.
44. Clancy CJ, Yu VL, Morris AJ, et al. Fluconazole MIC and the fluconazole dose/MIC ratio correlate with therapeutic response among patients with candidemia. Antimicrob Agents Chemother 2005;49(8):3171–7.
45. Schwarze R, Penk A, Pittrow L. Treatment of candidal infections with fluconazole in neonates and infants. Eur J Med Res 2000;5(5):203–8.
46. Driessen M, Ellis JB, Cooper PA, et al. Fluconazole vs. amphotericin B for the treatment of neonatal fungal septicemia: a prospective randomized trial. Pediatr Infect Dis J 1996;15(12):1107–12.
47. Watt KM, Benjamin DK, Cheifetz IM, et al. Pharmacokinetics and safety of fluconazole in young infants supported with extracorporeal membrane oxygenation. Pediatr Infect Dis J 2012;31(10):1042–7.
48. Celik IH, Demirel G, Oguz SS, et al. Compassionate use of voriconazole in newborn infants diagnosed with severe invasive fungal sepsis. Eur Rev Med Pharmacol Sci 2013;17(6):729–34.
49. Doby EH, Benjamin DK, Blaschke AJ, et al. Therapeutic monitoring of voriconazole in children less than three years of age: a case report and summary of voriconazole concentrations for ten children. Pediatr Infect Dis J 2012;31(6):632–5.

50. Karlsson MO, Lutsar I, Milligan PA. Population pharmacokinetic analysis of voriconazole plasma concentration data from pediatric studies. Antimicrob Agents Chemother 2009;53(3):935–44.
51. Santos RP, Sánchez PJ, Mejias A, et al. Successful medical treatment of cutaneous aspergillosis in a premature infant using liposomal amphotericin B, voriconazole and micafungin. Pediatr Infect Dis J 2007;26(4):364–6.
52. Frankenbusch K, Eifinger F, Kribs A, et al. Severe primary cutaneous aspergillosis refractory to amphotericin B and the successful treatment with systemic voriconazole in two premature infants with extremely low birth weight. J Perinatol 2006; 26(8):511–4.
53. Muldrew KM, Maples HD, Stowe CD, et al. Intravenous voriconazole therapy in a preterm infant. Pharmacotherapy 2005;25(6):893–8.
54. Manzoni P, Benjamin DK, Franco C, et al. Echinocandins for the nursery: an update. Curr Drug Metab 2013;14(2):203–7.
55. Chen SC, Slavin MA, Sorrell TC. Echinocandin antifungal drugs in fungal infections: a comparison. Drugs 2011;71(1):11–41.
56. Hope WW, Mickiene D, Petraitis V, et al. The pharmacokinetics and pharmacodynamics of micafungin in experimental hematogenous Candida meningoencephalitis: implications for echinocandin therapy in neonates. J Infect Dis 2008; 197(1):163–71.
57. Benjamin DK, Smith PB, Arrieta A, et al. Safety and pharmacokinetics of repeat-dose micafungin in young infants. Clin Pharmacol Ther 2010;87(1):93–9.
58. Hope WW, Smith PB, Arrieta A, et al. Population pharmacokinetics of micafungin in neonates and young infants. Antimicrob Agents Chemother 2010;54(6): 2633–7.
59. Kawada M, Fukuoka N, Kondo M, et al. Pharmacokinetics of prophylactic micafungin in very-low-birth-weight infants. Pediatr Infect Dis J 2009;28(9):840–2.
60. Smith PB, Walsh TJ, Hope W, et al. Pharmacokinetics of an elevated dosage of micafungin in premature neonates. Pediatr Infect Dis J 2009;28(5):412–5.
61. Heresi GP, Gerstmann DR, Reed MD, et al. The pharmacokinetics and safety of micafungin, a novel echinocandin, in premature infants. Pediatr Infect Dis J 2006; 25(12):1110–5.
62. Saez-Llorens X, Macias M, Maiya P, et al. Pharmacokinetics and safety of caspofungin in neonates and infants less than 3 months of age. Antimicrob Agents Chemother 2009;53(3):869–75.
63. Cohen-Wolkowiez M, Benjamin DK, Piper L, et al. Safety and pharmacokinetics of multiple-dose anidulafungin in infants and neonates. Clin Pharmacol Ther 2011; 89(5):702–7.
64. King KY, Edwards MS, Word BM. Hepatitis associated with micafungin use in a preterm infant. J Perinatol 2009;29(4):320–2.
65. Smith PB, Steinbach WJ, Cotten CM, et al. Caspofungin for the treatment of azole resistant candidemia in a premature infant. J Perinatol 2007;27(2):127–9.
66. Andes D, Diekema DJ, Pfaller MA, et al. In vivo comparison of the pharmacodynamic targets for echinocandin drugs against Candida species. Antimicrob Agents Chemother 2010;54(6):2497–506.
67. Andes DR, Diekema DJ, Pfaller MA, et al. In vivo pharmacodynamic target investigation for micafungin against Candida albicans and C. glabrata in a neutropenic murine candidiasis model. Antimicrob Agents Chemother 2008;52(10):3497–503.
68. Queiroz-Telles F, Berezin E, Leverger G, et al. Micafungin versus liposomal amphotericin B for pediatric patients with invasive candidiasis: substudy of a randomized double-blind trial. Pediatr Infect Dis J 2008;27(9):820–6.

69. Wagstaff AJ, Faulds D, Goa KL. Aciclovir. A reappraisal of its antiviral activity, pharmacokinetic properties and therapeutic efficacy. Drugs 1994;47(1): 153–205.
70. James SH, Kimberlin DW, Whitley RJ. Antiviral therapy for herpesvirus central nervous system infections: neonatal herpes simplex virus infection, herpes simplex encephalitis, and congenital cytomegalovirus infection. Antiviral Res 2009; 83(3):207–13.
71. Whitley RJ. The use of antiviral drugs during the neonatal period. Clin Perinatol 2012;39(1):69–81.
72. Kimberlin DW, Jacobs RF, Weller S, et al. Pharmacokinetics and safety of extemporaneously compounded valacyclovir oral suspension in pediatric patients from 1 month through 11 years of age. Clin Infect Dis 2010;50(2):221–8.
73. Hintz M, Connor JD, Spector SA, et al. Neonatal acyclovir pharmacokinetics in patients with herpes virus infections. Am J Med 1982;73(1A):210–4.
74. Yeager AS. Use of acyclovir in premature and term neonates. Am J Med 1982; 73(1A):205–9.
75. Kimberlin DW, Lin CY, Jacobs RF, et al. Safety and efficacy of high-dose intravenous acyclovir in the management of neonatal herpes simplex virus infections. Pediatrics 2001;108(2):230–8.
76. Sampson MR, Bloom BT, Lenfestey RW, et al. Population pharmacokinetics of intravenous acyclovir in preterm and term infants. Pediatr Infect Dis J 2014; 33(1):42–9.
77. Kimberlin D, Powell D, Gruber W, et al. Administration of oral acyclovir suppressive therapy after neonatal herpes simplex virus disease limited to the skin, eyes and mouth: results of a phase I/II trial. Pediatr Infect Dis J 1996;15(3):247–54.
78. Kimberlin DW, Whitley RJ, Wan W, et al. Oral acyclovir suppression and neurodevelopment after neonatal herpes. N Engl J Med 2011;365(14):1284–92.
79. Haefeli WE, Schoenenberger RA, Weiss P, et al. Acyclovir-induced neurotoxicity: concentration-side effect relationship in acyclovir overdose. Am J Med 1993; 94(2):212–5.
80. Rabalais GP, Nusinoff-Lehrman S, Arvin AM, et al. Antiviral susceptibilities of herpes simplex virus isolates from infants with recurrent mucocutaneous lesions after neonatal infection. Pediatr Infect Dis J 1989;8(4):221–3.
81. Tiffany KF, Benjamin DK, Palasanthiran P, et al. Improved neurodevelopmental outcomes following long-term high-dose oral acyclovir therapy in infants with central nervous system and disseminated herpes simplex disease. J Perinatol 2005;25(3):156–61.
82. Nassetta L, Kimberlin D, Whitley R. Treatment of congenital cytomegalovirus infection: implications for future therapeutic strategies. J Antimicrob Chemother 2009;63(5):862–7.
83. Acosta EP, Brundage RC, King JR, et al. Ganciclovir population pharmacokinetics in neonates following intravenous administration of ganciclovir and oral administration of a liquid valganciclovir formulation. Clin Pharmacol Ther 2007; 81(6):867–72.
84. Kimberlin DW, Acosta EP, Sánchez PJ, et al. Pharmacokinetic and pharmacodynamic assessment of oral valganciclovir in the treatment of symptomatic congenital cytomegalovirus disease. J Infect Dis 2008;197(6):836–45.
85. Whitley RJ, Cloud G, Gruber W, et al. Ganciclovir treatment of symptomatic congenital cytomegalovirus infection: results of a phase II study. National Institute of Allergy and Infectious Diseases Collaborative Antiviral Study Group. J Infect Dis 1997;175(5):1080–6.

86. Zhou XJ, Gruber W, Demmler G, et al. Population pharmacokinetics of ganciclovir in newborns with congenital cytomegalovirus infections. NIAID Collaborative Antiviral Study Group. Antimicrob Agents Chemother 1996;40(9):2202–5.
87. Trang JM, Kidd L, Gruber W, et al. Linear single-dose pharmacokinetics of ganciclovir in newborns with congenital cytomegalovirus infections. NIAID Collaborative Antiviral Study Group. Clin Pharmacol Ther 1993;53(1):15–21.
88. Kimberlin DW, Lin CY, Sánchez PJ, et al. Effect of ganciclovir therapy on hearing in symptomatic congenital cytomegalovirus disease involving the central nervous system: a randomized, controlled trial. J Pediatr 2003;143(1):16–25.
89. Oliver SE, Cloud GA, Sánchez PJ, et al. Neurodevelopmental outcomes following ganciclovir therapy in symptomatic congenital cytomegalovirus infections involving the central nervous system. J Clin Virol 2009;46(Suppl 4):S22–6.
90. Lestner JM, Smith PB, Cohen-Wolkowiez M, et al. Antifungal agents and therapy for infants and children with invasive fungal infections: a pharmacological perspective. Br J Clin Pharmacol 2013;75(6):1381–95.

Antibiotic Stewardship

Reassessment of Guidelines for Management of Neonatal Sepsis

C. Michael Cotten, MD, MHS*

KEYWORDS

• Antibiotics • Neonatal sepsis • Management • Guidelines

KEY POINTS

- The collective concerted efforts to reduce risk of early onset group B streptococcus since 1996, which have included use of antibiotics for large number of women and infants, have been successful.
- Information is emerging indicating that exposures to antibiotics may increase risk of future health problems, especially in preterm infants.
- Antibiotic stewardship is a current goal of the Centers for Disease Control and Prevention.
- Clinicians struggle with the decision to empirically treat well-appearing infants with risk-factors with antibiotics.
- Emerging large scale use of electronic health records may better inform the risk-benefit calculations that clinicians consider in deciding on use of empirical antibiotics for early onset sepsis.

DEFINING THE PROBLEM: EARLY ONSET SEPSIS

Epidemiologists define early onset sepsis (EOS) as culture positive infections occurring the first 3 postnatal days.[1,2] The Centers for Disease Control and Prevention (CDC) defines early onset group B streptococcus (GBS) disease as blood or cerebral spinal fluid culture-proven infection occurring in the first 7 postnatal days.[3,4] The National Institute of Child Health and Human Development's (NICHD) definition of EOS also requires that the infection be treated with antibiotics for 5 or more continuous days.[2] However EOS is defined, the obstetric and pediatric communities have collaborated to greatly reduce the risk of the major cause of EOS in term infants, GBS (*Streptococcus agalactiae*), since the CDC's first guidelines to reduce the risk were published in 1996.[3] At the time the first guidelines emerged, the incidence of

Disclosure: None.
Neonatology Clinical Research, Box 2739 DUMC, Durham, NC 27710, USA
* 2424 Erwin Road, Suite 504, Durham, NC 27705.
E-mail address: michael.cotten@duke.edu

EOS in the United States was 3 to 4 cases per 1000 live-born infants.[5] With guideline modifications in 2002 and 2010 strongly recommending universal screening, fine-tuning of culture methods, and intrapartum antimicrobial prophylaxis (IAP) drug choice when the mother is penicillin allergic, the incidence of EOS has decreased to 0.3 per 1000.[2,4,6] GBS remains the leading cause of EOS in term infants, whereas *Escherichia coli* is most prevalent among premature infants.[2,7]

At a population level, the 2- to 10-fold reduction in prevalence of EOS since 1996 is remarkable.[2,8,9] The guidelines have saved lives. However, the guideline-based strategies that have led to this reduction have contributed to 30% of mothers in the United States receiving antibiotics during labor.[8,10,11] On the neonatal side, single-center experiences and population estimates based on clinicians following the guidelines since the first were published indicate that 15% to 20% of term infants (more than 500,000 infants per year in the United States), most of whom are asymptomatic, are evaluated with screening blood tests for EOS and many also receive empirical antibiotics.[11–13]

RISKS OF ANTIBIOTICS: WHY BE CAUTIOUS?

Adherence to the CDC's guidelines has resulted in significant decreases in EOS; but antibiotic exposures, in the absence of an identified infection to treat, do not seem to be totally without risk. The emerging evidence for risk provides a rationale for identifying mechanisms to limit antibiotic exposure initiation to infants at highest risk while missing extremely few if any infants with evolving infection and limiting the duration of antibiotics for those whose evolving clinical picture indicates an extremely low likelihood of infection. Aminoglycosides are among the most commonly used antimicrobials for the prevention and empirical treatment of EOS and have the potential to cause renal and ototoxicity.[14,15] Among premature infants, the duration of the initial empirical course is associated with later-onset infection, necrotizing enterocolitis, and death.[16–18]

In a Swedish cohort, antibiotic exposure in the neonatal period was associated with almost triple the odds of later wheezing in infants 33 weeks of age and older.[19] In a Dutch cohort, the use of neonatal antibiotics was associated with changes to the microbiome, which in turn were associated with atopic symptoms (eczema and wheeze).[20,21] Although the information linking antibiotic exposure to wheezing and atopy via the microbiome is intriguing and biologically plausible, and animal studies have demonstrated the strong influence of neonatal antibiotics on later gut microbiome and respiratory outcomes,[22,23] the investigators of meta-analyses of the cohort studies associating neonatal antibiotic exposures with later wheezing in children find that the associations are subject to bias and recommend caution before justifying the limitation of antibiotics for the purpose of avoiding asthma at the current stage of evidence accumulation.[24,25] More immediately, clinicians and the community at large share the concern that overall use of antibiotics contributes to the development of resistant organisms, making careful and selective use of antibiotics to the highest-risk patients a universal goal. Antibiotic stewardship is the third of 4 core activities identified by the CDC to limit the development of antimicrobial-resistant organisms: (1) prevent infections, preventing spread; (2) tracking resistance patterns; (3) improving use of antibiotics; and (4) developing new antibiotics and diagnostic tests.[26]

REVIEW OF PAST AND CURRENT CENTERS FOR DISEASE CONTROL AND PREVENTION GUIDELINES

The third and most recent iteration of the CDC's guidelines to prevent GBS perinatal disease was published in 2010.[4] The CDC's initial and subsequent guidelines were the combined efforts of the CDC and numerous professional societies and experts in obstetrics, pediatrics, and microbiology.[3] The first guidelines suggested obstetric caregivers choose between a solely risk factor–based approach to the use of IAP or a universal screening of mothers plus risk factors–based approach to the use of IAP. In 2002, the CDC recommended universal culture-based screening of all pregnant women at 35 to 37 weeks' gestation to optimize the identification of women who should receive IAP.[27]

The CDC's third and most recent version of the guidelines has been endorsed by the American College of Obstetricians and Gynecologists, the American Academy of Pediatrics (AAP), the American College of Nurse-Midwives, the American Academy of Family Physicians, and the American Society for Microbiology.[4] Most of the changes between the second and third version of the guidelines deal with the antepartum approach to the mother and the laboratory methods used for the identification of GBS and testing for antimicrobial sensitivities. Although the CDC's initial guidelines recommended penicillin as the ideal choice for IAP for GBS because penicillin has a narrower spectrum of antimicrobial activity and, therefore, might be less likely to select for resistant organism than ampicillin, one clinical trial found that penicillin and ampicillin administered intravenously intrapartum were associated equally with the presence of ampicillin-resistant gram-negative organisms on postpartum vaginal-perineal culture.[4,28] The CDC now defines adequate IAP as greater than 4 hours of intravenous penicillin, ampicillin, or cefazolin before delivery.[4]

The CDC's 2010 guidelines also include a revised algorithm for the management of newborns with respect to the risk for early onset GBS disease that, if followed, could reduce antibiotic exposures among asymptomatic infants with risk factors compared with the earlier guidelines (**Fig. 1**). The 2010 guidelines state that the algorithm applies to all newborns, not just term and near-term infants. One very strong point made in the guidelines is that infants with signs of sepsis should receive a full diagnostic evaluation and receive antibiotic therapy pending the results.[4] The full diagnostic evaluation includes a blood culture, a complete blood count (CBC) including differential and platelet count, a chest radiograph if respiratory signs are present, and a lumbar puncture if the newborn is stable enough to tolerate the procedure and sepsis is highly suspected. Empirical therapy should include antimicrobial agents active against GBS (including intravenous ampicillin) as well as other organisms that might cause neonatal sepsis, such as E coli.

Well-appearing infants whose mothers had been identified as having chorioamnionitis, a difficult clinical diagnosis to make but one associated with 2- to 3-fold increase in odds of EOS,[12,29] should have diagnostic tests including a CBC and a blood culture and be started on empirical antibiotics while awaiting culture results. In the CDC's 2010 algorithm, the asymptomatic infants whose mothers were diagnosed with chorioamnionitis are the only asymptomatic infants that are to receive empirical antibiotics. The CDC's guidelines acknowledge the poor positive predictive value of the CBC indices, particularly when the CBC is obtained at birth compared with results from samples obtained between 6 and 12 postnatal hours; but even results obtained at 6 to 12 hours are poor predictors of positive cultures.[11,30,31] Although the CDC recommends that the CBCs and differentials and platelet counts are examined, they provide no guidance on normal ranges or advice on what clinicians should do with the results. For newborns whose mothers had chorioamnionitis and are started on empirical antibiotics, no guidance on how the results should influence the duration of antibiotics if the culture remains negative is provided.[4]

For infants with risk factors other than chorioamnionitis, the CDC's 2002 guidelines[32] recommended broad use of a "limited evaluation," which included a blood

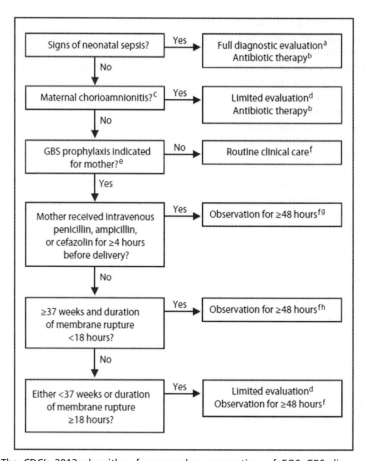

Fig. 1. The CDC's 2012 algorithm for secondary prevention of EOS GBS disease among newborns. [a] Full diagnostic evaluation includes a blood culture, a complete blood count (CBC) including white blood cell differential and platelet counts, chest radiograph (if respiratory abnormalities are present), and lumbar puncture (if patients are stable enough to tolerate procedure and sepsis is suspected). [b] Antibiotic therapy should be directed toward the most common causes of neonatal sepsis, including intravenous ampicillin for GBS and coverage for other organisms (including *Escherichia coli* and other gram-negative pathogens) and should take into account local antibiotic resistance patterns. [c] Consultation with obstetric providers is important to determine the level of clinical suspicion for chorioamnionitis. Chorioamnionitis is diagnosed clinically and some of the signs are nonspecific. [d] Limited evaluation includes blood culture (at birth) and CBC with differential and platelets (at birth and/or at 6–12 hours of life). [e] Indications for intrapartum prophylaxis to prevent early onset group B streptococcal (GBS) disease. [f] If signs of sepsis develop, a full diagnostic evaluation should be conducted and antibiotic therapy initiated. [g] If 37 weeks' gestation or greater, observation may occur at home after 24 hours if other discharge criteria have been met, access to medical care is readily available, and a person who is able to comply fully with instructions for home observation will be present. If any of these conditions are not met, the infant should be observed in the hospital for at least 48 hours and until discharge criteria are achieved. [h] Some experts recommend a CBC with differential and platelets at 6 to 12 hours of age. (*From* Verani JR, McGee L, Schrag SJ. Prevention of perinatal group B streptococcal disease–revised guidelines from CDC, 2010. MMWR Recomm Rep 2010;59:22.)

culture at birth and a CBC with differential and platelet count at birth and/or at 6 to 12 postnatal hours. All infants born to mothers with inadequate IAP were to have the limited evaluation. In the 2010 guideline, the CDC recommends that well-appearing infants who are 37 weeks' or more gestation whose mothers had an indication for GBS prophylaxis but received inadequate or no IAP can be managed with observation alone for 48 hours or more without diagnostic tests. For infants with inadequate IAP who are less than 37 weeks' gestational age or for infants of any gestational age whose membranes were ruptured 18 hours or more before delivery, the CDC recommends observation for 48 hours or more plus the limited evaluation but no empirical treatment unless there are clinical signs of sepsis. If signs develop, a full evaluation should be undertaken. For well-appearing late preterm infants who are 35 to 36 weeks' gestation whose mothers received adequate IAP, the CDC's 2010 guidelines do not recommend diagnostic evaluations. Evidence for these last 2 recommendations, both regarding preterm infants, arises from "opinions of respected authorities based on clinical or laboratory experience, descriptive studies, or reports of expert committees."[4]

AMERICAN ACADEMY OF PEDIATRICS COMMITTEE ON THE FETUS AND NEWBORN

In 2011, the AAP published an overall agreement with the CDC's guidelines.[33] Although the AAP's 2011 paper reviewed and summarized the CDC's guidelines, in 2012, the AAP's Committee on the Fetus and Newborn (COFN) took a step further and published a clinical report with a goal to "provide a practical and, when possible, evidence-based approach to the management of infants with suspected or proven early-onset sepsis."[34] The report provided a valuable and thorough review of the background behind the CDC's guidelines to reduce GBS EOS; information about the accuracy, reliability, and validity of the various diagnostic strategies for EOS; as well as a review of treatment strategies for EOS. The COFN's report included recommendations for the use of diagnostic tests and empirical treatment and also important variations from the CDC's guidelines and made a first attempt at giving guidance for the duration of empirical antibiotics in infants without signs of infection whose mothers had risk factors but whose cultures remained negative.

The first departure from the CDC's guidelines was the COFN's recommendation that preterm infants born to mothers with chorioamnionitis, rupture of membranes of 18 hours or more, or inadequate IAP have laboratory examinations drawn plus empirical treatment of a minimum of 72 hours. The COFN based this variation, which increased the number of infants to be treated compared with the CDC, on the higher risk of infection in premature infants compared with term infants when any of these risk factors were present.[35]

In addition to the guidance for starting empirical antibiotics in premature infants, the COFN provided 2 algorithms to apply to asymptomatic infants whose mothers had risk factors for EOS, one for infants less than 37 weeks' gestation and one for infants aged 37 or more weeks whose mothers had chorioamnionitis. In the algorithm for premature infants, those with maternal risk factors (chorioamnionitis or prolonged rupture of membranes 18 hours or more or inadequate IAP) should have screening laboratory examinations, including blood culture at birth and a CBC and differential plus/minus a c-reactive protein (CRP) between 6 and 12 postnatal hours, and initiation of empirical antibiotics. If the culture was positive, antibiotics should continue; if the blood culture was negative and the infant remained well, antibiotics should stop. If the blood culture was negative and the infant was well, but the 6- to 12-postnatal hour laboratory examinations were abnormal, the COFN recommended continuation of empirical antibiotics without a recommended duration. Similarly, for infants who are 37 weeks' or more gestation whose mothers were diagnosed with chorioamnionitis, cultures should be drawn at birth, screening tests should be drawn between 6 and 12 postnatal hours, and empirical antibiotics started, similar to the CDC's 2010 guidelines. Antibiotics would be continued in well-appearing infants if the culture was positive or if the culture was negative but the laboratory data were abnormal and the mother had received antibiotics during labor and delivery. As with the premature infants with abnormal screening tests, neither the duration of this continuation of empirical antibiotic treatment nor guidance on the degree of variance from normal to define abnormal screening laboratory results were provided.[34]

IMMEDIATE RESPONSE TO THE COMMITTEE ON THE FETUS AND NEWBORN'S 2012 GUIDELINES

The pediatric community responded to the COFN's clinical report with 4 letters to the editor.[9,36–38] The writers pointed out that the approach to the asymptomatic premature infant whose mother had chorioamnionitis, prolonged rupture of membranes, or inadequate IAP differed from the CDC's approach, which included only screening laboratories. The COFN's strategy would lead to more empirical antibiotic use than following the CDC's guideline. The writers also expressed concern that the COFN's suggestions would increase the duration of empirical antimicrobial courses in well-appearing infants based on tests with poor positive predictive value. The writers also pointed out the potential of biomarker tests other than the CBC and differential and CRP that could have value.[9,36–38] One writer offered the suggestion of assessing maternal temperature instead of trying to define chorioamnionitis, referring to the development of an online EOS risk calculator based on the assessment of 350 cases of EOS matched 3:1 with controls taken from a population of more than 600,000 infants born at 34 weeks or more at 14 California and Massachusetts hospitals.[9,11]

In the immediate response to these letters, the COFN's authors identified the number of days of empirical antibiotics an asymptomatic infant born to a woman treated with antibiotics for chorioamnionitis or for EOS risk factors should receive if the laboratory studies were abnormal as a major area of uncertainty in the prevention of EOS.[39] They modified their stance on continuing antibiotics when the results were abnormal and maintained their stance on treating premature infants with mothers with risk factors. Modifying the stance on continuation of antibiotics when laboratory results are abnormal they stated: "We would not treat a well-appearing, asymptomatic term infant with a negative blood culture longer than 48–72 hours, whose mother was treated for chorioamnionitis, even when the infant's laboratory data are abnormal."[39] They cited the CDC's 2010 guidelines report as providing rationale for this approach (ie, a normal physical examination at 48 to 72 hours in an otherwise well infant should exclude the possibility of EOS).[4] For premature infants, the COFN justified the recommendation for empirical therapy initiation for asymptomatic preterm infants whose mothers had risk factors with the fact that the preterm infants are at a higher risk of EOS than term infants with maternal risk factors.[35] The COFN's response to the query on potential biomarkers was that more study was needed before widespread adoption and, although they liked the potential to use the risk-of-EOS calculator, which included maternal temperature during labor to quantify the risk rather than the categorical definition of chorioamnionitis, and acknowledged its use would likely decrease the number of sepsis evaluations in the late preterm and term populations,[11] they thought it should be validated in more studies. In summary, they said that the COFN's revised algorithms would be forthcoming.[39]

THE NEXT ROUND

In 2013, before the publication of the COFN's revised algorithms published in June 2014, Brady and Polin[40] wrote independently with the purpose "to clarify AAP policy" on EOS, acknowledging the differences between the CDC's 2010 guidelines and the COFN's 2012 clinical report.[34,40] They reinforced the revised guidance on antibiotic duration provided in the response to the letters that followed the COFN's 2012 clinical report's guidance, which emphasized continuing empirical antibiotics based on persistently abnormal physical examination findings rather than laboratory values.[40] They pointed out that the COFN's 2012 clinical report noted that in some situations, approaches that differed from the 2010 CDC Guidelines could be altered, and may depend on local practice and resources. The 2013 commentary by Brady and Polin[40] states that the guidelines from the COFN and CDC concur in 2 situations: (1) symptomatic infants should be treated with broad-spectrum antibiotics and (2) healthy-appearing term and preterm infants whose mothers had chorioamnionitis should have a blood culture at birth, have empirical treatment started, and have laboratory examinations drawn between 6 and 12 postnatal hours (a CBC with differential plus/minus CRP); but the CDC did not offer guidance on what to do with the laboratory results.[40]

The COFN and CDC still differed in the approach to 2 situations. First, for well-appearing term infants whose mothers did not have chorioamnionitis but who had an indication for IAP and were inadequately treated, the CDC and COFN agree that these infants can be observed without additional testing if rupture of membranes (ROM) is less than 18 hours. The COFN thinks infants who are 35 and 36 weeks' gestation can be treated similarly. Differences between the CDC and COFN arise if ROM is 18 hours or more and IAP is inadequate. The CDC's guidelines recommend a limited evaluation, which would include a CBC with differential at birth or 6 to 12 postnatal hours and hospital observation for 48 hours.[4] The COFN recommends observation for 48 hours, without the laboratory tests, unless close observation is not possible.[40] The second area of discrepancy is for well-appearing infants less than 37 weeks' gestation whose mothers did not have suspected chorioamnionitis but had another indication and did not receive adequate IAP. The CDC recommended a limited evaluation (blood culture and CBC) and observation in the hospital for 48 hours, whereas the COFN recommended a CBC plus/minus CRP obtained between 6 and 12 postnatal hours and only obtaining a blood culture if antibiotics were to be started because of abnormal laboratory values. This statement seems to differ from the algorithm in the COFN's 2012 clinical report, which provides guidance for infants less than 37 weeks' gestation with inadequate IAP, including obtaining laboratory tests, a blood culture, starting empirical antibiotics (while obtaining the culture and awaiting laboratory results), and continuing antibiotics if the laboratory results were abnormal.[35,40]

The final recommendation in the 2013 commentary by Brady and Polin[40] points out that the CDC did not address the duration of empirical antibiotic treatment. The COFN made their initial recommendations based on laboratory testing results and then reiterated their written response to the community comments on their clinical report: "healthy-appearing infants without evidence of bacterial infection should receive broad-spectrum antimicrobial agents for no more than 48 hours. In small premature infants some may continue antibiotics for up to 72 hours while awaiting bacterial culture results."[40] There was no further discussion or a definition of the levels of laboratory values to consider abnormal or whether the abnormal laboratory values should be considered evidence of infection that could drive clinicians to continue empirical treatment and how many more days of empirical antibiotics should be continued.

IMPACT ON PRACTICE AND THE LATEST WORD FROM THE COMMITTEE ON THE FETUS AND NEWBORN

Clinicians may feel the need to use the CBC and differential and other biomarker tests, such as CRP, because of the potential for false-negative results from blood cultures, especially in cases when the blood sample volume is low or when intrapartum antibiotics have been administered.[35,41] When laboratory values, particularly the CBC, differential, and CRP, are measured in cases of asymptomatic infants born to mothers with risk factors, the prevalence of abnormal results can be quite high. Jackson and colleagues[42] reported on 2427 neutrophil counts and ratios of immature to total neutrophil (I:T) obtained during the first 24 postnatal hours from 856 infants born to mothers diagnosed with chorioamnionitis. Ninety-seven percent of symptomatic infants had abnormal neutrophil counts; 99% of the asymptomatic infants had an abnormal neutrophil count, immature neutrophil count, or I:T ratio.[42]

More recently, Kiser and colleagues[43] reported their center's experience managing infants whose mothers had chorioamnionitis. Their local guideline resembled the algorithm for the management of infants born to mothers with chorioamnionitis provided by the COFN in 2012, with the inclusion of continuing antibiotics to 7 days in asymptomatic infants who had abnormal CBC or CRP results. Of the 554 infants studied, 4 (0.7%) had positive cultures and 22 (4%) were treated for sepsis based on clinical signs without a positive culture. One hundred twelve (20.2%) asymptomatic infants were treated with prolonged antibiotics based on abnormal laboratory data. Most of the infants also had spinal taps, and none had a positive cerebrospinal fluid culture.

Following up on the pledge to provide revised algorithms and concurrent in the issue of *Pediatrics* that included Kiser and colleagues'[43] report, Drs Polin, Watterburg, Benitz, and Eichenwald[44] wrote a commentary on the "Conundrum of Early-Onset Sepsis." The researchers acknowledge that deciding how best to evaluate and treat an infant at risk for EOS is exemplary of every clinician's never-ending dilemma of dealing with the real world where decisions for individual patients are made absent informative results from high-quality randomized trials. To that point, they summarize Kiser and colleagues'[43] finding that, based on an algorithm similar to the COFN's 2012 algorithm and consistent with Jackson and colleagues'[42] earlier report, many asymptomatic term infants born to women with chorioamnionitis would receive prolonged antibiotic courses, counter to the COFN's revised statement that healthy-appearing infants with negative cultures should receive no more than 48 to 72 hours.[40,43,44] They further clarified that healthy-appearing infants with negative cultures should have antibiotics stopped "even when the infant's laboratory results are abnormal."[39,44] For Kiser and colleagues'[43] cohort, this could have decreased the percentage of infants treated for greater than 48 hours from 24% to 4%.[44] Polin and colleagues[44] go on to make several conclusions from the accumulating evidence and experience, including that the physical examination is as good or better than most laboratory tests in "ruling in or ruling out sepsis," and that "commonly used laboratory tests have a limited positive predictive accuracy and should never be used as a rationale to continue treatment in an otherwise healthy term infant at 48–72 hours of life."[44] They cite the 2012 clinical report[34] for the conclusion that "laboratory tests should never be used," although that report included the algorithm that guided clinicians to continue treatment if the laboratory values collected between 6 and 12 postnatal hours were abnormal.

The authors of this most recent commentary then makes 3 suggestions for the management of newborns suspected of EOS: (1) antibiotics may be discontinued by 48 hours in well-appearing term newborns born to women with chorioamnionitis; (2) longer (to 72 hours) empirical treatment might be considered for premature infants or infants with abnormal screening studies; and (3) lumbar punctures are recommended in cases whereby the blood culture is positive, the infant does not improve on appropriate antimicrobial coverage, or the clinician views the infant as having a high probability of sepsis because of clinical signs or abnormal laboratory data.[44] So with this latest update, the author allows (without recommending) the laboratory values to influence the decision to treat longer than 48 hours and whether a spinal tap is done or not.

WHERE DO WE GO NEXT?

The COFN panel acknowledges that they are breaking new ground with their evolving recommendations on the duration of empirical therapy and the lack of strong data to support their decisions.[44] We await either cohort study data or randomized trials of the COFN's 2012 clinical report approaches, like Kiser and colleagues'[43] cohort study, versus the COFN's 2012 in-reply approaches, which, for the most part, disregard the ancillary tests. Choosing an outcome of greatest importance that is feasibly measured (more likely hospital readmissions rather than wheezing at school age) but has a low incidence (4 of 404 readmitted for fever or suspected sepsis in Jackson and colleagues'[42] cohort study) will make such a study challenging. For a study to have 90% power to detect a difference between a 1% rehospitalization rate for suspected infection in infants managed with a strategy of giving empirical antibiotics for longer than 2 to 3 days versus 3% among infants managed with an approach that stopped empirical antibiotics after 48 hours regardless of laboratory values like the more recent modified recommendation[39,44] with an alpha of 0.05, 1028 infants would be needed for each study arm. Not insurmountable, but this type of study may be hard to do given the strength of entrenched local opinion on a specific clinical approach and the challenges of achieving equipoise among clinicians and families agreeing to enroll their newborn into the study and not entrusting their own doctor with the decision.

In addition to the duration of antibiotics questions, alternatives to the CDC and COFN's algorithms to obtain diagnostic tests based on the risk factors inclusive of chorioamnionitis and start treatment warrant some discussion. Chorioamnionitis can be a subjective definition, and obstetricians wishing to maximize the likelihood that mothers and infants stay together and get discharged to home in the first postnatal day may avoid classification of a mother as having chorioamnionitis.[9,12] Escobar and colleagues[12] and Puopolo[9] acknowledge this clinical reality and propose that we adopt a multifactor assessment approach that includes the objective measure of maximum maternal temperature in labor in calculating the odds ratios for sepsis in infants. Clinicians could use the calculated odds ratio based on the Web-available tool that is the product of their cohort study to develop an individualized approach for each infant, incorporating known, objective maternal risk factors. This clinical tool is available as an online tool: http://www.dor.kaiser.org/external/DORExternal/research/InfectionProbabilityCalculator.aspx.[6,9,12]

Finally, all the investigators of the commentaries, guidelines, and clinical reports agree that infants with signs of infection deserve treatment, even when intrapartum antibiotics were used. Escobar and colleagues[12] reported much higher odds of EOS among symptomatic versus asymptomatic infants evaluated for EOS, but the asymptomatic infants with risk factors still had higher odds of EOS than the overall population rate.[12] That said, most clinicians would agree that for term and later preterm infants, there is some tolerable duration of signs to resolve that would allow for not treating, especially in the absence of risk factors. In the last report by Polin and colleagues,[44] they say, "Symptomatic neonates without risk factors for infection (who improve over the first 6 hours of life) may not require treatment, but must be monitored closely."[44] The severity of the clinical signs must also be considered and a shorter duration tolerated before empirical antibiotics are started when a variation from the expected norms are extreme.

SUMMARY

Since their inception in 1996, the guidelines aimed at preventing perinatally acquired GBS, and indirectly EOS, have led to a significant reduction in EOS and EOS-related mortality. In their 2010 iteration, the CDC's guidelines have narrowed the categories of infants who receive empirical antibiotics from prior versions and continue to recommend laboratory tests in the evaluation of infants at risk for EOS. The COFN has taken steps into the less-charted waters of the duration of empirical antimicrobial therapy for suspected EOS but, more recently, have reconsidered the reliance of abnormal laboratory test results to drive the duration of empirical antibiotics beyond 48 to 72 postnatal hours. Undoubtedly, the guidelines from the CDC and the COFN will continue to adapt to emerging evidence on the contributions of novel biomarkers as we learn more about the intricacies of the newborn's response to infection.[45–47] While we await the future guidelines and better predictive value from novel biomarker tests and combinations of risk factors and biomarker levels, following the COFN's most recent compilation of recommendations, basing the initiation of treatment on the presence and persistence of signs of infection and basing the duration of treatment primarily on the presence of signs in the absence of positive cultures seem reasonable. The ancillary tests may inform clinicians and provide rationales for closer observation and even longer empirical treatment when clinical signs are equivocal or complete resolution is delayed.

REFERENCES

1. Manual of operations Vermont Oxford Network Database. Part 2 data definitions and data forms for infants born in 2013. 2013. Available at: https://public.vtoxford.org//wp-content/uploads/2014/03/Manual-of-Operations-Part-2-17_1.pdf. Accessed October 5, 2014.
2. Stoll BJ, Hansen NI, Sanchez PJ, et al. Early onset neonatal sepsis: the burden of group B Streptococcal and E. coli disease continues. Pediatrics 2011;127:817–26.
3. Prevention of perinatal group B streptococcal disease: a public health perspective. Centers for Disease Control and Prevention. MMWR Recomm Rep 1996;45:1–24.
4. Verani JR, McGee L, Schrag SJ. Prevention of perinatal group B streptococcal disease–revised guidelines from CDC, 2010. MMWR Recomm Rep 2010;59:1–36.
5. Schuchat A, Zywicki SS, Dinsmoor MJ, et al. Risk factors and opportunities for prevention of early-onset neonatal sepsis: a multicenter case-control study. Pediatrics 2000;105:21–6.
6. Mukhopadhyay S, Puopolo KM. Risk assessment in neonatal early onset sepsis. Semin Perinatol 2012;36:408–15.
7. Bauserman MS, Laughon MM, Hornik CP, et al. Group B Streptococcus and Escherichia coli infections in the intensive care nursery in the era of intrapartum antibiotic prophylaxis. Pediatr Infect Dis J 2013;32:208–12.
8. Weston EJ, Pondo T, Lewis MM, et al. The burden of invasive early-onset neonatal sepsis in the United States, 2005-2008. Pediatr Infect Dis J 2011;30:937–41.
9. Puopolo KM. Response to the American Academy of Pediatrics, Committee on the Fetus and Newborn statement, "management of neonates with suspected or proven early-onset bacterial sepsis". Pediatrics 2012;130:e1054–5 [author reply: e1055–7].

10. Van Dyke MK, Phares CR, Lynfield R, et al. Evaluation of universal antenatal screening for group B streptococcus. N Engl J Med 2009;360:2626–36.
11. Puopolo KM, Draper D, Wi S, et al. Estimating the probability of neonatal early-onset infection on the basis of maternal risk factors. Pediatrics 2011;128: e1155–63.
12. Escobar GJ, Li DK, Armstrong MA, et al. Neonatal sepsis workups in infants >/=2000 grams at birth: a population-based study. Pediatrics 2000;106:256–63.
13. Mukhopadhyay S, Eichenwald EC, Puopolo KM. Neonatal early-onset sepsis evaluations among well-appearing infants: projected impact of changes in CDC GBS guidelines. J Perinatol 2013;33:198–205.
14. Hsieh EM, Hornik C, Clark RH, et al. Best Pharmaceuticals for Children Act—Pediatric Trials Network. Medication use in the neonatal intensive care unit. Am J Perinatol 2014;31:811–22.
15. McCracken GH Jr. Aminoglycoside toxicity in infants and children. Am J Med 1986;80:172–8.
16. Cotten CM, Taylor S, Stoll B, et al. Prolonged duration of initial empirical antibiotic treatment is associated with increased rates of necrotizing enterocolitis and death for extremely low birth weight infants. Pediatrics 2009;123:58–66.
17. Alexander VN, Northrup V, Bizzarro MJ. Antibiotic exposure in the newborn intensive care unit and the risk of necrotizing enterocolitis. J Pediatr 2011; 159:392–7.
18. Kuppala VS, Meinzen-Derr J, Morrow AL, et al. Prolonged initial empirical antibiotic treatment is associated with adverse outcomes in premature infants. J Pediatr 2011;159:720–5.
19. Alm B, Erdes L, Mollborg P, et al. Neonatal antibiotic treatment is a risk factor for early wheezing. Pediatrics 2008;121:697–702.
20. Penders J, Thijs C, Vink C, et al. Factors influencing the composition of the intestinal microbiota in early infancy. Pediatrics 2006;118:511–21.
21. Penders J, Thijs C, van den Brandt PA, et al. Gut microbiota composition and development of atopic manifestations in infancy: the KOALA Birth Cohort Study. Gut 2007;56:661–7.
22. Ly NP, Litonjua A, Gold DR, et al. Gut microbiota, probiotics, and vitamin D: inter-related exposures influencing allergy, asthma, and obesity? J Allergy Clin Immunol 2011;127:1087–94 [quiz: 1095–6].
23. Russell SL, Gold MJ, Willing BP, et al. Perinatal antibiotic treatment affects murine microbiota, immune responses and allergic asthma. Gut Microbes 2013;4:158–64.
24. Heintze K, Petersen KU. The case of drug causation of childhood asthma: antibiotics and paracetamol. Eur J Clin Pharmacol 2013;69:1197–209.
25. Penders J, Kummeling I, Thijs C. Infant antibiotic use and wheeze and asthma risk: a systematic review and meta-analysis. Eur Respir J 2011;38:295–302.
26. Antibiotic resistance threats in the United States. CDC morbidity and mortality weekly report 2013. Available at: http://www.cdc.gov/drugresistance/threat-report-2013/index.html. Accessed October 5, 2014.
27. Schrag S, Gorwitz R, Fultz-Butts K, et al. Prevention of perinatal group B streptococcal disease: revised guidelines from CDC. MMWR Recomm Rep 2002; 51(RR–11):1–22.
28. Edwards RK, Clark P, Sistrom CL, et al. Intrapartum antibiotic prophylaxis 1: relative effects of recommended antibiotics on gram-negative pathogens. Obstet Gynecol 2002;100:534–9.
29. Alexander JM, McIntire DM, Leveno KJ. Chorioamnionitis and the prognosis for term infants. Obstet Gynecol 1999;94:274–8.

30. Christensen RD, Rothstein G, Hill HR, et al. Fatal early onset group B strepto-coccal sepsis with normal leukocyte counts. Pediatr Infect Dis 1985;4:242–5.
31. Newman TB, Puopolo KM, Wi S, et al. Interpreting complete blood counts soon after birth in newborns at risk for sepsis. Pediatrics 2010;126:903–9.
32. Schrag S, Gorwitz R, Fultz-Butts K, et al. Prevention of perinatal group B strepto-coccal disease: revised guidelines from CDC. MMWR 2002;51(No. RR-11):1–22.
33. Baker CJ, Byington CL, Polin RA. Policy statement-recommendations for the prevention of perinatal group B streptococcal (GBS) disease. Pediatrics 2011; 128:611–6.
34. Polin RA. Management of neonates with suspected or proven early-onset bacterial sepsis. Pediatrics 2012;129:1006–15.
35. Ottolini MC, Lundgren K, Mirkinson LJ, et al. Utility of complete blood count and blood culture screening to diagnose neonatal sepsis in the asymptomatic at risk newborn. Pediatr Infect Dis J 2003;22:430–4.
36. Cotten CM, Benjamin DK Jr, Smith PB, et al. Empirical antibiotic therapy for suspected early-onset bacterial sepsis. Pediatrics 2012;130:e1052–3.
37. Sukumar M. Need clarification on "abnormal labs". Pediatrics 2012;130:e1055.
38. Sise ME, Parravicini E, Barasch J. Urinary neutrophil gelatinase associated lipocalin identifies neonates with high probability of sepsis. Pediatrics 2012; 130:e1053–4.
39. Polin RA, on behalf of the Committee on Fetus and Newborn. In reply. Pediatrics 2012;130:e1055–7.
40. Brady MT, Polin RA. Prevention and management of infants with suspected or proven neonatal sepsis. Pediatrics 2013;132:166–8.
41. Schelonka RL, Chai MK, Yoder BA, et al. Volume of blood required to detect common neonatal pathogens. J Pediatr 1996;129:275–8.
42. Jackson GL, Engle WD, Sendelbach DM, et al. Are complete blood cell counts useful in the evaluation of asymptomatic neonates exposed to suspected cho-rioamnionitis? Pediatrics 2004;113:1173–80.
43. Kiser C, Nawab U, McKenna K, et al. Role of guidelines on length of therapy in chorioamnionitis and neonatal sepsis. Pediatrics 2014;133:992–8.
44. Polin RA, Watterberg K, Benitz W, et al. The conundrum of early-onset sepsis. Pediatrics 2014;133:1122–3.
45. Srinivasan L, Harris MC. New technologies for the rapid diagnosis of neonatal sepsis. Curr Opin Pediatr 2012;24:165–71.
46. Wynn JL, Cvijanovich NZ, Allen GL, et al. The influence of developmental age on the early transcriptomic response of children with septic shock. Mol Med 2011; 17:1146–56.
47. Shah BA, Padbury JF. Neonatal sepsis: an old problem with new insights. Virulence 2014;5:170–8.

Index

Note: Page numbers of article titles are in **boldface** type.

A

AAP. *See* American Academy of Pediatrics (AAP)
Acyclovir
   dosing in infants, 185–187
American Academy of Pediatrics (AAP)
   COFN of, 199–204
Amphotericin B deoxycholate
   dosing in infants, 179–182
Amphotericin B lipid complex
   dosing in infants, 179–182
Ampicillin
   dosing in infants, 168–169
Anidulafungin
   dosing in infants, 184–185
Antibiotic(s)
   in bacterial meningitis in infants management, 37
   broad-spectrum
      in premature infants, 108
   for CA, 160–161
   dosing of. *See* Antibiotic dosing
   novel
      for staphylococcal infections in infants, 126
   risks associated with, 196
Antibiotic dosing
   in infants, **167–176**
      ampicillin, 168–169
      clindamycin, 169–171
      introduction, 167–168
      meropenem, 171
      metronidazole, 172
      piperacillin/tazobactam, 172–174
Antibiotic stewardship, **195–206**
   AAP COFN on, 199–204
   CDC on, 196–199
Antifungal dosing
   in infants, **177–185**
      echinocandins, 184–185
      introduction, 177–179
      polenes, 179–182
      triazoles, 182
Antimicrobial agents. *See* Antibiotic(s)

Clin Perinatol 42 (2015) 207–216
http://dx.doi.org/10.1016/S0095-5108(15)00010-X
0095-5108/15/$ – see front matter © 2015 Elsevier Inc. All rights reserved.

Antistaphylococcal penicillin
    in infants, 124
Antiviral dosing
    in infants, **185–189**
        acyclovir, 185–187
        ganciclovir, 187–188
        introduction, 177–179
        valacyclovir, 185–187
        valganciclovir, 187–188
Astrovirus
    NEC due to, 141

B

Bacteremia
    UTIs in infants and, 21
Bacteria
    NEC due to, 134–138
        atypical bacteria, 138
        gram-negative bacteria, 137–138
        gram-positive bacteria, 135–137
Bacterial meningitis
    described, 30
    in infants, **29–45**
        causes of, 31
        clinical presentation of, 33
        in developed countries, 30–31
        in developing countries, 31
        diagnosis of, 33–36
            ancillary tests in, 35
            CSF parameter interpretation in, 35
            lumbar puncture in, 33–37
        epidemiology of, 30–31
        introduction, 30
        long-term outcomes of, 38
        pathogenesis of, 32–33
        prevention of, 38–40
        risk factors for, 33
        treatment of, 37–38
Birth weight
    candidiasis related to, 107
Bloodstream infections (BSIs), **1–16**
    causative agents, 6–8
        Candida spp., 8
        CoNS, 6–7
        Enterococcus spp., 7
        gram-negative organisms, 7
        S. aureus, 7
    control and prevention of, 10
    definitions of, 2
    described, 1

epidemiology of, 2
incidence of, 2
introduction, 1
resistance to, 8–10
risk factors for, 3–6
    central lines, 3–5
    medications, 5
    NICU environment, 5–6
BPD. *See* Bronchopulmonary dysplasia (BPD)
Brain disease
    CA and, 159
Broad-spectrum antibiotics
    candidiasis related to, 108
Bronchopulmonary dysplasia (BPD)
    CA and, 160
BSIs. *See* Bloodstream infections (BSIs)

C

CA. *See* Chorioamnionitis (CA)
Candida spp.
    BSIs due to, 8
    NEC due to, 141
Candidiasis
    in premature infants, **105–117**
        background of, 105–106
        diagnosis of, 109–111
        microbiology of, 109
        pathogenesis of, 106
        risk factors for, 106–109
            broad-spectrum antibiotics, 108
            central venous catheters, 108
            NICU environment, 107–108
            prematurity and birth weight, 107
        treatment of, 111–112
Candiduria
    treatment of, 22
Caspofungin
    dosing in infants, 184–185
CDC. *See* Centers for Disease Control and Prevention (CDC)
Centers for Disease Control and Prevention (CDC)
    in antibiotic stewardship, 196–199
Central line(s)
    BSIs related to, 3–5
Central line–associated blood stream infections (CLABSIs), 3–5
    epidemiology of, 2
    incidence of, 2
Central nervous system (CNS)
    bacterial meningitis of
        in infants, 33

Central venous catheters
    candidiasis related to, 108
Cerebrospinal fluid (CSF) parameters
    interpretation of
        in bacterial meningitis in infants diagnosis, 35
Children
    drugs in
        mechanisms for study of, 168
Chorioamnionitis (CA), **155–165**
    defined, 155–157
    management of, 160–161
    in neonates, **155–165**
        outcomes of, 158–160
            BPD, 160
            brain disease, 159
            lung disease, 159
            neonatal sepsis, 158
            preterm birth, 158
            respiratory distress syndrome, 159–160
        pathophysiology of, 157–158
CLABSIs. *See* Central line–associated blood stream infections (CLABSIs)
Clindamycin
    dosing in infants, 169–171
    for staphylococcal infections in infants, 125
Clostridia spp.
    NEC due to, 136–137
CMV. *See* Cytomegalovirus (CMV)
CNS. *See* Central nervous system (CNS)
Coagulase-negative *Staphylococcus* (CoNS)
    BSIs related to, 6–7
    clinical manifestations of, 123
    diagnosis of, 123
    epidemiology of, 121–122
COFN. *See* Committee on the Fetus and Newborn (COFN)
Committee on the Fetus and Newborn (COFN)
    of AAP, 199–204
CoNS. *See* Coagulase-negative *Staphylococcus* (CoNS)
Coronavirus
    NEC due to, 140
Cronobacter sakazakii
    NEC due to, 137–138
CSF. *See* Cerebrospinal fluid (CSF)
Cytomegalovirus (CMV)
    NEC due to, 139–140
    perinatal, **61–75**
        clinical correlation, 64–70
        diagnostics in, 67–70
        discussion, 71–72
        introduction, 61–62
        prevalence/incidence of, 63–64
        prevention/treatment of

infant interventions for, 66–67
maternal interventions for, 64–66
vaccines for
maternal
research related to, 70–71

D

Drug(s)
BSIs due to, 5
in children
mechanisms for study of, 168
E
Early onset sepsis (EOS)
described, 195–196
Echinocandins
dosing in infants, 184–185
Empirical therapy
for staphylococcal infections in infants, 126
Enterococcus spp.
BSIs related to, 7
Enterocolitis
necrotizing. See Necrotizing enterocolitis (NEC)
Enteroviruses
NEC due to, 140–141
EOS. See Early onset sepsis (EOS)
Escherichia coli
NEC due to, 138
UTIs in infants due to, 18

F

Fluconazole
dosing in infants, 182–183
Fungus(i)
NEC due to, 141

G

Ganciclovir
dosing in infants, 187–188
GBS. See Group B streptococcus (GBS)
Gram-negative organisms
BSIs related to, 7
Group B streptococcus (GBS) vaccine
in bacterial meningitis in infants prevention, 38–40

H

Hepatitis
B, 92–94
clinical correlation, 93
described, 92

Hepatitis (*continued*)
    diagnosis and treatment of, 93–94
    discussion, 93–94
    epidemiology of, 93
    transmission/pathogenesis of, 92–93
  C, 94–95
Herpes simplex virus (HSV)
  described, 48
Herpes simplex virus (HSV) infection
  maternal
    clinical features of, 49–50
    terminology related to, 49
  mother-to-child transmission of
    prevention of, 52–53
    risk factors for, 50–51
  neonatal, **47–59**
    clinical features of, 51–52
    described, 48
    epidemiology of, 48–49
    introduction, 47–48
    treatment of, 53–56
HIV
  NEC due to, 141
HIV infection
  perinatal, 88–92
    described, 88
    diagnosis and treatment of, 89–92
    discussion, 89–92
    epidemiology of, 88–89
    transmission/pathogenesis of, 89
HSV. *See* Herpes simplex virus (HSV)

I

Infant(s)
  antibiotic dosing in, **167–176**. *See also* Antibiotic dosing, in infants
  antifungal dosing in, **177–185**. *See also* Antifungal dosing, in infants
  antiviral dosing in, **185–189**. *See also* Antiviral dosing, in infants
  bacterial meningitis in, **29–45**. *See also* Bacterial meningitis, in infants
  premature
    candidiasis in, **105–117**. *See also* Candidiasis, in premature infants
  staphylococcal infections in, **119–132**. *See also* Staphylococcal infections,
    in infants
  uncircumcized
    UTIs in, 19
  UTIs in, **17–28**. *See also* Urinary tract infections (UTIs), in infants
Infection(s). *See also specific types*
  bloodstream, **1–16**
  staphylococcal
    in infants, **119–132**
  TORCH, **77–103**

K

Klebsiella spp.
    NEC due to, 138

L

Linezolid
    for staphylococcal infections in infants, 125–126
Liposomal amphotericin
    dosing in infants, 179–182
Lumbar puncture
    in bacterial meningitis in infants diagnosis, 33–37
Lung disease
    CA and, 159

M

Medication(s). *See* Drug(s)
Meningitis
    bacterial
        in infants, **29–45**. *See also* Bacterial meningitis
    neonatal
        prevention of, 38–40
    UTIs in infants and, 21
Meropenem
    dosing in infants, 171
Methicillin resistance
    in staphylococcal infections in infants, 123–124
Metronidazole
    dosing in infants, 172
Micafungin
    dosing in infants, 184–185

N

NEC. *See* Necrotizing enterocolitis (NEC)
Necrotizing enterocolitis (NEC)
    infectious causes of, **133–154**. *See also specific causes, e.g.,* Bacteria
        bacteria, 134–138
        fungi, 141
        introduction, 133–134
        viruses, 138–141
Neonatal intensive care unit (NICU)
    BSIs due to, 5–6
    candidiasis in, 107–108
Neonatal sepsis
    CA and, 158
Neonate(s)
    CA in, **155–165**. *See also* Chorioamnionitis (CA)
    HSV infection in, **47–59**. *See also* Herpes simplex virus (HSV) infection, neonatal

NICU. *See* Neonatal intensive care unit (NICU)
Norovirus
    NEC due to, 139

P

Parvovirus B19, 86–88
    clinical correlation, 87
    described, 86
    diagnosis and treatment of, 87–88
    discussion, 87–88
    transmission/pathogenesis of, 86–87
Penicillin
    for staphylococcal infections in infants, 124
Piperacillin/tazobactam
    dosing in infants, 172–174
Polene(s)
    dosing in infants, 179–182
Premature infants
    candidiasis in, **105–117**. *See also* Candidiasis, in premature infants
Preterm birth
    CA and, 158
Pseudomonas spp.
    NEC due to, 138
Pyuria
    defined, 21–22

R

Renal abnormalities
    UTIs in infants due to, 19
Respiratory distress syndrome
    CA and, 159–160
Rotavirus
    NEC due to, 138–139
Rubella, 85–86

S

Sepsis
    early onset, 195–196
Staphylococcal infections
    in infants, **119–132**
        clinical manifestations of, 123
        diagnosis of, 123
        epidemiology of, 120–122
        introduction, 119–120
        resistance to, 123–124
        treatment of, 124–126
Staphylococcus spp.
    coagulase-negative. *See* Coagulase-negative *Staphylococcus* (CoNS)

S. aureus
    BSIs due to, 7
    clinical manifestations of, 123
    diagnosis of, 123
    epidemiology of, 120–121
S. epidermidis
    NEC due to, 135–136
Steroid(s)
    antenatal
        for CA, 161

T

TORCH infections, **77–103**. *See also specific infections, e.g.,*
    Toxoplasmosis
    HBV, 92–94
    HCV, 94–95
    introduction, 77–78
    parvovirus B19, 86–88
    perinatal HIV infection, 88–92
    rubella, 85–86
    toxoplasmosis, 78–82
    Treponema pallidum, 82–85
Toxoplasmosis, 78–82
    clinical correlation, 81–82
    described, 78
    diagnosis and treatment of, 82
    discussion, 82
    epidemiology of, 80–81
    transmission/pathogenesis of, 78–80
Treponema pallidum, 82–85
    clinical correlation, 83–84
    described, 82–83
    diagnosis and treatment of, 84–85
    discussion, 84–85
    epidemiology of, 83
    transmission/pathogenesis of, 83
Triazole(s)
    dosing in infants, 182–184

U

Uncircumcized infants
    UTIs in, 19
Urinary tract infections (UTIs)
    in infants, **17–28**
        causes of
            E. coli, 18
            maternal history of UTIs, 19–20
            renal abnormalities, 19
            uncircumcized males, 18–19

Urinary (*continued*)
    clinical correlations, 20–21
    concomitant bacteremia and meningitis, 21
    diagnosis of, 21–22
    epidemiology of, 17–20
    in first three days of life, 17
    introduction, 17
    recurrence of, 23
    risk factors for, 17–20
    treatment of, 22–23
  maternal history of
    UTIs in infants related to, 19–20
UTIs. *See* Urinary tract infections (UTIs)

V

Vaccine(s)
  CMV
    maternal
      research related to, 70–71
    GBS
      in bacterial meningitis in infants prevention, 38–40
Valacyclovir
  dosing in infants, 185–187
Valganciclovir
  dosing in infants, 187–188
Vancomycin
  for staphylococcal infections in infants, 124–125
Vancomycin resistance
  in staphylococcal infections in infants, 124
Varicella zoster virus (VZV) infection
  perinatal, **61–75**
    discussion, 71–72
    introduction, 63
    prevalence/incidence of, 63–64
    prevention/treatment of
      infant interventions for, 66–67
      maternal interventions for, 64–66
Virus(es)
  NEC due to, 138–141
    astrovirus, 141
    CMV, 139–140
    coronavirus, 140
    enteroviruses, 140–141
    HIV, 141
    norovirus, 139
    rotavirus, 138–139
Voriconazole
  dosing in infants, 183–184
VZV infection. *See* Varicella zoster virus (VZV) infection

Moving?

Make sure your subscription moves with you!

To notify us of your new address, find your **Clinics Account Number** (located on your mailing label above your name), and contact customer service at:

Email: journalscustomerservice-usa@elsevier.com

800-654-2452 (subscribers in the U.S. & Canada)
314-447-8871 (subscribers outside of the U.S. & Canada)

Fax number: 314-447-8029

Elsevier Health Sciences Division
Subscription Customer Service
3251 Riverport Lane
Maryland Heights, MO 63043

ELSEVIER